UNDERSTANDING PAIN

UNDERSTANDING PAIN

What You Need to Know to Take Control

ALAN D. KAYE, MD, PhD, AND
RICHARD D. URMAN, MD, MBA,
EDITORS

The Praeger Series on Contemporary Health and Living
Julie K. Silver, MD, Series Editor

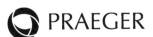 PRAEGER

AN IMPRINT OF ABC-CLIO, LLC
Santa Barbara, California • Denver, Colorado • Oxford, England

Library of Congress Cataloging-in-Publication Data

Understanding pain : what you need to know to take control / Alan D. Kaye, and Richard D. Urman, editors.
   p. cm. — (The praeger series on contemporary health and living)
   Includes bibliographical references and index.
   ISBN 978–0–313–39603–8 (hardcopy : alk. paper) — ISBN 978–0–313–39604–5 (ebook)
1. Pain—Treatment—Popular works. I. Kaye, Alan David. II. Urman, Richard D.
RB127.U535   2011
616′.0472–dc23   2011031286

ISBN: 978–0–313–39603–8
EISBN: 978–0–313–39604–5

15 14 13 12 11   1 2 3 4 5

This book is also available on the World Wide Web as an eBook.
Visit www.abc-clio.com for details.

Praeger
An Imprint of ABC-CLIO, LLC

ABC-CLIO, LLC
130 Cremona Drive, P.O. Box 1911
Santa Barbara, California 93116-1911

This book is printed on acid-free paper ∞

Manufactured in the United States of America

I dedicate this book to my mother, Florence Susan Feldman, for showing me her pain and how to live with it. Also, I thank my mother for encouraging me to go to medical school and to complete a pain fellowship to help others in pain, to understand their problems, and to help treat and overcome their ailments. I also thank all of my pain teachers along the way with a special note of appreciation to the great pain doctors at Texas Tech Health Sciences Center in Lubbock.
ADK

I wish to dedicate this work to my patients who inspired me to write this book. I would like to acknowledge all my mentors and trainees at Harvard Medical School for bringing in new perspectives and giving me opportunities to both learn and teach. Finally, a very special thanks to the following people in my life who have been supportive throughout: my parents, Dennis and Tanya, and my wife, Dr. Zina Matlyuk-Urman.
RDU

CONTENTS

Part II: Specific Painful Conditions and Treatment Options

Contents

Series Foreword

Contemporary Health and Living

Over the past 100 years, there have been incredible medical breakthroughs that have prevented or cured illness in billions of people and helped many more improve their health while living with chronic conditions. A few of the most important 20th-century discoveries include antibiotics, organ transplants, and vaccines. The 21st century has already heralded important new treatments including such things as a vaccine to prevent human papillomavirus (HPV) from infecting and potentially leading to cervical cancer in women. Polio is on the verge of being eradicated worldwide, making it only the second infectious disease behind smallpox to ever be erased as a human health threat. Pain is a complex condition that is often ignored or undertreated.

In this series, experts from many disciplines share with readers important and updated medical knowledge related to diagnosing and treating pain. All aspects of health are considered, including disease-specific subjects and preventive medical care. Disseminating this information will help individuals to improve their health, researchers and doctors to determine where there are gaps in our current knowledge, and policy makers to assess the most pressing needs in health care.

Series Editor Julie K. Silver, MD
Assistant Professor
Harvard Medical School
Department of Physical Medicine and Rehabilitation

PART I

Introduction

1

HISTORICAL PERSPECTIVE ON TREATING PAIN

Ike Eriator, MD, MPH, Daniel S. Reynolds, MD,
and Joe Cook, MPH

INTRODUCTION

Natural human birth is usually done in pain. Death is often in pain. Between these two landmarks, a great deal of time is also spent in pain. John Dryden, a 17th-century writer, noted that "of all the happiness that mankind can get, it is not in pleasure, but in rest from pain." Albert Schweitzer, a 20th-century theologian and physician, noted that pain was a "more terrible lord of mankind than even death itself."

Today, pain remains a leading public health problem and a significant source of personal and family suffering across different cultures and geographical boundaries. It is the oldest medical problem, and it remains a universal affliction for mankind. Alternative therapies, assisted suicide, substance abuse, narcotic regulation, disability, and compensation issues are all strongly related to pain and to pain relief. The largest numbers of people utilizing complementary and alternative medicine today are patients with pain. Considering the effects of pain on society, community, family, and individuals, the World Health Organization in 1997 made the "alleviation of pain, the reduction of suffering, and the provision of palliative care for those who cannot be cured" its sixth global priority. The U.S. Congress mandated the 10-year period, January 1, 2001, to December 31, 2010, as the decade of "Pain Control and Research," making pain management second only to the brain as a medical area to be so recognized. Improved terminal (e.g., end-of-life) pain management has been listed as one of the top 20 chronic medical problems for the focus of the U.S. government and private health care organizations in order to have the broadest impact on patients, families, and communities.

Throughout history, the spiritual, social, and political meaning of pain defined the suffering of individuals. The word "pain" originates from the Latin word "*poena*," which refers to punishment. Through the ages, some people have achieved absolution through punishment for their sins or the sins of the people. In the Christian doctrine, pain is the means of purification and redemption, endowed with divinity by the suffering of Christ. The first of the four noble truths in Buddhism is that life is suffering. The Quran makes clear that man was created into a life of pain, toil, and trial. In many primitive cultures, treatment of pain included rituals to frighten pain-inflicting spirits out of the sufferer's body, including things such as dance and music, animal sacrifice, and even application of electric eels to injured body parts.

With such dominance of pain over mankind through the ages, it is no wonder that human beings, since the dawn of history, have sought and used agents that assuage pain. The Egyptian papyri dating back to 4000 BC contains information on pain treatment. In ancient China, pain was viewed as an imbalance between the yin and the yang. The practice of acupuncture today still strives to adjust the balance between these energies. The oldest of the sacred books of India, the Rig-Veda, which was probably written as far back as 4000 BC, described several agents including analgesics and anesthetics still in use. At the temple of Aesculapius, the Greek god of medicine, patients with pain would sleep, and in the night, the god, in conjunction with priests and physicians, would bring about a cure using potions, bandages, and physical procedures as well as mystical and transcendental energies. Hippocrates, an ancient Greek physician and his disciples paid great attention to the problem of pain. They experimented with medications including opium, mandrake, and hemlock. They employed cooling techniques and physiotherapy. To alleviate the pain of surgery, they would sometimes produce unconsciousness by compressing the carotid arteries (the word carotid comes from Greek for deep sleep). Hippocrates was also known to advise women in childbirth to chew willow bark, which contains a form of salicylic acid, the parent compound of modern aspirin.

NARCOTICS

Narcotics are often used in reference to medications that work like morphine. *Opioid* is the more scientific term for this group of pain medications. Opium is the dried extract obtained from the poppy fruit and contains natural medicines like morphine and codeine. The evidence for use of opium dates back to the Assyrian "poppy" art from 4000 BC. The Sumerians cultivated the poppy plants and isolated opium from the capsule of the fruits. They called opium "gil" (meaning joy), and the plant "hul gil" (meaning plant of joy). For about 3,000 years, opium was used as a means of assuaging pain as well as achieving sleep and dreams, and this is the origin of the phrase "pipe dreams." Galen described opium confections, which were quite popular in Rome and were even hawked by shopkeepers and itinerant quacks. Paracelsus (1493–1541 AD), a Swiss Renaissance physician, carried opium in the pommel of his saddle, referring to it as the "stone of immortality." The compounding of tincture of opium is attributed to him, which was called "laudanum" (meaning "something to be praised"). Thomas Sydenham, an English physician, in 1680 wrote that, "Among the remedies which it has pleased Almighty God to give to man to relieve his sufferings, none is so universal and so efficacious as opium."

In the initial part of the 19th century, two important developments opened up a new era of possibilities. First, Friedrich Wilhelm Serturner, a German pharmacist, described the isolation (from opium) of "the alkaloidal principle," which from his experiments he named morphine after the Greek god of dreams. Second, the widespread adoption of the hypodermic syringe occurred. Opium and morphine were among the first drugs to be administered by this method, and the developments were regarded as "the greatest boon given to medicine since the discovery of chloroform." Florence Nightingale, a celebrated English nurse, noted during her illness that "nothing did me any good, but a curious little new fangled operation of putting opium under the skin which relieved one for 24 hours." During the American Civil War (1861–1865), soldiers were given syringes and taught how to dose themselves. Morphine preparations were used indiscriminately and turned many veterans into addicts. In fact, addiction for some time was known as "soldier's disease."

Opium and morphine were incorporated into multiple remedies, including those that were claimed to cure the opium habit and alcoholism. The medical profession's need for something that worked was a major stimulus for the opium market. Opium was often referred to as "G.O.M."—"God's Own Medicine"—and was used in treating ailments as widely varied as anemia, angina pectoris, diabetes, insanity, menstrual cramps, tetanus, nymphomania, vaginismus, and vomiting in pregnancy. In the United States, the Ebert prescription survey in 1885, which reviewed about 15,700 prescriptions, showed quinine and morphine as the most frequently used agents in medicines. Opium and morphine were also incorporated in multiple remedies for children including the famous "Dover's powder," "Brown mixture," and "Mrs. Winslow's Soothing Syrup." These remedies were instrumental in the passage of the first Pure Food and Drug Act in 1906, which ended the availability of opioids as over-the-counter medications in the USA and introduced the first legally enforceable pharmacopoeia of the United States.

The use of opium soared largely due to medical prescribing. The dark side of this use was also clearly evident at the time in London, where the opium dens were a constant feature of Victorian life. Some doctors were concerned that opium created dependency and that opium users, when deprived even for a single day, "became languid, dejected and uneasy." Edward Levinstein (1831–1882) described morphine addiction in *The Morbid Craving for*

Morphia. The withdrawal features including stomach cramps, diarrhea, sleeplessness, nervousness, pupillary dilatation, and gooseflesh led to the term "cold turkey."

The family burden of opioid addiction at that time may be gleaned from the autobiographical play *Long Day's Journey into Night,* by Eugene O'Neill. Set in August 1912, the powerlessness, doubts, and sorrow caused by the mother's addiction to morphine were such that the author could not bear the publication of the book in his own lifetime. The shame often felt by such addicts and their families helped to trigger the demand for severe laws to curtail both medical and nonmedical use of narcotics.

This was a major contributing factor in the development of the Harrison Narcotic Control Act in 1914, which was the first legislation regulating the production, import, and distribution of opioid medications in the United States. It became illegal for practitioners to supply addicts with narcotics. Soon thereafter, violation of the rule resulted in the arraignment of about 25,000 physicians, 3,000 of whom served prison terms. Consequently, many physicians withdrew from prescribing narcotics. This era continued for many decades, highlighted by the regulatory "War on Drugs." Psychotherapy or surgery became the available options for treating chronic non-cancer pain. Neurosurgeons would tie, cut, or crush the nerves transmitting the pain, but the procedures were often too disabling.

The search for a safer analgesic (e.g., painkiller) without addictive properties led to the production of diacetylmorphine (heroin) in the late 19th century. Ironically, it was described as a safe preparation with many of the virtues and none of the dangers of morphine. It was also said to be free of addictive properties and was even recommended for the treatment of morphine addiction! In 1939, meperidine (Demerol) was discovered. Again, it was initially thought to be nonaddictive and it soon became the most popular opioid analgesic in the United States. However, with clinical usage, the growing number of people addicted to this new medication soon convinced the Bureau of Narcotics of its addictive potential. Nalorphine was produced in 1942 as the first drug to reverse the effects of the narcotic. Its development was a pharmacological milestone in the history of medicine. It was used as an antidote for the effects of morphine in the early 1950s. Further research resulted in the discovery of the "pure" antidote, naloxone, as well as other related antidotes such as pentazocine, butorphanol, and buprenorphine. Other synthetic narcotics soon followed.

In 1946, methadone was introduced. The abstinence syndrome seen with methadone was different from that of the natural alkaloids, in that the onset was slower and its intensity was less. In 1949, methadone was shown to be effective for addicts who were withdrawing from heroin. By 1950, oral methadone was established at U.S. Public Health Service hospitals for the treatment of opioid abstinence syndrome. In the 1950s, the American Medical Association came out with a position statement indicating that the use of narcotics to treat addicts on an outpatient basis was substandard therapy.

In the mid-20th century, the major sites in the brain and spinal cord where opioids work were localized. The brain's own narcotic-like substances (called enkephalins) and the receptors on which opioids in general acted were also discovered. The widespread use of epidural and spinal narcotics soon followed. By acting directly on the sites with these receptors, these routes provided means of decreasing the amount of such medications used to achieve pain control by 10 to 100 times when compared to the intravenous injection route.

In 1982, the World Health Organization published guidelines, now known as the "WHO Ladder," for the treatment of cancer pain. The decades of opioid restriction lasted until the 1980s. By then, a pathologist in Michigan was helping patients with intractable pain (that could not get adequate treatment) to end their lives. In addition, there were small studies showing that opioids were helpful for some patients with non-cancer pain. Many pain professional organizations supported the need for a wider use in such patients, in the so-called "War on Pain." Pain became the fifth vital sign in many major hospitals in the 1990s. The Joint Commission mandated pain assessment and treatment, and the U.S. Congress passed an act declaring the decade from 2001 to 2010 as the "Decade of Pain Control and Research." By the middle of the first decade of the 21st century, the sales of pain medications had more than tripled, and at the same time, misuse of opioid medications had reached an epidemic proportion.

CANNABIS (MARIJUANA)

Cannabis (marijuana), like narcotics, also has been used and misused for thousands of years for social entertainment and as folk medication. Queen Victoria used it for her menstrual cramps. Purification of the plant product led to the discovery of the active agents called cannabinoids. Similar compounds produced by the brain for its internal activities as well as special receptors for the natural and synthetic cannabis-like substances have also been discovered.

ASPIRIN-LIKE MEDICATIONS

Aspirin and similar medications (often referred to as "NSAIDs, which stands for "nonsteroidal anti-inflammatory drugs") are commonly used today. They help with pain, fever, and inflammation. Like the narcotics, they were originally used in the form of plant preparations. Hippocrates and Galen recommended the use of the willow bark. The crude herbal preparation was used for about 2,000 years. It was only in the 19th century that the active agent was extracted from the willow bark. Aspirin was synthesized from salicylic acid and introduced in 1899 and was very effective for pain and fever. By the end of World War I, it had supplanted the narcotics for treating mild to moderate pain. It was not until 1971 when it was demonstrated that aspirin-like medications work by influencing the production of certain chemicals called prostaglandins. The cyclooxygenase (COX-2) enzyme—responsible for the production of the prostaglandin leading directly to inflammation and pain—was discovered in 1988. The COX-2 selective inhibitors are a form of aspirin-like medications with special selectivity for this enzyme, and are associated with reduced risk of peptic ulcer compared to the regular members like aspirin. Celecoxib (e.g., Celebrex), the first member of this special group, was introduced in 1999 and quickly became the most frequently prescribed new medication in the United States at the time. Some members of this group, such as rofecoxib (e.g.,Vioxx), were later shown to significantly increase the risk of heart attack and stroke. Vioxx was withdrawn from the market in 2004.

OTHER AGENTS AND THERAPIES

The history of pain treatment encompasses much more than those of narcotics and aspirin-like medications. New methods of analgesia started with the discovery of nitrous oxide (laughing gas) in 1772 and the description of its analgesic properties. It was used as an analgesic for dental extractions. Ether, "the sweet oil of vitriol," was synthesized in 1540 and used for toothache. In 1846, William Morton gave his famous demonstration of ether-induced general anesthesia. Due to the smell and low potency of ether, James Young Simpson introduced chloroform for childbirth in 1848, and surgery soon followed.[5] Surgical anesthesia remains one of the greatest revolutions of modern medicine.

Cocaine, which was extracted from the dried leaves of the coca plant, was the first local anesthetic to be used. It was used in the first spinal anesthesia in 1897. But cocaine had significant side effects with high doses or prolonged usage. Procaine (commonly known as Novocain) was synthesized in 1904 as a safer alternative. It is the oldest man-made local anesthetic that is still in clinical use. It was used for serial nerve blocks in the early part of the 20th century. Dr. Emery Rovenstine became the first anesthesiologist to open a nerve block clinic for pain relief in 1936.

Dr. Henry K. Beecher, an anesthesiologist, observed during the Second World War that seriously wounded soldiers complained of less pain compared to his civilian patients. To account for the emotional and cognitive components of pain, he introduced the concepts of placebo response and randomized trial of analgesic agents, and these had spread to modern medicine at large. Meanwhile, in the United Kingdom, another physician, Dr. Cicely Saunders, solidified the concept of managing "total pain" by recognizing the physical, mental, social, and spiritual distress that is associated with pain. She used strong narcotics like morphine, in combination with other agents like gin and cocaine (Brompton's cocktail), to maintain the quality of life for the dying patients. Saunders is best known for her role in the development of hospice and palliative care in modern medicine. Dr. John Bonica, an anesthesiologist like Henry Beecher, treated soldiers and veterans of the Second World War. Intrigued by the benefits of informal collaboration with an orthopedic surgeon, a neurosurgeon and a psychiatrist, he established a multidisciplinary pain clinic in 1947. He also advocated for an interdisciplinary pain field. His magnum opus *The Management of Pain*, published in 1953, gathered together the available information on the causes, diagnosis, and treatment of human pain.

The gate control theory, published in 1965, indicated that painful sensation can be "crowded out" in "competition" for transmission within the nervous system by other sensations (namely vibration, touch, etc.). This led to the successful application of transcutaneous electrical nerve stimulation (TENS) devices and implantable spinal cord stimulators, which are now in widespread use. The new theory also incited more discussion about pain treatments, including psychological treatment options. In 1970, Wilbert Fordyce, a clinical psychologist, introduced operant conditioning in the treatment of chronic pain, using rewards to help patients learn to self-manage pain and resume normal activities. This has further developed into the cognitive and biofeedback modalities commonly used today.

THE SILENT EPIDEMIC

Pain remains the most common reason for seeking medical attention. On the average, 15–30 percent of Americans experience chronic pain annually. About 50 million are totally or partially disabled due to chronic pain. Chronic pain is more common in women, people with lower socioeconomic status, and in the older age group.

The National Institutes of Health estimated that the United States spends about $100 billion annually on medical expenses, lost wages, lost productivity, and other costs related to pain. Among the workforce, about 12.7 percent of employees lose productive time due to pain, resulting in a loss of about 4 billion workdays annually and a $61.2 billion loss in productivity. Seventy-three percent of Americans fear inadequate pain relief at the end of life, and 69 percent of cancer patients surveyed would consider suicide if they felt their pain was inadequately controlled.

Surgery is the most common cause of acute (e.g., new onset) pain in the United States, leading to the hospitalization of about 41.5 million Americans each year. The majority of patients report moderate to severe pain after surgery, despite the availability of modern treatments and techniques. In hospitalized patients, pain is associated with increased recovery time, length of stay, and worse treatment outcomes. It is not surprising that 57 percent of patients who are about to undergo surgery described pain as their greatest concern.

Back pain is the most expensive of all musculoskeletal conditions in the industrialized countries. Four out of five people in the United States will have low back pain at some point in their lifetime. The majority of people will recover, usually within six weeks. Between 2 and 5 percent of the adult population of the United States has a disabling low back pain at any given time. Currently, back problem is the primary cause of disability in persons under the age of 45 years. One in 25 people will change jobs or retire early due to low back pain. The direct cost in the occupational setting is jeopardizing workers' compensation benefits in some countries. One multinational study showed that the rate of back surgery in the United States is five times that in Sweden, and there was no evidence of positive effects on back function, pain level, or work.

The Pendulum Swings

In pain management, quite a lot has unfolded in the last few decades. Basic research on mechanisms of pain has advanced significantly. Clinical treatment of pain has progressed from the use of morphine in treating cancer pain being called "unfortunate" in the 1940s all the way to hydrocodone becoming the most commonly prescribed medication in the United States. But with the improvement in treatment availability, the pendulum is swinging back, and some of the age-old problems are beginning to resurface. As of 2005, unintentional overdosing was second only to motor vehicle crashes as a cause of untimely death in the United States. For every fatal overdose, there were seven cases of nonfatal overdoses among patients on long-term narcotics for non-cancer pain. Many abusers are getting the medications from close relatives. The Food and Drug Administration has introduced Risk Evaluation and Mitigation Strategies (REMS) to ensure that the benefits of the drugs continue to outweigh the risks.

Concluding Remarks

The world of pain management has come a long way. The result of this long journey can be measured by the current status of pain. Today, the burden of pain in the community has been recognized, or is being recognized. The impetus and use of complementary (alternative) treatment modalities are gaining ground. Nerve blocks are being done using x-rays to guide and improve accuracy. Basic scientific research is elucidating the genetic basis of pain and the variation in responses. Many states and accreditation agencies have established practice standards for pain management. From the Assyrian poppy act all the way to the isolation of microscopic particles in the body responsible for pain signals and use of PET Scan to detect brain-related pain activities, mankind has seen a tremendous amount of progress. But narcotics remain the bedrock for the control of severe pain. Narcotics and aspirin-like medications still constitute 95 percent of the analgesics in use today. Potent analgesics without addiction continue to elude pain practitioners and researchers. History is remarkable for its ability to repeat itself. Paradoxically, its light is often on the stern, shining on the waves behind us. History clearly shows that we must carefully balance the benefits of the treatment with the side effects. Managing pain remains a continuing challenge. But our ability to help those suffering from pain continues to improve with each passing era and the emerging theory and technology.

REFERENCES

Adams, K., and Corrigan J. M. (eds.): Priority areas for quality improvement. In: *Priority areas for national action: Transforming health care quality.* Washington, DC: Institute of Medicine, National Academy of Sciences, 2003, pp. 41–114.

Eriator, I. I.: Opioid use in the United States. *Federal Practitioner,* 2003; 20 (11): 50–64.

Hansson, T. H. and Hansson, E. K.: The effects of common medical interventions on pain, back function, and work resumption in patients with chronic low back pain: A prospective 2-year cohort study in six countries. *Spine,* 2000; 25: 3055–3064.

Kuehn, B. M.: Alarming nonfatal overdose rates found for opioids, sedatives and tranquilizers. *JAMA,* 2010; 303: 2020.

Meldrum, M. L.: A capsule history of pain management. *JAMA,* 2003; 290: 2470 – 2475.

Porter, R.: Medicine, state and society. In: *The greatest benefit to mankind.* London: Harper Collins, 1997, pp. 628–667.

Stewart, W. F., Ricci, J. A., Chee, E., Morganstein, D., and Lipton, R.: Lost productive time and cost due to common pain conditions in the US workforce. *JAMA,* 2003; 290: 2443–2454.

Wall, P.: How treatment works. In: *Pain, the science of suffering.* New York: Columbia University Press, 2000, pp. 107–124.

OTHER RESOURCES

https://dawninfo.samhsa.gov/default.asp: Provides information on misuse of pain medi
-cations.

http://www.painpolicy.wisc.edu/: Provides information on public policies and statistics.

2

HOW TO CHOOSE A PAIN PRACTITIONER WHO IS RIGHT FOR YOU

Rinoo V. Shah, MD, MBA, and Alan D. Kaye, MD, PhD

Selecting an appropriate health care provider is the first step in taking control of your pain. So, do your homework before you make an appointment to see a particular practitioner or agree to undergo a treatment. The purpose of this chapter is to guide you when making a choice among the myriad number of pain treatment providers.

An early pioneer in pain medicine, Dr. John Bonica, is quoted as saying, "Pain is a major concern influencing every aspect of life. It is the most common symptom of disease, which compels patients to seek medical advice. Whereas acute symptomatic pain serves the useful purpose of warning, chronic pain is a malefic force that imposes severe emotional, physical, and economic stresses on the patient."

Since pain is complex and affects many aspects of a person's life, there are providers who specialize in treating these different aspects. Patients are bombarded with seductive marketing practices that highlight the problems of pain. A number of these treatments may or may not work. In a perfect world, a patient may be able to review the choices available to him or her and make an informed decision. The world is not perfect, but ordinary. Information is not transparent, and the patient has to rely on the advice of the health care worker. The world is a difficult—not ordinary—place for chronic pain patients. Their desperation adversely affects their choices and decision making. They may become fearful, nervous, distrustful, and angry. This can alter a patient's judgment and behavior. This type of behavior, unfortunately, can create a rift between the patient and the health care provider. This rift can cause further alienation and desperation. The patient may then begin to distrust advice that may be medically sound and seek therapies that are heavily weighted toward hope.

People do not make decisions like computers do. We have built-in biases that influence how we make decisions. In an ideal world, a visit to the best physician in the world should not be affected by whether the physician's personality dovetails with your own personality. In the real world, patients value "subjective" as much as "objective" measures. Empathy, dedication, and concern are important personality traits that patients value highly. Most formal organizations that evaluate physicians neglect these "softer" measures. Licensing boards and medical societies (physician trade organizations) focus on objective measures. For example, a medical license board wants to know whether the physician graduated from an accredited medical school; whether the physician was sued; or whether the physician committed a crime. These organizations rely on a combination of fact checking and voluntary reporting. This is a time-consuming and detailed process, but effective at verifying a physician's credentials.

The Internet has empowered patients to express opinions about physicians. Social media and patient websites clearly emphasize "softer" measures. Some websites such as Angie's List allow participants to rate their experience with different physicians. RateMds.com is another website where patients can rate their doctor on qualities such as knowledge, helpfulness, punctuality, and overall quality. PatientsLikeMe.com is a website/online community where patients with certain chronic disorders, such as fibromyalgia, can share opinions on treatments. They can receive feedback. Yelp.com is a website that ranks restaurants and entertainment venues, but they have a section on doctors and health care providers. There are many websites, blogs, and social media outlets that address, in a relatively simple format, "Can you recommend a good physician or procedure for my pain?" The caveat is that an opinion will vary from person to person. You may still like a movie, despite negative reviews. You may like a physician, even if another patient disapproves of that physician.

We know that a number of our physician colleagues review their online profiles. Physicians, like all people, respond to incentives. Many strive to improve their online profiles, in a manner that will make their patients happy. Many physician employers value patient satisfaction surveys and conduct annual reports on their physicians. Some organizations link a physician's income to success on these surveys. Electronic health records will give patients a further leg up in taking control of their health care. A patient can voice concerns about their health care, with greater ease. As information becomes more fluid and transparent, patients will be able to act in their own best interests. With electronic or "portable" records, second opinions become easier. Your physician will naturally be more accountable. Information on the Internet can give meaningful feedback to a physician. Many times this information can surprise or offend a doctor. The doctor may or may not wish to take corrective action. The adage "The customer knows best" can be transformed into "The patient knows best." With the ever-present Internet, this adage comes with teeth!

Medical education has historically emphasized patient satisfaction, physician empathy, and attention to a patient's needs. Unfortunately, there is a disconnect between these noble ideals and the reality of a busy practice. There was no way to monitor how physicians could improve their "bedside manner." The Internet makes physicians accountable. "Niceness," courtesy, and empathy are now incentives and goals that doctors pursue.

Physicians are concerned, however, that a patient's opinion may not accurately reflect their lifelong commitment to the practice of medicine. Physicians may practice medicine appropriately, but this may not meet the expectations of a patient. Just as there is cyber-bullying, a single angry patient with a computer can damage a physician's reputation. The Internet may not capture the opinions of patients who do not consider themselves technologically savvy. A small group of patients on the Internet may not reflect the breadth and number of opinions expressed privately. This is known as a selection bias. The loudest opinion may not be the correct opinion. Reputation and trust are the cornerstones of a therapeutic relationship between a patient and physician. Pain physicians may see a chronic pain patient several times a year, for the rest of their lives! Patients should carefully evaluate "subjective" information and ask their doctor about their online profiles. A face-to-face interaction is often the best way to build or end a doctor-patient relationship.

Now we shall discuss some objective measures that patients should expect of their physician.

1. *First and foremost, your physician should have an active license to practice medicine.* Licenses are granted by each state. Each state has a medical board that decides who gets to practice medicine in that state. For instance, if you see a physician in an office in New York City, the physician must have an active and current license in New York State. A physician must maintain an active license before evaluating you. Most states require physicians to renew their license every two years. In order to maintain the license, the physician must truthfully answer a series of questions regarding their moral conduct, capacity to be a law-abiding citizen, and continuing education. The initial licensure process is very detailed, time consuming, and expensive. Maintaining a license is not time consuming. However, medical boards share information and may conduct audits to ensure physician honesty during the renewal process. The goal of the licensing board is to protect the public. It is very hard to get a license, but very easy to lose it. The medical licensing boards have significant power and investigate patient complaints. Many have become more accessible to the public, by providing toll-free numbers and websites. The medical boards are very approachable to patients. Each state has a medical board with a different threshold for investigating complaints. Any complaint of a moral transgression, such as intoxication or inappropriate sexual conduct, is taken very seriously. No patient should be afraid of contacting the board. On the other hand, complaints such as prolonged office wait times might not be investigated. A medical board investigation is very thorough and involves several experts. Often, the outcome of this investigation is published. Malpractice information may be made available by the medical

board. Sometimes a medical board may suspend or terminate a physician's license. This is reserved for the most serious grievances. So, contact your state medical board. Just type the name of your state, followed by medical board or physician licensing board, on an Internet search engine. You can then search for your physician's medical board profile. Alternatively, call your phone company—a medical board is typically located within your state's capital.

2. *Board certification is extremely important.* These medical boards are different from those run by the states. A state medical board determines if a physician is qualified to practice medicine, but that physician can theoretically practice any procedure. Board certification establishes whether the physician meets the competency requirement to practice their specialty. Even if a physician is licensed by their state's medical board, the physician cannot say that he or she is board certified. Board certification is an honor and privilege granted to specific physicians. These physicians have to complete advanced training (residency or fellowship training) that is accredited. The American Council of Graduate Medical Education (ACGME) is the main organization responsible for accrediting these training programs. There are many opportunities for physicians to get training after medical school. This training might not be accredited by the ACGME. If a physician gets training outside of the ACGME, then a patient should inquire about their clinical experience. Board certification typically requires completion of an ACGME training program and the completion of an examination. A specialized medical society is granted the power to decide who is board certified in their specialty. Only these physicians can state that they are board certified. Usually this is a straightforward issue. For instance, the American Board of Physical Medicine and Rehabilitation decides who can become board certified in the medical specialty of physical medicine and rehabilitation. The American Board of Anesthesiology determines who can become board certified in the medical specialty of anesthesiology. Both these boards require completion of a residency program, several difficult examinations, evidence of moral character, and compliance with the law. This is a very rigorous process.

As medicine grows and further specializes, new board certification opportunities arise. Physicians of different specialties may wish to seek board certification in these new specialties. This is the case with Pain Medicine and Palliative Medicine. Physicians who have already finished residency training may not be able to go back into training. They may be "grandfathered," or they may have to take an alternative path to demonstrate that they are qualified to practice this new specialty. Physicians in residency training may have to undertake a fellowship, after their residency is finished. After the new specialty matures and fellowship training programs become established, the "grandfather" option will close. Thereafter, all physicians will have to complete a formal training program, such as an accredited ACGME fellowship. Physicians who complete a fellowship are a unique bunch. They have opted to take a significant pay cut, move their families for one year (pain medicine fellowships), and become "demoted" to a trainee status. They could have gone on to practice, but opted to tough it out through a formalized fellowship program.

Pain management fellowships developed over the past two decades. The number of "fellows" in training has hovered in the range of 220–240 per year.

In this day and age, pain management fellowships are extremely competitive. Older physicians, e.g., in their 50s, may never have had access to fellowships. Younger physicians, e.g., in their 20s or early 30s, have access to fellowships. Physicians in their mid-30s to 40s are "in between." So, it is understandable if a 60-year-old pain physician is not fellowship trained. A 30-year-old physician that practices pain without a fellowship, quite simply, "didn't make the cut." The pathway to board certification in pain medicine is significantly easier for someone who completes an ACGME fellowship than it is for someone without a fellowship. Ask your doctor if they completed an ACGME-accredited pain fellowship. Many established pain practices seek out fellowship and board certified physicians. Many hospitals require board certification and may require a fellowship for certain advanced pain management procedures.

There are many excellent pain physicians who are not fellowship trained or board certified. This continues to be a bone of contention, among those who didn't complete an ACGME fellowship. However, "excellent" is a subjective adjective. Completion of an ACGME-accredited pain fellowship and board certification in pain medicine are objective honors. Our personal preference is to seek out an ACGME pain fellowship and board certified pain specialist, if they are younger than 45. If they are older than 45, then seek out a pain physician who is board certified.

The American Board of Medical Specialties and the American Council of Graduate Medical Education offers information about training after medical school. The American Board of Medical Specialties allows patients to check if their doctor is board certified.

3. *Physicians have to face additional hurdles to practice.* Hospitals and outpatient surgery centers have specialized committees that decide which physicians can practice at these facilities. Likewise, insurance companies will evaluate physicians using their own criteria. If a physician has privileges at a hospital or is enrolled in a health insurance plan as a provider, (s)he has crossed the threshold for these institutions. You can contact your health insurance company or local hospital to determine if the physician is on their panel (insurance company) or medical staff (hospital).

4. *Physicians may have conflicts of interest.* Sometimes a "conflict of interest" may exist to provide patient convenience. For instance, a "one-stop shop" for pain management may offer physical therapy, x-rays, lab analysis, procedures, and psychological counseling. Many of these services are integrated. Patients have to understand that there may be financial incentives at work, whether it is a large nonprofit organization or a solo practice. There is a raging debate about whether or how much financial incentives influence physicians. Patients have a right to know if there is a financial conflict of interest. This may also apply to the procedure you are getting. Physicians are not required to disclose such information, except in a few states. Patients can ask. Many device and drug companies are moving toward increased transparency in these financial disclosures. Some physicians are voluntarily restricting access of drug representatives, for instance. There are arguments for and against the influence of financial incentives on physicians prescribing medications or recommending treatment. You may wish to ask your physician about these conflicts. This applies to nonphysician health care providers as well. The Association for

Medical Ethics is one organization that tackles the problem of financial incentives in medicine. Many societies do not subscribe to this view, but have increasingly required financial disclosure from physicians that publish articles or serve on committees/directorships.

5. *Malpractice information is available through some medical board websites.* In New Jersey, for example, physicians are required to report lawsuits and the outcomes of these lawsuits. This is a very contentious issue, since many physicians claim that most lawsuits are frivolous. Plaintiffs' attorneys, in contrast, believe this is a patient safety issue, and malpractice is a negative indicator of physician performance. Lawsuits are far more common than disciplinary proceedings by a state medical board or specialty medical society. The goals are different. The state medical board wants to safeguard the public's safety, but a lawsuit is to provide restitution for a patient. Medical disciplinary proceedings may be a better indicator of public endangerment, as compared to a malpractice lawsuit. Malpractice lawsuits tend to be less transparent than medical board proceedings. Complications can occur with any procedure, and a malpractice lawsuit doesn't imply that the physician is bad. Physicians should carry malpractice insurance.

6. *There are alternative certification boards.* The American Board of Interventional Pain Physicians (ABIPP) is a medical specialty board providing "Board Certification in Interventional Pain Management and Competency Certification in Controlled Substance Management, Competency Certification in Coding, Compliance, and Practice Management and Competency Certification in Fluoroscopic Interpretation and Radiological Safety." Their mission statement is "To advance the practice of interventional pain management and bring to the profession the highest quality possible in education in interventional techniques." The actual practice of interventional pain management requires knowledge about regulations governing medical care, risks associated with narcotic prescriptions, patient safety, and risk management. Physicians must have good technical skills and a full understanding of pain management procedure devices. There was no formal mechanism to test physicians on these skills, until ABIPP. The ABIPP certificate is available only to certain board-certified physicians licensed in the United States. ABIPP hopes to gain recognition by the American Board of Medical Specialties. Hence, physicians who are diplomates of ABIPP have paid money and studied to take a voluntary examination!

   The American Board of Pain Medicine (ABPM) is another certification society. ABPM administers a psychometrically developed and practice-related examination in the field of pain medicine to qualified candidates. Physicians who have successfully completed the ABPM credentialing process and examination will be issued certificates as specialists in the field of pain medicine and designated as Diplomates of the American Board of Pain Medicine. The ABPM has gained approval in a few states, such as California and Florida, to allow their diplomates to advertise themselves as "board certified." The ABPM hopes to gain recognition by the American Board of Medical Specialties, but this has not yet occurred.

   State medical boards are very strict in terms of "board certification." If a physician advertises that they are board certified, this board must be recognized by their state medical board. The American Board of Medical Specialties can help determine if your physician is board certified in pain medicine. If the physician advertises board certification and this board is not recognized by their state medical board, the physician can face disciplinary action.

7. *Research and publications demonstrate a physician who has taken time out of their daily practice, in order to give back to the field of medicine.* Physicians are very busy, and publishing is a voluntary effort. A peer-reviewed publication by a physician is an honor. "Peer-reviewed" means that esteemed colleagues in the physician's field rate this physician's research and writing. If this is accepted, the work is published. The peer review process is conducted in a "blind" fashion to minimize conflicts of interest. Physicians cannot "lobby" to have their research published.

Any physician who publishes in the peer-reviewed literature is distinguished among colleagues. Very savvy patients can search a physician's publications to get opinions on a particular treatment. The National Library of Medicine has a wonderful search engine, known as PubMed. A patient can type the name of the physician or medical problem on PubMed (http://www.ncbi.nlm.nih.gov/pubmed) and get an extensive list of research that has been published. This can be quite daunting, even for physicians. Most of the articles are in medical jargon. If your physician has published peer-reviewed research, you should take pride in having a physician that has made a remarkable accomplishment.

Different pain physicians have different practice philosophies. The waiting room will give you a clearer idea of a physician's philosophy. I learned this from a patient! Patients tell us other practitioners' offices were full of patients who were heavily sedated and fatigued. Locally, these physicians are known to prescribe strong sedatives and high-dose narcotics. Other physicians have a practice focusing on mobility, wellness, motivation, and pain relief. The waiting room analysis was enough for this patient to come to our practices. Pain, unlike other medical specialties, is based on a disease process. Most other specialties focus on a specific organ system. So, it is hard to pigeonhole a pain physician into a specific box as to what they do.

Here are some general guidelines:

1. *Pain Specialist:* These providers may have additional training in anesthesiology, physiatry, neurology, or another specialty. Pain management doesn't yet have a dedicated residency training program. Pain physicians deal with chronic pain. They will listen to your story and ask specific questions about your pain. They usually conduct an exam. They may review your imaging studies, labs, and other tests. They may recommend a treatment. These treatments include medications, painkillers, physical therapy, nerve blocks, surgery, or psychological counseling. Since there are special rules governing potent painkillers, such as morphine, the pain practitioner may have you sign a special agreement. This is known in lay terms as a "drug agreement"; this outlines your doctor's and your responsibilities with the use of prescription pain killers and sedatives (controlled substances). You may have to undergo urine drug testing and you may

be called in to count your pills. You may be confronted, by your doctor, about anonymous phone calls regarding your use of painkillers. The American Society of Interventional Pain Physicians focuses on "promoting the development and practice of safe, high quality, and cost-effective interventional pain management techniques." This society has developed a number of evidence-based guidelines on the practice of interventional pain, on the appropriate use of opioids in chronic pain, and the responsible practice of interventional and medical pain management. The American Academy of Pain Medicine and the American Pain Society are other societies involved in education, research, promotion, and practice of pain management.

2. *Physiatry (Physical Medicine and Rehabilitation):* This is a medical specialty. A practitioner must be a physician, not a physical therapist. These physicians gain extensive experience in the nonsurgical treatment of musculoskeletal disorders. They have experience in neurological disorders, amputations, prostheses, and special nerve evaluation procedures. They receive extensive training on dealing with disabilities and on treatments to improve a patient's function and mobility. This broad swath of experience is useful in helping chronic pain patients improve from a functional standpoint. The American Academy of Physical Medicine and Rehabilitation is a good resource for this specialty.

3. *Anesthesiology:* Anesthesiologists pioneered the field of pain management. They have extensive experience in the use of pain medications, nerve blocks, and sedation, and in the management of vital functions such as airway breathing and circulation. They have pioneered a number of invasive procedures for pain relief, particularly in the acute setting (immediately following surgery). According to the American Society of Anesthesiology, "Anesthesiologists are primarily responsible for the safety and well-being of patients before, during and after surgery. This may include: 1. Placing the patient in the state of controlled unconsciousness called 'general anesthesia'; 2. Providing 'regional anesthetics,' in which only a portion of the body is made numb; 3. Administering sedation when indicated for the relief of pain or anxiety." Anesthesiologists play a critical role in and outside the operating room.

4. *Neurology:* These physicians have extensive experience in the diagnosis and treatment of neurological disorders. According to the American Academy of Neurology, "A neurologist is a medical doctor with specialized training in diagnosing, treating, and managing disorders of the brain and nervous system."

5. *Neurosurgery:* These surgeons perform spine and peripheral nerve surgeries for pain relief. Surgery can benefit a limited number of patients. Most neurosurgeons prefer to have a pain specialist manage their pain patients for the long term; they like to limit their role to managing the aspects of surgical care. A pain specialist may work closely with a neurosurgical colleague, particularly with chronic spinal pain problems. Some surgeries for pain relief are becoming minimally invasive. These surgeries are less traumatic and promote faster recovery. As these surgeries become less invasive, there is a growing overlap in terms of which physicians perform these procedures. For instance, a certain type of video camera assisted removal of a "ruptured" disc (endoscopic discectomy) is increasingly being performed by well-trained interventional pain specialists. This is a recent development, but historically, surgery of the spine has been dominated by neurosurgeons. There are a few conditions that require

relatively urgent neurosurgical evaluation—these are rare conditions that can rapidly cause nerve, spinal cord, or brain damage. Most chronic pain conditions evaluated by a neurosurgeon have failed already conservative care. Surgery for most chronic pain conditions is optional (elective). Many surgeons will clearly advise that there is no guarantee of a cure.

6. *Orthopedic Surgery:* Orthopedic surgeons deal with bone, joint, muscle, ligament, and tendon problems. Collectively, these musculoskeletal problems are very common. Orthopedic surgeons may subspecialize in specific body areas, such as the spine or hand. They typically limit their role to surgery and surgical decision making. They can use their skills to diagnose and treat orthopedic problems. Orthopedic surgeons spend a large amount of their time giving nonsurgical advice—a visit to an orthopedic surgeon doesn't necessarily mean surgery.

7. *Spine specialist or back pain specialist:* This is a catch-all moniker. These specialists may or may not be physicians. If they are physicians, they may or may not be surgeons. Spine care has grown by leaps and bounds over the past 20 years. The greatest innovation in this field has been the cross collaboration between health care providers with different backgrounds. The North American Spine Society is an excellent resource for patients with spine pain problems.

There are a number of other specialists that may be involved in your care, depending on the location of the pain problem. Your pain specialist may seek their input as part of a comprehensive approach to care. As medicine becomes more specialized, multiple providers may be involved in your care.

There are many nonphysician providers involved in the treatment of pain. These include: acupuncturists, chiropractors, physical therapists, occupational therapists, massage therapists, and psychologists. These providers are an important part of the "conservative approach" to pain. None of these practitioners can perform medical procedures, such as an injection or surgery. They have a limited scope in terms of which services they can provide. This scope is defined by their licensing boards and specialty societies. The goal of these providers is to reduce pain and improve function. Some would consider them as part of the holistic approach to treating pain.

Conclusion

Pain is very complex and demands a multidisciplinary approach. The sad reality is that there is no cure. The focus is on reducing pain and improving function. Patients should seek out providers that have objective evidence of their competency—e.g., license, specialty fellowship training, board certification, and publications. Patients should seek out providers with positive subjective attributes. Although there are numerous rating sites and forums, a face-to-face interaction is the best way to decide. A pain patient may have to see multiple specialists and undergo multiple procedures. This can be frustrating, but patients should engage their health care provider to determine if the treatment makes sense.

3

DEFINING PAIN AND UNDERSTANDING TYPES OF PAIN

Eun Jung Yi, MD

INTRODUCTION

Chronic pain is now an epidemic. The annual cost of chronic pain in the United States is at least $100 billion. Surprisingly, pain affects more Americans, approximately 76 million, than any other common conditions such as diabetes and heart disease. It also accounts for the highest number of doctor visits. Furthermore, Americans over 65 years of age use more medications to control pain than other age groups. The most common pain syndromes according to the National Institute of Health Statistics survey in 2006 include low back pain (27%), headache (15%), and neck pain (15%). If you are experiencing any of these three syndromes, clearly you are not alone.

WHAT IS PAIN?

The sensation of pain is a self-preservation mechanism. Pain notifies us of a physical insult to our bodies that requires attention. From this experience, we learn to avoid the particular conditions that cause pain and to increase awareness of the affected area of our body. Everyone experiences pain at one time or another in their lives, but it is unlikely to be experienced the same way by everyone. The degree of pain perceived is subjective. This is because each one of us has a different pain threshold—the point at which we feel that a certain sensation becomes painful. In addition, pain tolerance levels also differ among us. Pain tolerance is the maximum level of pain a person can tolerate. So, excruciating pain for one person may not be extremely painful at all to another. What this means is that there is no objective measurement for pain beyond the patient's own description. Part of the reason why there is so much variation in our experiences is our biological mechanisms that modify pain signals by decreasing or increasing pain perception in our bodies. The pain experience is truly personal and complicated.

In the allopathic medical community, a standard definition of pain is: "an unpleasant sensory and emotional experience associated with actual or potential tissue damage or described in terms of damage." Let us take a closer look into this definition. Pain includes both physical sensation and emotions. The painful physical sensation is any perceived noxious stimuli such as a paper cut. Pain can be initiated by a noxious sensation, but it can also be accentuated or initiated from cognitive and behavioral activities. Some emotions affecting pain include anxiety, fear, and depression. These feelings may arise when we experience pain, whether it is ongoing or short lasting. We can begin to feel anxious or fearful about experiencing pain and about having another painful event. Continuing with the earlier example, if we were collating papers and had a paper cut halfway through the activity, we may be more cautious of our hand movements as we are anxious not to have another cut. We may even place rubber thimbles on our fingers to protect our fingertips. Perhaps we may be so fearful of a paper's edge barely grazing our hand that this causes us to be hypersensitive to the feeling of the paper and may even cause us to feel a slight bit of pain. To some readers, this may be a description of an exaggerated response to a paper cut. Another example may be getting a vaccine shot or your blood drawn when you are fearful of needles. Anticipating pain from a shot may cause us to flinch in pain when only the needle point barely contacts our skin. If the pain is ongoing for months, it is not uncommon to also experience depression in addition to the anxiety and fear that may arise. As one can see, the medical definition of pain encompasses a spectrum of emotional stimuli as well as physical experience.

How Do We Process Pain?

The sensation of pain is transmitted from the peripheral nervous system (your nerves) to the central nervous system (your brain), where it is processed, and a response is transmitted back from your brain to your nerves. For example, if one stubbed a toe, pain is felt near the injured toe. Thereafter, a natural reaction would be holding onto that painful toe. Particular nerves called A and C nerve fibers start the chain reaction that involves many nerves that transmit painful sensation to the brain to be processed. These nerves communicate directly to another set of nerves located in the spinal cord, specifically the dorsal horn. From this area, pain signals reach various parts of the brain. There are regions of the brain that differentiate between pain and other types of sensation such as itchiness. Other regions of the brain manage coping aspects of pain perception. In addition, there are other areas of the brain that send anti-pain signals that dampen pain. So once the stubbed toe pain signal is processed in the brain, the sensation starts to diminish with the anti-pain signals. Of course, as discussed earlier, the degree of pain is a personal experience, and the degree of dampening is individual. Although the sensation of stubbing one's toe may be the same action, the reception of this sensation in our bodies is widely different from the way the pain signals are processed in our brain.

Types of Pain

Categorizing pain is helpful in determining effective treatments. There are many ways to describe types of pain, from sensation types to chronologic types. Typically, pain is described by the type of sensation. Sometimes certain types of sensations are more affiliated with a persistent type of pain rather than with temporary pain, which we will describe later in this section. First, we will begin with nociceptive pain. This type of pain is generated by stimulation of the nociceptors on the A and C nerve fibers in the peripheral nervous system as discussed in the section above, hence its name. Perceived noxious stimulation includes thermal pain (e.g., burn from a stove), mechanical pain (e.g., cutting), and chemical pain (e.g., acid on skin). Further categories within nociceptive pain include somatic (e.g., musculoskeletal) and visceral (e.g., body organ) pain. Superficial somatic pain is sharp and clearly located on the body, for instance a paper cut on your finger. Deep somatic pain can also be sharp but is often aching and emanating from bones, tendons, or muscles such as the postsurgical pain from knee surgery. Visceral pain describes an ache from organs such as bowel cramping or that from a gallbladder stone. This type of pain is often located in a vague location rather than a distinct spot.

Another type of sensation causing pain occurs with nerve injury. When this occurs, it may generate neuropathic pain. This type of pain is most often described as a burning or electric sensation. Most of the time, neuropathic pain can be resolved and is self-limiting if an underlying disease is resolved such as the sharp nerve pain from shingles. Sometimes though, neuropathic pain can persist and evolve into a different pain syndrome such as in postherpetic neuralgia, which can occur after exposure to shingles in some individuals.

Besides categorizing various types of pain by specific sensation, pain can also be categorized by whether it is acute (e.g., short term) or chronic (e.g., long term). Sometimes a distinct process occurs that changes the character of the initial acute pain, and this can develop into a persistent painful state of being. In general, one suffers from chronic pain when the physical pain persists for more than the expected period of healing and can develop into a chronic condition that causes continuous or recurring pain. Some common chronic pain complaints include headache, neck pain, low back pain, and arthritis pain.

Chronic pain usually develops over three to six months. When an acute injury occurs, inflammation develops. Inflammation is caused by a multitude of different biological signals released from cells involved in the healing process of bodily injury. Once the healing is completed, the acute pain resolves.

However, inflammation may also affect the brain's ability to process pain and measure its intensity. This process then increases the likelihood of chronic pain. The perception of pain can change from the physical location in the body to within the brain such that the perception of pain can be enhanced with future injury. In fact, "hypersensitivity" can occur and pain sensed even though a given sensation may not normally be painful. There are several manifestations of this type of hypersensitivity to pain, including "allodynia," a painful sensation experienced with stimulation that is ordinarily not painful, such as light touch or mild temperature (similar in many ways to sunburn), and hyperpathia, an exaggerated pain response to a normally painful sensation.

How Does Chronic Pain Affect Us?

Chronic pain often interferes with quality of life. It can affect sleep patterns, mood, concentration, and overall enjoyment of life. Therefore, attainable therapeutic goals such as returning to work or a particular hobby can improve quality of life and decrease the disability caused by pain.

The pain experience includes cognitive, emotional, and behavioral components that can hinder your ability to positively adjust to pain. Preexisting negative beliefs and unrealistic expectations may enhance the pain state. Expectations such as returning to your usual functional ability and having a pain-free existence can be unrealistic. Over time, one may find that these unattainable expectations start to affect mood. Additionally, discouragement over functional ability may make one avoid all activities that may cause increased pain. These activities may include social functions, hobbies, or work. Unfortunately, as more activities are avoided, the more likely you are to start perceiving yourself as "deconditioned" or even disabled. With this mind-set, perception of self and one's life will become negatively influenced. Personal and work relationships may suffer as one begins to become angry, resentful, or deeply disappointed with life. In addition, persistent pain can make one tired, irritable, or depressed and cause difficulty concentrating. Pain can appear to be controlling one's life and may reinforce avoidance of social activities.

Understanding the type of pain one is experiencing may assist in advocating for a *multimodal* pain management plan to increase pain control, in adjusting expectations, to increase pain tolerance, to improve functional capacity, and to reclaim your life. Multimodal means applying multiple methods such as using medication along with physical therapy, injections, and emotional counseling.

How Does This Information Apply to the Daily Experience of Acute (New Onset) or Chronic Pain?

Given that there are many types of pain, and that each person can process and experience pain in different ways, there is no one foolproof method of pain management. Understanding the type of pain being experienced may assist in obtaining a broad-based pain management plan in hopes of increasing pain control and in adjusting expectations and improving daily function. Certain medications are more effective for particular types of pain, just as certain behavioral techniques are more effective when coping with chronic pain. Allopathic medical intervention (such as prescription for analgesics, and interventional pain-control techniques such as epidural steroid injections) is just one aspect of pain management. Because the pain experience includes a mental processing and emotional/behavioral component, pain psychology and occupational therapy can assist with minimizing the perceived disability and distress. This will likely contribute to increased quality of life. Furthermore, supplemental therapies such as physical therapy, massage, heat, and acupuncture may be helpful. These therapies will be addressed in later chapters of this book. Often your first interactions involving pain management will be with a primary care physician, who may consult pain medicine specialists for further therapies as warranted. It is important to effectively communicate with your medical provider to see if your particular pain symptoms/syndrome can be addressed in a multimodal and effective way.

ADDITIONAL RESOURCES

Green, C. R., K. O. Anderson, et al. (2003). "The Unequal Burden of Pain: Confronting Racial and Ethnic Disparities in Pain." *Pain Medicine* 4(3): 277–294.

International Association for the Study of Pain. (2009). "Coping with Pain." *Pain Clinical Updates* 17(5): 1–5.

National Centers for Health Statistics. (2006). *Chartbook on Trends in the Health of Americans 2006, Special Feature: Pain.*

National Institutes of Health. (September 4, 1998). *NIH Guide: New Directions in Pain Research*: 1. Bethesda, MD: National Institutes of Health.

Warfield, Carol, and Zahid Bajwa. (2004). *Principles and Practice of Pain Medicine.* 2nd edition. New York: McGraw-Hill.

4

THE EVALUATION: WHAT TO TELL THE DOCTOR

Brian Derhake, MD, MSc, and Jianguo Cheng, MD, PhD

INTRODUCTION

Brittany is a 16-year-old high school junior who has been suffering from left leg pain after she twisted her ankle four months ago. She was hoping that the pain would go away, but it did not. Indeed, her left leg became extremely sensitive, and even the slightest touch to the left leg would cause persistent, excruciating burning pain. She was no longer able to attend her volleyball practice and was increasingly concerned about her upcoming SAT test as she had missed many days of school due to the pain. She was very nervous when her family doctor told her she had to see a pain specialist as her orthopedic surgeon did not think she had a fracture. She was worried about whether the pain doctor could help her and whether the doctor could truly comprehend her pain and treat it effectively.

"What should I tell my doctor?" is one of the most common questions patients ask before visiting a pain physician. This chapter will answer some of these common questions. When arriving for an office visit, it is important to keep in mind that the patient and physician are a team, working together toward a common goal. Imagine a marching band trying to play without good communication from a field commander, or a football team trying to run an offense without the ability to receive plays from their coach on the sideline. Just as a good marching band or football team requires clear communication to accomplish their goals, patients and physicians need to have clear communication to accomplish the goal of mutual understanding and effective treatment of the pain.

Pain History

When arriving for an initial evaluation, patients are usually first greeted by a receptionist or another member of the front-office staff. This is a person on the team with many responsibilities, including identifying and checking in patients, ensuring patients' privacy, collecting insurance information, scheduling, and acting as an interface with the medical staff and the patients. It is often advisable to limit your conversation to these functions, and you should not feel compelled to explain your pain in front of the entire waiting room. More often than they would prefer, physicians find themselves running behind schedule, requiring patients to wait for longer than expected. In such instances, it is advisable to approach the front-office staff and inquire about the delay and remind her/him that you are waiting. Please keep in mind that many reasons can cause delays. Most commonly, the physician may have to spend extra time with a patient with unanticipated needs. Pain can be a very complex issue, and appropriate treatment of pain requires a level-headed and clear conversation between the patient and physician. One can certainly appreciate a physician who is willing to push back his day in order to meet the needs of his patients. It is important to communicate clearly and calmly so that everyone on the team can optimize his/her function toward the ultimate good of quality patient care.

After the initial interaction with the front-office staff, a patient will usually be taken back to an examination room. Oftentimes, a nurse, nurse practitioner, physician's assistant, resident physician, or fellow physician will arrive to take vital signs, document current medication usage, review allergies, etc. These valuable members of the medical team will report directly to your pain physician. In many practices, physicians rely on these members of the team to take an initial history and gather much of the information necessary for decision making. It is important to answer their questions as honestly and thoughtfully as if one were talking to the pain physician.

It is very helpful for a patient to have an updated list of all of the medications that are currently being taken or prescribed with dosing information, including strength of the medication and timing of administration. For example: Aspirin 325 mg, one pill by mouth daily. This should include over-the-counter medications, vitamins, and herbal supplements. For some patients, it may be easier to put all of the medication bottles in a bag and bring them to the office visit. This is certainly more helpful than arriving with an incomplete list or no list at all!

This is also an appropriate time to discuss any alcohol, tobacco, or illegal drug use. Patients are often hesitant to admit to their medical team when they are using these substances because of fear of legal action, inappropriate treatment by the physician, or decreased respect one may have for them. These fears are understandable but unnecessary. One must understand that a pain physician's job is to best treat each patient and help with their pain and overall health. Although not advised by physicians, it is understood that some patients "self-medicate" in order to cope with pain or other problems. It is critical that physicians know about every substance that a patient is taking, both legal and illegal, in order to avoid certain dangerous medication interactions and to prepare the most appropriate treatment plan.

Along with documentation of vital signs, medications, and allergies (remember to include medical, food, and environmental allergies), the nurse or other member of the medical team may ask about past medical, psychological, or surgical history. It is often tempting to edit one's history to the events that a patient thinks are pertinent. However, it is advisable not to delete anything from this portion of the history, as seemingly unimportant or unrelated events can often influence a physician's decision making and medication selection. Patients are encouraged to bring documentation of previous medical workups, such as MRI, CT, or x-ray exams. In addition to the reports of these, it is also advisable to bring a hard copy or a CD of the images, as many physicians prefer to view images for themselves. One should also bring reports of any other workups such as EMG, EEG, sleep studies, cardiac workups, stroke workups, etc.

A patient will be asked to describe the current painful condition or "chief complaint" that has brought him/her in for the office visit. There are two possible scenarios that can take place at this time. The first scenario is one where the inquiring medical professional needs only a short explanation of the patient's problem as can be summed up in one or two sentences. An example would be, "I have had pain in my lower back with radiation down my right leg for the past two months after hurting myself moving a bookcase." In this first scenario, the medical professional will then report this to the pain physician, who will take a more detailed history. A second possible scenario exists where the medical professional does, in fact, want a full report of the pain history. It is advisable to ask how much detail is needed at this stage of the evaluation.

When it comes to the full details of the pain history, the medical professional will often direct the conversation with specific questions about the inciting events, location, characteristics, timing, responses to treatment, etc. Patients are advised to answer the questions as specifically as possible without "veering off course" to other details. The reason for this approach is that most medical professionals have an ordered way in which they ask questions to more effectively document the encounter and make a diagnosis. Situations may even arise where a patient may be interrupted in answering a particular question. One should not take offense to the interruption, but realize that the medical provider is attempting to direct the conversation in a way that will more effectively lead to a correct diagnosis. At times, details that seem very important to a patient are in fact not very important medically. At other times, patients may be asked to give more detail about a seemingly unimportant piece of information. There will be a time for the patient to discuss additional concerns or ask questions about details of their pain condition, which may not have been included in the medical professional's inquiries.

The following list of inquiries is intended to give you an idea of how the evaluation will proceed. It is not intended for you to memorize or to cause anxiety related to "forgetting some of the details." One may find it helpful to consider the answers to some of these questions before the appointment, in order to more clearly and efficiently tell the doctor your pain history. Pain physicians and their staff will know which questions to ask, and may add or eliminate questions from the list as they see fit.

Some common pieces of information are often requested about a patient's pain. These include time of original onset of pain, factors leading to the initial onset of pain (such as motor vehicle accident, work-related injury, surgical pain, etc.), changes in the pain since the initial presentation, location of the pain and where it moves or radiates, description of the pain (such as: aching, dull, electrical, sharp, stabbing, shooting, radiating, throbbing, numb, tingling, hot, cold, severe, moderate, mild, etc.), severity of the pain (usually on a scale of 0 to 10, with 10 being the most severe pain one can imagine) and its impact on patients' daily life, work, and sleep pattern, whether the pain increases or decreases at certain times of day or night, and aggravating factors such as positional changes and physical activity. There will also be an inquiry about responses to previous treatment, such as hot or cold compresses, exercise, physical therapy, massage, chiropractic care, acupuncture, medications, and prior injections and/or surgeries.

PHYSICAL EXAMINATIONS

At some point during the discussion of a patient's history, a physical exam will be performed. Just as either the pain physician or a member of the medical team may take the entire history or part of the history, it is also possible that either the pain physician or a resident/fellow physician may perform the physical exam, in part or in whole. Remember to participate fully in any examination performed, even if not by the pain physician, because the results of the exam will be reported to the pain physician and will likely influence the diagnosis, and ultimately the treatment.

Along with the verbal history provided by the patient, the physical exam is one of the most important factors in leading to a diagnosis. The actual exam performed may be very extensive, including neurological and musculoskeletal exams. However, depending on the condition, the exam may be relatively short. A brief physical exam does not mean that the medical professional is somehow rushing or providing incomplete care. It simply means that the particular condition with which a patient has presented requires only a certain type or amount of examination to diagnose.

At times, certain components of the exam may be intended to reproduce the pain of which the patient complains. It is important to alert the medical provider when pain is produced by a certain component of the exam, as well as whether the pain is the same as the pain one usually experiences or whether the pain is new or somehow different. Remember, each individual is ultimately in control of his/her own body, and if a certain component of the exam is too painful or somehow unacceptable, a patient should mention this to the medical provider. Recognizing that the medical provider should be sensitive to and mindful of the impact of his/her exams, it is perfectly acceptable to refuse a portion of the physical exam because it is too painful or somewhat unacceptable. A patient should not be looked down upon or treated differently because of such refusal.

DIAGNOSIS

Remember that pain physicians and their staff members probably have treated many patients for acute and chronic pain. Based on detailed and accurate history, proper physical exam, and necessary laboratory studies such as radiological findings, pain physicians can usually make a diagnosis or narrow down to a short list of differential diagnoses. Many patients are relieved when they find out that the specialist has in fact seen, diagnosed, and treated their condition many times before.

Of course, there is always a possibility that a physician will not come to a definite diagnosis on the first office visit. Pain has many complicated mechanisms and associated environmental and psychosocial factors that contribute to its presentation. Physicians may request additional studies such as MRI, CT, or x-ray. They may also request consultation from specialists from other departments such as neurology, physical medicine and rehabilitation, psychiatry, psychology, or surgery. At times, they may need to perform certain diagnostic blocks or injections or prescribe a course of certain medications in order to more accurately determine the diagnosis. One should keep in mind that there might be several causes of pain in a particular patient and therefore several diagnoses.

Although uncommon, it is possible that a physician may not be able to provide a diagnosis or treat a particular painful condition, despite appropriate evaluation and his/her best efforts. In this situation, physicians are encouraged to explain their thoughts to the patient and honestly tell them the limitations either at the individual level or at the level of pain medicine. A patient should not be angry with a physician who is unable to give a definite diagnosis or manage a painful condition, but rather, should appreciate his/her honesty and efforts. At any point that the patient is under the care of a certain physician, it is always acceptable to request a second opinion or referral to someone who may be able to more accurately diagnose or treat a condition.

Throughout the history and physical portions of the office visit, it is important to remember the "team concept" mentioned at the beginning of this chapter. A physician and his associates can provide the most accurate diagnosis and treatment only if a patient effectively communicates and answers questions appropriately.

Treatment Options

The goal of treatment is to reduce severity of pain, improve quality of life, and enhance the level of function. Treatment options for a chronic pain patient are very broad and often include behavioral modification, exercise, physical therapy, acupuncture, biofeedback, relaxation, stress management, coping skills, trials of medications, various injections and nerve blocks, minimally invasive procedures, and even surgeries. The "multidisciplinary" approach of pain management is discussed in Chapter 5.

Physical therapy is one of the most important treatment options. Patients often notice a decrease in pain once they have increased muscle tone, flexibility, and range of motion. Sometimes, injections are given by a pain physician to reduce a patient's pain temporarily, so they can more fully participate in physical therapy.

The treatment option with which many patients are the most familiar is medication management. Over the last several years, the medical community has welcomed a number of new medications that have positively contributed to the management of pain. Academia and the pharmaceutical industry are working to provide better medications for the future. Unfortunately, the "magic pill" has not yet been invented to alleviate everyone's pain. For the time being, we rely on an assortment of medications with various mechanisms of action. Oftentimes, a physician might prescribe several different types of medications in order to treat the pain in various ways. Some medications may provide rapid onset of relief shortly after taking a pill, while others may take time to work. Some medications require titration to achieve an effect, meaning that small doses are given at first and then raised, as tolerated, over the course of weeks or months. A patient, who may not receive relief from the initial starting dose of a medication, may receive relief once the dose is increased. Almost all the medications have side effects that may be dose dependent. The goal of titration is to find an optimal dose that is effective and devoid of significant side effects. It is important to realize that most medications are not intended to cure painful conditions, but to improve the pain associated with them. Until the "magic pill" is invented, physicians and patients must rely on imperfect medications that may not fully eliminate pain but rather decrease the severity of pain. Further discussion of medications is included in Chapter 6, among others.

In regard to injections, many fellowship-trained pain physicians are competent in performing the procedures while recognizing the indications, contraindications, and potential complications. Oftentimes, patients prefer these "minimally invasive" procedures to manage their pain as opposed to surgeries. These minimally invasive techniques commonly involve the use of an x-ray or ultrasound machine to allow the physician to place a needle near the area of a specific nerve or focus of pain, at which point he/she can inject various types of medication to help alleviate the pain. Understandably, many patients are apprehensive of having these injections. However, the injections are not nearly as uncomfortable as anticipated for most patients because certain medications are usually given intravenously to decrease both pain and anxiety while the injections are performed. Further discussion of injections and minimally invasive techniques including epidural injections, radiofrequency ablation, cryoablation, intrathecal pumps, and spinal cord stimulators are discussed in later chapters of this book, particularly Chapters 26 and 27.

Prognosis

Of course, prognosis is linked to the type and severity of the patient's pain. Certain conditions are much more treatable than others. It is often difficult to predict how well a patient will respond to certain pain interventions. While some will respond dramatically to the first intervention or treatment provided, others will require multiple attempts and techniques to alleviate their pain. Patients must realize that complete alleviation of pain is often not possible with current treatment options. However, through a combined approach of interventional techniques, medications, and physical therapy, many patients report a significant improvement in overall pain and functionality.

Additional Resources

There are many resources available to the public. In general, it is recommended for patients to be educated about their medical conditions. Sometimes, patients attempt to diagnose themselves with information (whether true or false) they have read on various websites. One should keep in mind that although self-diagnosis is not advisable, a better understanding of your pain condition is encouraged. The Additional Resources below provide up-to-date, basic information to help patients become educated regarding their conditions.

http://www.mayoclinic.com
http://www.painfoundation.org
http://www.painmed.org
http://www.theacpa.org
http://www.webmd.com

5

Treating Pain as a Team (Multidisciplinary) Effort

Dmitri Souzdalnitski, MD, PhD, Matthew Hansen, MD, and Jianguo Cheng, MD, PhD

Introduction

Chronic pain is an albatross. It is a life-changing condition requiring patience, dedication, and steely resolve. Similar to other chronic illnesses, chronic pain may affect multiple organs and body systems, alter the musculoskeletal, neurological, cardiovascular, endocrine, and immune systems, and create stress so significant that it negatively impacts all aspects of life. It frequently awakens concealed diseases and brings about behavioral, occupational, and social disturbances. Seen in this light, it is easy to understand why many cases of chronic pain should be viewed as a disease itself rather than a constellation of symptoms. Consequently, it is not surprising that single modality treatment (monotherapy) often fails to meet patients' expectations. The belief in a "magic pill" or a "miracle procedure" is unrealistic. There is no panacea. We have not discovered the fountain of youth. The treatment of chronic pain requires the commitment of many towards the goals of one.

After the World Wars and during the dawn of the baby boomers, the battle against chronic pain was being fought with a judicious use of surgery and the indiscriminate application of bed rest. It took decades to realize that bed rest is often harmful for people with chronic (non-cancer) pain and years still to find other effective treatment combinations and restorative options. Over half a century ago, patients would roam from one doctor's office to the next looking for relief from their pain. This endless and ineffective wandering caught the eye of anesthesiologist Dr. John J. Bonica during his days at the Madigan Army

Hospital in 1944. He found that pain management at his institution was not optimal, despite the presence of highly experienced and capable colleagues, each of whom came from a variety of specialties and possessed diverse sets of clinical skills. Coming up with a simple yet revolutionary solution, Dr. Bonica invited his colleagues—an orthopedist, a neurosurgeon, an internist, a psychiatrist, and a radiation therapist—to meet regularly to discuss the difficult pain problems of their patients. This informal collaboration met with tremendous clinical success, prompting Dr. Bonica to organize the first multidisciplinary pain center in 1947. Bonica's idea was that even the most talented pain practitioner would be unlikely to have an extensive hands-on experience in all aspects of chronic pain. This brilliant epiphany reflects the reality of the multidimensional aspect of chronic pain.

At first glance, the benefit of Dr. Bonica's discovery seems obvious. Nevertheless, it took another 40 years for this vision to come to fruition. In fact, multidisciplinary pain teams have developed only recently. Regardless, the most effective approach to the management of chronic pain is through the use of a multidisciplinary team of specialists with a diverse range of skills and expertise.

SYMPTOMS

Unfortunately, there are many types of pain and immeasurable amounts of ways to experience them. Nociceptive pain is caused by actual damage to body tissue, such as a cut or fracture. Neuropathic pain is derived from an injury or dysfunction of the nerves, spinal cord, or brain. It is commonly associated with burning, tingling, and sensitivity to heat and cold. It is described as sharp, aching, or throbbing. Psychogenic pain originates from the mind and is experienced differently by every patient.

It is important to define and address psychosocial issues influencing chronic pain syndrome as early as possible. The most common type of psychological dysfunction associated with chronic pain is depression. Treatment of depression can also help insomnia, which is very common in chronic pain. With a multidisciplinary team approach, a psychiatrist or psychologist can assess personal, family, and community support and provide necessary therapies to improve psychological functioning and overall quality of life.

Multidisciplinary interventions should be considered as soon as chronic pain is diagnosed. This is because the chances of getting back to one's daily routine are higher with early and adequate pain management. Effective interventions are best carried out by a multidisciplinary team. Suffice it to say, a multidisciplinary evaluation is particularly recommended.

DIAGNOSIS

Sometimes it is difficult to localize the pain generator or identify the cause of the pain. Consultation with experts in pain management may help better understand the pain and provide new ways of thinking and treating the chronic pain condition. In many cases, proper referral can be very productive and beneficial to patients. In an expert's hand, proper diagnosis is often based on history, physical exam, and diagnostic studies. In this way, the cause of the pain may be revealed and an effective treatment plan may be formed.

An early return to work or school and the participation in productive activity is highly dependent on the adequate assessment of what a patient can and cannot do. Occupational and vocational rehabilitation counselors in a multidisciplinary pain management team often work closely with occupational therapy consultants to assess and treat physical impairment whenever possible.

Dependency on potent painkillers may become a problem of its own, particularly in patients with long-term opioid therapy. In fact, there is evidence that suggests long-term opioid usage can lead to an increased sensation of pain. The multidisciplinary approach to the use of opioids and other pain medications allows one to learn additional pain control tools and become less dependent on opioid medication. It may lead to successful weaning off of opioids and better pain control in many cases.

TREATMENT

Therapies, such as behavioral modification, physical therapy, home exercise, and pain medications, may be effective in many patients. Nonetheless, consultation to pain specialists with a multidisciplinary team is often a wise step in providing therapies allowing for greater pain relief and functional improvement. Effective communication amongst providers with different expertise is facilitated when a multidisciplinary team is working together on a regular basis. The "one-physician office" practice model is rarely adequate in such cases. A multidisciplinary team that works together can overcome individual limitations, allowing for the organization of individually structured exercise programs to reduce the individual's fear of repeat injury, teaching of proper body mechanics and postural awareness, and the use of alternative noninvasive pain-control therapies in addition to the medications and procedures that are often necessary. All of these are done in a cohesive way with an ultimate goal of reducing pain, improving quality of life, and enhancing functional recovery.

Referrals are frequently made by primary care physicians or family doctors. They may also come from the patient (self-referral), a pain management team member, or from a wide variety of other sources, including physicians of different specialties, other health care providers, attorneys, employers, and insurance carriers. Keep in mind that the most important member of the team is you, the patient. Specialists can only do so much. If the patient is not on the same page as the rest of the team, then the chance of success is minimal. Unfortunately, some patients may fear that their pain is imagined. Rest assured. Pain-related specialists know that pain is real, regardless of whether it is nociceptive, neuropathic, or psychogenic, and will work to control your symptoms and return you to a productive and rewarding lifestyle.

Most multidisciplinary teams deal with diverse chronic pain conditions, including chronic back or joint pain, fibromyalgia, pain caused by the nerves themselves (such as trigeminal neuralgia or diabetic neuropathy), phantom limb pain, complex regional pain syndrome I (e.g., reflex sympathetic dystrophy), CRPS II (causalgia), central (sometimes called "thalamic") pain, and facial, gastrointestinal, and other pains. There are even distinct multidisciplinary programs for the treatment of intractable headaches and cancer. In fact, many therapeutic techniques used in the management of chronic non-cancer pain syndromes may be effective for patients with cancer.

Similar to the multidisciplinary team approach, pain physicians themselves tend to come from diverse backgrounds and trainings. Before specializing in pain management, pain physicians may have been trained as anesthesiologists, internists, neurologists, psychiatrists, or physiatrists. The pain physician coordinates care for the patient, controlling symptoms with both medical management as well as interventional procedures. In order to improve patient care, the pain physician relies on a network of therapeutic options.

The pain psychologist is an important member of this network. Persistent pain lasting over six months may cause emotional and maladaptive behaviors necessitating expert consultation and treatment to manage specific problems caused by chronic pain disease, most commonly depression or insomnia. Psychological services include extensive evaluation and individual, family, and group psychotherapy with an emphasis on explaining the nature of unproductive responses to pain, teaching effective problem solving, behavioral modification, and stress management techniques. These services can reduce depression and anxiety, allowing for a more controlled behavioral response to pain. In addition, the pain psychologist can reduce the probability of treatment failure.

A psychologist may also use biofeedback equipment to educate patients on the nature of their body's response to pain, stress, and helplessness. Through visual and/or auditory feedback, this technology can help patients control the body systems intimately associated with the intensity of their pain (including muscle tension, breathing, perspiration, and others). Once patients observe how their own body responds to pain and stress, the psychologist can show them how to rework these functions through a variety of mind-body techniques.

Physical therapists instruct patients on restoring appropriate posture and biomechanical functions, providing gait training, helping with muscle strength, stability improvement, and organized cardiovascular fitness. Stretching of flexor muscles and strengthening of the extensor muscles are typically emphasized, as these exercises are among the most effective in chronic pain. Physical therapy is provided on both an individual and a group basis. Patients may be educated on using additional modalities at home. Common modalities include heat or cold packs, ultrasound, transcutaneous electrical neurostimulation (TENS), whirlpool, and massage.

Occupational therapists help develop a work simulation program for the patient, which may include a site visit to the workplace to which the patient intends to return. This worksite analysis allows for the observation and retraining of patients in the specific job-related tasks that they will need to perform. The occupational therapist is also responsible for ergonomic training. The goal of the occupational therapist is to provide a safe home and work environment, allowing the patient to overcome any personal handicaps and perform the activities of work, leisure, and daily living. Of note, there is a reasonable overlap between the duties of physical therapists and occupational therapists.

If a patient is unable to perform the duties required to work, a vocational counselor may be able to help. Vocational counselors perform comprehensive job analyses along with vocational evaluations to help patients choose a profession in light of their chronic pain condition. They also provide initial guidance for retraining or can refer the patient to a local official vocational rehabilitation agency. In addition, patients may act as a liaison with employers to facilitate their smooth transition back to work. The vocational counselor may not only mediate the patient's relationships with their employer, but also negotiate adjustments to the patient's job description if the patient returns to work with the same employer.

Other members in the multidisciplinary team of pain management include acupuncturists, Tai Chi masters, aquatherapists, therapeutic recreation specialists, chaplains, dieticians, chemical dependency counselors, substance abuse counselors, pharmacists, volunteers, and physicians of different specialties, such as orthopedists or rheumatologists. Additionally, the pain management specialists may consult alternative treatment providers, such as specialists in reflexology, yoga, meditation, reiki, chiropractics, balneotherapy (a special type of natural bath treatment), hypnosis, art therapy, music therapy, tribal healing, volunteer work, and health care resorts, among others.

There is an important distinction to be made between inpatient and outpatient multidisciplinary teams. Most patients are treated effectively in a collaborative outpatient multidisciplinary program as described above. An outpatient daily program is much more likely to be paid by insurance, since hospitalization can be very costly. In addition, this program can realistically simulate the ordinary activities of a patient's daily life, allowing for a smooth transition from the multidisciplinary program back into their normal lives. However, patients who require round-the-clock medical or nursing care, such as those with unstable medical illness requiring inpatient monitoring, or those who are not ambulatory or independent in the activities of daily living, may need inpatient multidisciplinary chronic pain treatment. In this case, the same services described above are available to the patients in a hospital setting, in large medical centers.

To begin inpatient therapy, insurance coverage is typically verified prior to initiation of the multidisciplinary team involvement. Once accomplished, medical records are requested and then reviewed by the multidisciplinary team in order to establish the patient's suitability for further evaluation. The patient would need to allow his or her referring physician to communicate to the inpatient multidisciplinary team, either verbally or by written authorization. The communication can be performed by discharge summary, telephone, or personal meetings with the goal of providing necessary information that will help in the continued management of the patient. If a patient is self-referred for a multidisciplinary team evaluation, it is important to make sure all the medical documentation is readily available, including the copies of studies with actual images, preferably on a CD. This will help speed up the evaluation and avoid excess risks and expenses associated with additional diagnostic evaluations.

In addition to existing medical documentation, individuals may be asked to fill out patient questionnaires before undergoing a consultation. Generally, the multidisciplinary intervention plan is generated on the basis of available medical documentation and the questionnaires at the time of referral. The main goal of the first consultation is to determine what needs to be done to help the patient, to reduce medical services, and to facilitate the patient's self-management. There is a small probability that the multidisciplinary team intervention may be initially postponed or declined. The first discussion at the multidisciplinary meeting will frequently contain useful suggestions for further management of the patient's chronic pain. The patient's primary care or family doctor, who will remain an integral part of the multidisciplinary pain management team, can effectively use these suggestions.

As mentioned previously, multidisciplinary care extends the expertise of the referring health care provider and will use all its diverse components to meet the pain management needs of the patient. The medical director of the multidisciplinary pain management team is typically a highly experienced physician who oversees and optimizes the care of the chronic pain. The medical director may be certified in a variety of disciplines, including physical medicine and rehabilitation, anesthesiology, neurology, rheumatology, occupational medicine, orthopedic surgery, neurosurgery, psychiatry, internal medicine, and others. Importantly, this physician possesses extensive expertise in the rehabilitation and treatment of pain disorders. The medical director is responsible for orchestrating the team's efforts to produce the maximum "bang for your buck," including safe use of diagnostic and therapeutic interventions, protecting patients from ill-informed, costly diagnostic or marginally effective treatment procedures.

The role of the nurse case manager is critical in the day-to-day monitoring of a patient's progress. These team members perform troubleshooting and provide ongoing communication with referral sources, employers, attorneys, health insurance providers, other health care providers, and patient families. Other responsibilities of the nurse case manager in the multidisciplinary pain management team include development of policies and procedures, quality assurance, and collection and maintenance of patient data.

The assumption that chronic pain affects not just the patient, but the patient's family and members of their social circle, makes the role of the team's social worker indispensable. Ideally, family members provide strong support for the patient's behavioral adaptation to chronic pain. However, this is not always the case. With permission, the social worker will assess the patient's interactions with their family, loved ones, and close members of their community as an important part of the evaluation and treatment process.

Prognosis

Professional clinical studies unquestionably support not only the efficacy, but also the cost-effectiveness of the team effort in pain management. A quantitative review of 65 studies in 1992 found a multidisciplinary approach to be effective in reducing medication use, reducing emotional distress, reducing health care utilization, increasing both the ability to return to work and physical activity levels, and closing disability claims as compared to monotherapy or no treatment at all. In addition, multidisciplinary teams were found to be six times more cost-effective than surgery performed for chronic pain.

Despite an excess of compelling evidence that team efforts are better for patients than monotherapy, barriers to successful implementation of the multidisciplinary approach are the same now as they were in the last century. Most patients and third-party payers unrealistically expect multidisciplinary teams to completely resolve the pain. Some patients and insurers consider the emphasis on independency of a chronic pain patient, behavioral modification, family and community involvement, rehabilitation and retraining (key elements of the team effort philosophy) to be inadequate. For many, it is difficult to accept the fact that curing chronic pain is generally not possible. Nonetheless, the multidisciplinary team effort, if applied early in the course of the disease, may prevent major structural and functional changes, allowing for a fruitful and prosperous life.

Additional Resources

Desirable Characteristics for Pain Treatment Facilities. http://www.iasp-pain.org. Last accessed 09/23/2010.

Mahoney, Diana. Multidisciplinary Approach Helps in Chronic Pain (Multidisciplinary Pain Management Program). *Internal Medicine News*, 37 (16): 20 (1). August 15, 2004.

Potash, Shana. Team Approach to Pain Relief. *NIH MedlinePlus: The Magazine.* Fall 2007. http://www.nlm.nih.gov/medlineplus/magazine/issues/fall07/articles/fall07pg23.html. Last accessed 05/23/2011.

Stanton-Hicks, Michael. *The Cleveland Clinic Guide to Pain Management.* Kaplan Publishing, 2009.

6

MEDICATIONS USED TO MANAGE PAIN

Kay Yeung, MD, and Justin Hata, MD

Medications used to relieve pain and/or discomfort are called *analgesics*. Similar to all medications, each and every analgesic (or, "pain reliever") has benefits and risks. There are many different kinds of pain medications, and each medicine may have a slightly different effect on each person. Some types of pain may respond better to certain medications than others. For instance, pain due to arthritis may respond better to nonsteroidal anti-inflammatory drugs (NSAIDs), such as ibuprofen, than it would to acetaminophen (Tylenol).

Three main categories of medications will be presented here: (a) non-opioid (non-narcotic) analgesics—acetaminophen and NSAIDs; (b) opioid (narcotic) analgesics; and (c) coanalgesics (combined non-opioid and opioid drugs).

NON-OPIOID PAIN MEDICATIONS

The non-opioid pain medications most often used are the nonsteroidal anti-inflammatory drugs (NSAIDs) and acetaminophen (Tylenol) for treating pain related to surgery, trauma, arthritis, and cancer. NSAIDs are generally better at treating pain caused by inflammation than acetaminophen because acetaminophen lacks the ability to reduce inflammation. All NSAIDs have properties that help relieve pain, decrease inflammation, and reduce fever. When NSAIDs are combined with other pain medicines, they can act cooperatively together and create more pain relief than when either is used alone.

Acetaminophen (Tylenol)

Acetaminophen is a medication used to treat pain. It actually differs from the rest of the NSAIDs because it lacks anti-inflammatory effects. Compared to aspirin, acetaminophen does not damage the gastric lining. Acetaminophen is a frequently used pain medication because it is a readily available over-the-counter (OTC) medication that does not require a prescription from a physician. It is a popular alternative to aspirin and other NSAIDs because it lacks the side effects commonly associated with NSAIDs (increased risk of bleeding, stomach ulcers, kidney damage). Acetaminophen is broken down in the liver and can cause significant harm to the liver if taken in amounts that exceed the maximum total daily dose. Drugs or other substances, like alcohol, can increase the risk of liver damage if taken together with acetaminophen.

NSAIDs

NSAIDs are drugs that cause analgesia (pain relief), reduce inflammation and can reduce fevers. They can be categorized into drugs that are (a) nonspecific inhibitors of COX (enzymes that regulate various bodily functions such as inflammation), or (b) selective COX-2 inhibitors. NSAIDs work by blocking the body's response to painful stimuli.

The following are subcategories of NSAIDs and their common drug names. We have included brand and generic names, as well as useful comments about common reasons for taking the drug and possible safety concerns.

- *Diflunisal (Dolobid):* This may be better tolerated by the stomach than other NSAIDs
- *Acetic acid derivatives: Indomethacin, sulindac, tolmetin.*
  - Indomethacin (Indocin): Its use is limited due to the higher frequency of side effects.
- *Propionic acid derivatives: Ibuprofen, naproxen, fenoprofen, ketoprofen, diclofenac.*
  - These include common OTC formulations such as ibuprofen (Motrin, Advil), naproxen (Aleve/Naprosyn), fenoprofen (Nalfon), ketoprofen (Orudis), flurbiprofen (Ansaid), oxaprozin (Daypro).
- *Diclofenac:* Flector Patch 1.3% is a patch that is placed on the skin. This form of diclofenac is commonly used for acute pain due to minor sprains, strains and contusions. Voltaren gel 1% is very effective for muscle strain, spasm and other musculoskeletal conditions. It is spread on the skin over the affected painful area, with extremely good results.
- *Pyrrolopyrrole:* Ketorolac (Toradol) is available as an injection or a pill. The pain-relieving properties are much more potent that its anti-inflammatory properties, but use is typically limited to five days of treatment.
- *Carboxylic acids*
  - *Acetylated:* Aspirin (Acetylsalicylic acid) is one of the oldest non-opioid oral analgesics, invented in 1897. Aspirin is well absorbed by the stomach and small intestines, but can cause gastric disturbance and bleeding. Aspirin has been associated with Reye's syndrome. This is a dangerous condition associated with the use of aspirin during a viral illness in children that may result in seizures, coma, and sometimes death. Aspirin has largely been replaced by newer NSAIDs for the treatment of pain.

○ *Nonacetylated, Salicylate salts:* sodium salicylate, salicylamide, diflunisal, choline magnesium trisalicylate, and salsalate: These analgesics produce fewer GI (gastrointestinal) side effects than aspirin.

- *COX-2 Selective NSAIDs (celecoxib, rofecoxib, valdecoxib, parecoxib):* COX-2 selective inhibitors provide similar pain relief as the nonselective NSAIDs with less risk of GI ulceration and bleeding. The risk of acute heart attacks and strokes may be increased in patients treated chronically with selective COX-2 inhibitors. Of these, only celecoxib (Celebrex) is currently available in the United States.

Examples of commonly used non-opioid analgesics are shown in Table 6.1.

Table 6.1
Selected Non-Opioid Analgesics

Drug	Average Dose (mg)	Dose Interval (hours)	Maximum Daily Dose (mg)	Comments
Acetaminophen (Tylenol)	500–1,000	4–6	4,000	
Salicylates				
Salicylates Acetylated (Aspirin)	500–1,000	4–6	4,000	Should not be given to children under 12 with possible viral illness, risk of Reye's syndrome.
Salicylates-Modified Diflunisal (Dolobid)	1,000 initial, 500 subsequent	8–12	1,500	Dose in the elderly 500–1,000 mg/day.
Salicylates salts Choline magnesium trisalicylate (Trilisate, Tricosal)	1,000–1,500	12	2,000–3,000	Unlike aspirin and NSAIDs, does not affect clotting.
NSAIDs				
Ibuprofen (Motrin, Advil)	200–400	4–6	2,400	
Naproxen (Naprosyn, Naprolan)	500 initial, 250 subsequent	6–8	1,500	
Naproxen sodium OTC (Aleve)	220	8–12		

Table 6.1 (Continued)

Drug	Average Dose (mg)	Dose Interval (hours)	Maximum Daily Dose (mg)	Comments
Ketoprofen OTC (Actron)	12.5–25	4–6		
Indolacetic acid Indomethacin (Indocin)	25	8–12	200	High incidence of GI and CNS side effects.
Ketorolac (Toradol)	30 or 60 mg Intramuscular (IM) or 30 mg IV (intravenous) or IM; 10 mg pill	6	150 first day, 120 thereafter	Limit to 5 days of treatment. May cause renal failure in dehydrated patients. Elderly limit to 10–15 mg IM/ IV every 6 hours.
Diclofenac potassium (Cataflam)	50	8	150	

OPIOID (NARCOTIC) ANALGESICS

Opioids are another class of medications that is commonly utilized to alleviate pain. There are two main categories: long-acting opiates and short-acting opiates. Long-acting opiates are used in patients with chronic pain because they provide a more balanced and continuous level of medicine in the blood.

Short-Acting Opioids

Short-acting opioids are typically used for acute (recent onset) or breakthrough pain. Short-acting opioids are often used in combination with other agents such as acetaminophen, aspirin, or NSAIDs to improve its efficacy. Using a combination allows the patient to use fewer opioid medications and thus have less potential for negative side effects from opioids. Some opioids have pain-relieving properties due to their ability to stimulate natural opioid receptors and other receptors. Two examples are tramadol or methadone.

Commonly used short-acting opioids include the following: oxycodone, hydrocodone, codeine, and tramadol.

Opioids are associated with negative side effects including constipation, nausea, vomiting, sedation, respiratory problems, itching, addiction, physical dependence, and tolerance. Caution should be used in patients with a history of breathing problems, asthma, and liver failure.

Tramadol (Ultram, Ultracet): Tramadol has several effects, which make it very useful in helping to treat pain associated with osteoarthritis, fibromyalgia, low back pain, and diabetic neuropathy (nerve pain). The typical starting dose is 50 mg every 4–6 hours. Tramadol may be useful in some types of nerve pain. Common side effects include nausea, dizziness, somnolence, and headache. In less than 1 percent of users, it has been shown to cause seizure activity. The risk of this is increased if there is a history of alcohol abuse, head injury, stroke, or decreased kidney function. Patients who take medications that alter serotonin levels in the body should avoid taking tramadol.

Codeine: Most of the codeine used in the United States is produced from morphine, but in other countries, codeine is a widely used, naturally occurring opioid found in opium. For the treatment of tension headache, codeine is frequently combined with acetaminophen, butalbital, and caffeine. It is also used to relieve coughing in some cold or cough syrup formulations. Tylenol #3 with codeine is a common preparation used for pain.

Oxycodone: Oxycodone is a semisynthetic opioid processed from an organic chemical found in the opium plant. It is 1.5 times as potent as morphine. Oxycodone is a good choice for mild to moderate pain, for acute pain after a dental procedure, or for chronic low back pain.

There are short- and long-acting forms of oxycodone. The short-acting form is called oxycodone, Oxy IR, or Roxicodone. Oxycodone can also be combined with acetaminophen (Percocet, Endocet, or Roxicet) or with aspirin (Percodan or Endodan). There is a long-release formulation of oxycodone called Oxycontin. The advantage is that it lasts longer, and thus patients need to take it less frequently. The advantages of the sustained-release oxycodone is that there are no active metabolites, it takes less time for it to act, and the pain relief effects lasts longer. Oxycontin is typically taken every 12 hours. Oxycodone may be associated with fewer side effects (hallucinations, dizziness, and itching) than morphine.

Oxycodone is metabolized by the liver. About 10 percent of the population has low levels of certain liver enzymes, and may require higher-than-usual doses to get the same pain-relieving effect. There are also certain medications that interact with oxycodone. Caution should be used in patients also taking certain types of antidepressant and antipsychotic medications. The dose of oxycodone should be decreased in patients with kidney disease.

Meperidine (Demerol): This is a common medication given orally or by an injection into the muscle, but the popularity has decreased due to potential toxicity to the nervous system. This medication is weaker than morphine, but takes effect sooner and lasts a shorter time. There is less sedation and less itching associated with its use. Side effects include depressing heart function and causing low blood pressure when changing from a sitting/lying down position to standing. Meperidine is broken down in the body into normeperidine, which is neurotoxic if it builds up, especially if you have kidney disease.

Normeperidine toxicity can cause involuntary twitching of muscles, seizures, and subtle mood changes. Meperidine for long-term use is not recommended, since normeperidine toxicity can even occur in patients with normal kidney function. Caution should be used if patients are also taking monoamine oxidase inhibitors or selective serotonin reuptake inhibitors (types of antidepressant medications), tramadol, or methadone.

Hydrocodone: The hydrocodone/acetaminophen combination is also known as Vicodin. Other names for this combination include: Norco or Lortab. Like oxycodone, peak concentrations are reached within one to two hours. The hydrocodone abuse potential is similar to oxycodone.

Propoxyphene (Darvon, Darvocet): Propoxyphene is similar in strength to aspirin. It is often used in the treatment of headaches when combined with aspirin and caffeine. If this combination is taken daily, it may cause headaches to occur if it is stopped. Thus, combinations of propoxyphene, aspirin, and caffeine should be used for a limited amount of time only. There are also numerous side effects and precautions associated with this medication. Caution should be used in patients with liver disease. Side effects include dizziness, nausea, vomiting, and sedation. If accidental excessive amounts are ingested, more serious side effects can occur such as seizures and irregular cardiac rhythms, and the heart can even stop. When used with other drugs that also depress the central nervous system, like sedatives, muscle relaxants, antidepressants, or tranquilizers, the combined effect may cause increased risk of more depressant effects of propoxyphene. Accidental ingestion of large quantities of propoxyphene can be fatal. Because of concerns regarding side effects of propoxyphene containing compounds (e.g., Darvon and Darvocet), it was recently removed from the market in the United States.

Table 6.2 shows commonly prescribed opioid medications for moderate pain.

Longer-Acting Opioids

Morphine: Morphine is the original and standard opioid pain medication from which opioid strength comparisons are made. The oral form is available as sustained release (SR) or immediate release (IR). The sustained-release form is given every 8 to 24 hours with the following as examples: MS Contin, Oramorph, Kadian, and Avinza. Morphine is slower to take effect, but lasts longer compared to other opioids. Morphine should be used cautiously in patients with liver and kidney disease.

Hydromorphone: Also known as Dilaudid, it is available as both a short-acting (IR) and a long-acting pain medication. Hydromorphone is stronger than morphine. It starts acting 30 minutes after taken in pill form. Hydromorphone is associated with less frequent side effects (nausea, itching, sedation, nausea, and vomiting) compared to morphine. Hydromorphone is broken down by the liver, and it may build up to dangerous levels if the patients have

Table 6.2
Oral Opioids Commonly Used for Moderate Pain

Name	Starting Dose Adults (mg)	Precautions/Contraindications
a. Morphine-like (mu agonists)		
Codeine	30–60	Mostly combined with nonopioid analgesics. Around 10% lack enzyme needed to make codeine active. May cause nausea and constipation more often.
Oxycodone (Percocet)	5	Mostly combined with non-opioid analgesics.
Meperidine (Demerol)	50	Metabolites may accumulate with repetitive dosing. Can cause CNS excitation. Avoid if kidney disease or taking monoamine oxidase inhibitors. Do not use for more than 1–2 days.
Propoxyphene (Darvon, Darvocet)	65–130	Metabolite accumulation with repetitive dosing. Overdose is complicated by convulsions. Not recommended for older adults or patients with renal disease. Removed from the market in the USA in 2010.
Hydrocodone (Vicodin)	5–10	Mostly combined with non-opioid analgesics (Vicodin).
b. Weak mu agonist and monoamine reuptake inhibitor		
Tramadol (Ultram)	50–100	Increased risk of seizures.

kidney disease. These side effects can include seizures, involuntary muscle twitching, and pain from sensations that normally do not cause pain.

Methadone: The name methadone comes from its chemical structure name (6-di*meth*ylamino-4,4-*di*phenyl-3-heptan*one*). Despite its reputation, methadone has several advantages including low cost, activity within 30 minutes, and multiple receptor sites of action, and it does not have known breakdown products that cause toxicity to the nervous system. This last feature is important for patients requiring high doses of opioids. Otherwise, possible side effects could include sedation, confusion, hallucinations, and involuntary muscle twitching. Methadone works on a variety of receptors that make it a good medication for patients who develop tolerance and dependence of opioids and thus need higher and increasing doses of opioids to get the same pain-relieving result. Methadone is also helpful in neuropathic pain. Neuropathic pain is pain from nerve damage, injury, or dysfunction, which may present as pain that is described as burning, shooting, tingling, or numbness. For pain relief, methadone is often used every four to eight hours. Methadone can be used once a day for methadone maintenance therapy to prevent the onset of opioid withdrawal syndrome. Methadone is broken down in the body by the liver. Methadone can interact with other drugs that share the same liver enzymes. Interactions can occur with drugs such as phenytoin, St. John's wort, rifampin, and carbamazepine. The acid in the stomach can affect the absorption of methadone. Patients taking Protonix or omeprazole to decrease stomach acid will absorb more methadone. Methadone can be used in patients with kidney failure on dialysis. Unlike other sustained release opioids, methadone can be broken in half or chewed.

Table 6.3 depicts commonly prescribed opioids for severe pain.

Fentanyl: For chronic pain, a Fentanyl Duragesic patch can be used to deliver medication through the skin. The patch should be placed on the upper body, on a hairless flat surface area without any open wounds. An area like the arm or abdomen with more fatty tissue for the drug to deposit is better than the upper

Table 6.3
Opioids Used for Severe Pain, Starting Oral Dosages

Name	Brand Names	Starting Oral Dose Adults (mg)	Comments	Precautions and Contraindications
Morphine	MS Contin MS IR Duramorph Avinza Kadian Oramorph-SR	15–30	Standard used to compare other opioids.	Sustained release (MS Contin, Oramorph SR) releases drug over 8–12 hours.
Hydromorphone (Dilaudid)	Dilaudid	4–8	Slightly shorter duration than morphine.	
Hydrocodone	Norco, Lortab, Hycodan, Vicodin			
Oxycodone	Oxycontin, OxyFAST, Roxicodone Percocet Tylox	10–20		
Methadone		5–10	Long lasting.	Accumulates with repeated dosing, caution in older adults.

chest, especially if you can feel the ribs underneath. The Fentanyl Duragesic patch slowly delivers medicine continuously and is left on and replaced every three days. The patch contains four layers: (1) an outer layer that prevents drug loss or moisture from penetrating; (2) a layer that contains fentanyl in gel form mixed with other chemicals that aid in absorption; (3) a rate-controlling membrane that helps to slowly release the drug; and (4) a silicone adhesive layer that sticks to the skin. Advantages include less constipation than with other opioids that are taken by mouth. It is also good for patients who cannot tolerate eating or who have chronic nausea and vomiting. The Fentanyl patch has slow absorption and therefore can take an average of 13 hours before blood levels are high enough to provide pain relief. After taking the patch off, it may take up to 16 hours before the blood levels of fentanyl drop by 50 percent. Patients should avoid submerging the patch in hot water, cutting the patch in half, or using a heating pad over the patch. This can cause more of the drug to be released all at one time, causing overdose or even death. It should not be used over broken skin because this can affect the rate of drug absorption. Common side effects include those related to the adhesive: skin redness, itching, and occasional formation of a pustule (an inflamed collection of pus in the top skin layers).

OTHER NON-OPIOID CLASSES OF PAIN MEDICATIONS

There are a number of other drug classes that may complement the effects of opioids or NSAIDs by either enhancing the pain-relieving effects, having independent analgesic activity in certain situations, or counteracting the side effects of the opioids. For neuropathic pain, medicine such as tricyclic antidepressants, gabapentin, lidocaine patch 5%, opioids, and tramadol can be effective.

Tricyclic Antidepressants

Tricyclic antidepressants (TCAs: amitriptyline, desipramine, imipramine, nortriptyline) have been used to treat neuropathic pain. The pain-relieving effects are seen at lower dosages than that recommended for treating depression. It is often taken at night to take advantage of its sedating side effects. Amitriptyline can have side effects such as dry mouth, urinary retention, constipation, delirium. TCAs are relatively contraindicated in patients with coronary disease, since it can worsen ventricular arrhythmias.

Antiepileptics

Antiepileptics include Gabapentin (Neurontin), Carbamazepine (Tegretol), Oxcarbazepine (Trileptal), Topiramate (Topamax), Sodium valproate (Depakote or Depacon), Phenytoin (Dilantin), and Lamotrigine (Lamictal).

Membrane stabilizers are a category of medications used to treat "nerve" pain. Injury to the tissue can cause changes in the way the nervous system responds to stimuli. Pain nerve fibers affected by tissue injury may have increased sensitivity. Sensations or stimuli that would normally be painless would then cause pain, like wind blowing across the arm, water from the shower, or a light touch. This is called allodynia. Neuropathic pain refers to a state of pain related to situations that cause the abnormal pain signals. Some common causes of neuropathic pain include trigeminal neuralgia, intercostal neuralgia, complex regional pain syndrome (CRPS or RDS), central poststroke pain, HIV-associated polyneuropathy and diabetic peripheral neuropathy. In neuropathic pain, there is an increase in the excitability of ion channels. Medications for nerve pain are aimed at decreasing the activity at these ion channels. The categories of membrane stabilizers include sodium channel blocker, anticonvulsants (phenytoin, carbamazepine, oxcarbazepine, valproic acid, lamotrigine, topiramate, Levetiracetam), local anesthetics (lidocaine, mexilitene), and calcium channel blockers (Gabapentin, Lyrica).

Calcium Channel Blockers: Gabapentin and Lyrica

Gabapentin has been useful in neuropathic pain. The usual initial dose is 100–300 mg at bedtime. This is gradually increased to a maximum of up to 4,800 mg a day divided into three doses during the day. Side effects include fatigue, somnolence, and dizziness. The dose should be reduced in kidney disease. Pregabalin (Lyrica) is newer on the market and has been used for fibromyalgia, postherpetic neuralgia, and diabetic neuropathy.

Anticonvulsants

Phenytoin (Dilantin): This has been used in the treatment of diabetic neuropathy although it is not a first-choice treatment, since there are conflicting results on its effectiveness. Side effects include somnolence, giddiness, slowing of thought, thickening of the gums, and coarsening of facial characteristics. Phenytoin activates a group of liver enzymes called P450. Thus phenytoin may interact and decrease the effectiveness of other medications including meperidine, mexilitine, haloperidol, lamotrigine, and carbamazepine.

Carbamazepine (Tegretol): This medication is primarily useful in treating trigeminal neuralgia (tic doloreux), poststroke pain, postherpetic neuralgia, and diabetic neuropathy. Side effects include nausea, vomiting, and sedation. Patients on long-term treatment with carbamazepine should have blood tests every two to four months, since there is an increased risk of having decreased production of blood elements.

Oxcarbazepine: This is similar to carbamazepine, but it is less likely to cause CNS side effects like dizziness or blood abnormalities. Thus, the advantage over carbamazepine is that repeated blood test monitoring is generally not necessary. However, a decrease in blood sodium levels may develop, which will result in dizziness and somnolence. In several countries, this is the drug of choice for trigeminal neuralgia.

Lamotrigine (Lamictal): This medication has been used for trigeminal neuralgia, especially for cold-induced pain. It can be beneficial when carbamazepine does not help. It also has a role for prevention of trigeminal neuralgia in susceptible patients. Lamotrigine has been considered for patients with HIV-associated nerve pain. The most common side effect is a rash, especially in pediatric patients when lamotrigine is combined with valproic acid. The efficacy of lamotrigine is decreased when used in conjunction with phenytoin and carbamazepine.

Topiramate (Topamax): This medication acts on multiple sites. Topiramate has been studied in patients with diabetic neuropathy. Its effectiveness is still being investigated. It should be used in conjunction with other membrane stabilizer agents if it is used for pain management. Side effects include sedation. It may also cause kidney stones and certain eye disorders.

Local Anesthetics

Local anesthetics are used in neuropathic pain to treat postherpetic neuralgia, trigeminal neuralgia, radiculopathies (pinched nerves), and peripheral neuropathies (e.g., seen in diabetes). It is used to block the firing of abnormal nerves, but does not block normally conducting nerves.

Lidocaine: Lidocaine can be given through the IV, with the dose based on a person's weight. Lidocaine is a medication that can affect heart rhythms and slow the heart rate. Therefore, an EKG is indicated if lidocaine is used long term. Side effects of lidocaine include dizziness, blurred vision, and seizures.

Commonly, a 5 percent skin patch (transdermal) is used and has been beneficial in patients with postherpetic neuralgia, post-thoracotomy pain, intercostal (rib) neuralgia, musculoskeletal conditions, and meralgia parasthetica (pain over the lateral thigh from nerve injury).

Mexilitene: Mexilitene can be considered the oral version of lidocaine since it is also prevents irregular heart rhythms. Mexilitine can be used for diabetic neuropathy, thalamic stroke pain, and spasticity. Side effects include somnolence, irritability, blurred vision, and nausea. Patients taking this medication should have their blood tested on a regular basis.

Antispasmodic Agents—Baclofen (Lioresal)

Baclofen binds to the so-called $GABA_B$ receptors in the body and decreases the release of neurotransmitters. Basically, it depresses nerve activity. Baclofen may be helpful in reducing spasms at night to allow patients to sleep better. Baclofen is indicated to treat spasticity, especially in patients with spinal cord injury or multiple sclerosis. Baclofen comes in 10 or 20 mg tablets and can be titrated to a maximum dose of 80–100 mg if needed and tolerated. Sleepiness and dizziness are the most frequent side effects. In larger doses, confusion and hallucinations may appear.

Skeletal Muscle Relaxants

Spasticity is an involuntary increase in muscle tone occurring during a muscle stretch. Common drugs used to reduce spasticity can act centrally to enhance the inhibitory transmission of nerves. The following will be discussed: tizanidine, cyclobenzaprine, chlorzoxazone, soma, and methocarbamol. Benzodiazepines (such as Valium) will be discussed in the next section.

Tizanidine (Zanaflex): This is a newer muscle relaxant that may be used to treat spasticity and rheumatologic conditions related to painful muscle spasms. It can also be effective as an antispastic agent in patients with multiple sclerosis, spinal cord injury, motor neuron disease, and stroke. Tizanidine is comparable to baclofen, but causes less muscle weakness. When compared with diazepam, tizanidine is similar in effect and causes less sedation. Overall it is better tolerated than diazepam and baclofen, but it may be more expensive. Side effects include: headache, digestive disturbance, somnolence, dry mouth, and hallucinations.

Cyclobenzaprine Hydrochloride (Flexeril): This can help relieve local skeletal muscle spasms without interfering with muscle strength. It acts primarily on the brain. It acts similarly as tricyclic antidepressants. Cyclobenzaprine improves symptoms of skeletal muscle spasm, reduces local pain and tenderness, and helps with range of motion. It is recommended for short-term use only (2–3 weeks). The effectiveness for long-term use has not been extensively studied. Common side effects include drowsiness, dizziness, and dry mouth. Interactions may occur if patients are taking monoamine oxidase inhibitors (type of antidepressant).

Chlorzoxazone (Paraflex or Parafon Forte): It is believed that chlorzoxazone acts on the spinal cord, where it inhibits nerve pathways involved with increased muscle tone. Chlorzoxazone is recommended for short-term use in muscle spasms related to acute, painful musculoskeletal conditions. Side effects may include digestive disturbance, dizziness, drowsiness, and liver toxicity.

Carisoprodol (Soma): Soma produces muscle relaxation, but some of its effect may be caused by its sedative effects. It is recommended for the relief of discomfort and pain in acute musculoskeletal conditions, but not indicated to treat spasticity. The most frequent side effect is drowsiness, tremor, irritability, insomnia, confusion, discoordination of muscle movements, and disorientation. Rarely, a patient may experience increased heart rate and low blood pressure when changing from a sitting to standing position.

Methocarbamol (Robaxin, Robaxisal): Methocarbamol is primarily used to relieve discomfort associated with acutely painful musculoskeletal conditions. The mechanism is unclear, although it is believed to act as a primary nervous system depressant. Side effects may include drowsiness, lightheadedness, nausea and dizziness.

Benzodiazepines—Diazepam (Valium), Lorazepam (Ativan), Clonazepam (Klonopin)

Diazepam and less often clonazepam are used as muscle relaxants. Diazepam is most effective in patients with spinal cord disease and injury, and occasionally helpful in alleviating local muscle spasms and pain due to inflammatory joint disease and pinched nerves (radiculopathy). Diazepam produces decreased tone in the muscles, but often produces decreased muscle strength and has side effects of sleepiness, dizziness, sedation, confusion, memory loss, and increased reaction time. Side effects may be even more prevalent if used along with other nervous system–acting drugs like baclofen, barbiturates, and opioids. Dependence may develop with long-term use, and stopping it right away may cause withdrawal symptoms such as seizures and delirium (confusion).

Topical Agents—Capsaicin Cream, EMLA

Capsaicin is an enzyme found in hot peppers that depletes a substance in pain nerves that relay pain signals. It is applied on the skin surface as a cream or solution and has been used effectively in neuropathic pain and arthritic pain. Initially when applied, there is some burning, but most patients become tolerant to this effect. However, some patients cannot tolerate the drug.

Another topical local anesthetic used is called EMLA cream, made of prilocaine and lidocaine (two local anesthetics). Oftentimes this cream is used in children during IV placement. In large amounts over 600 mg, it can cause toxicity. Finally, lidocaine is a local anesthetic previously discussed that can be used on the skin to help with pain related to postherpetic neuralgia.

CONCLUSION

Medications are the mainstay of both acute and chronic pain because most of these are relatively inexpensive, convenient for patients and families, non-labor intensive, and often effective. Overusing medications is discouraged, but medications for pain should be used when it is indicated and under the direction of a physician.

There are many negative effects to the undertreatment of pain including poor healing, weakness, muscle breakdown, increased risk of blood clots due to immobility, and stress hormone effects. Pain can also impair effective breathing, increase salt and water retention, decrease gut mobility, impair immune responses, and increase blood pressure. Psychologically, pain can cause anxiety, depression, and sleep deprivation.

Medications together with other therapies may decrease pain and improve overall health and well-being.

ADDITIONAL RESOURCES

Everyday Health (http://www.everydayhealth.com)
WebMD: http://www.webmd.com

7

SPECIAL CONCERNS REGARDING COMMONLY PRESCRIBED DRUGS

*Adam M. Kaye, PharmD, FASCP, FCPhA,
and Alan D. Kaye, MD, PhD*

Throughout this book, analgesics (painkillers) are described in various treatment regimens for a broad range of conditions. With this in mind, we feel it is important to devote another chapter focused entirely on analgesic medications. This chapter was written by a well-known, experienced pain physician who is also a pharmacologist and a pharmacist that has extensive experience educating pain patients.

Traditionally, acute (new onset) and chronic pain have been poorly treated by physicians, possibly due to concern by physicians of addiction and risk of toxicities. Acute pain usually is a symptom of a disease and self-limiting, while chronic pain persists beyond the usual course of an ailment and itself becomes the disease. In recent years, both the acute and chronic management of pain have emerged as a unique aspect of medicine. Newer treatment options have also improved the success of pain management (analgesia) for many patients by increasing the duration and potency of pain relief available. Doctors who treat pain successfully often rely on patients self-reporting assessments to assist them in adjusting pain treatment. Patients can help physicians treat their pain by assisting in the monitoring of their pain relief with each medication and reporting adverse effects promptly. Long-term treatment with an opiate (narcotic) medication requires a so-called "opiate contract" signed by the patient and the practitioner. Frequently, these patients suffer from pain associated with musculoskeletal conditions (pain in the muscles, joints, and bones) or cancer. Patients with musculoskeletal pain often require treatment with analgesics for either intermittent pain exacerbations or constant disabling pain. It is well described that continued opioid treatment in these patients must be contingent on treatment compliance and achievement of functional improvement goals.

Typical options for non-cancer pain treatment for most patients involve "morphine-like" or opioid and "anti-inflammatory," or NSAID medications. These medications are available in various different oral and topical (skin) formulations. Furthermore, these medications are available in immediate- and extended-release formulations. The successful selection and adjustments of these therapies can not only reduce pain and suffering, but also improve quality of life and emotional well-being.

Successful pain relief usually involves, in part, using a few different medications of various strengths and durations of actions to provide an effective regimen for their condition. Most patients have a combination of dull to severe pain that occurs constantly, along with sudden peaks of exacerbations that often occur after certain activities that require quick-onset medications. Specific medications are available to provide immediate, but often temporary pain relief, while other medications can provide a longer duration of pain relief, often with a slower onset of action. An understanding of the medication options available, along with knowledge of the patient's daily pain occurrences, allows for the creation of an effective pain regimen. Some of these medicines will have "IR" in their name, which means immediate release. Others will have "SR" or "CR," which means sustained release or controlled release. It is important to understand that each drug has a "half-life," which is the time in which it takes half the drug to leave the body, and is an indication of how long the drug will have its effect. For example, though both medications are considered analgesic pain medications, Percocet has a half-life of 3–4 hours, while methadone has a half-life of 23 hours. It takes 5–6 half-lives for a drug to totally be eliminated from your body. Doctors must also anticipate potential common adverse side effects, including sedation, constipation, and nausea, and help you reduce or minimize complications with the medications.

NSAID MEDICATIONS

Medications usually started for acute pain such as that seen with an acute injury, such as a fall or a motor vehicle accident, include the nonsteroidal anti-inflammatory drugs (NSAIDs). This class of drugs is also called "non-opioid," which means it is free of any morphine-like ingredients. While drugs in this class of medications work well for some by reducing swelling, pain, spasm, and other processes, the "ceiling" effect or the "maximum relief available" to be provided is often limited to less severe pain.

The NSAID class of drugs is not known to cause any tolerance or dependency. Examples of commonly used NSAIDs include aspirin, ibuprofen, naproxen, ketoprofen, indomethacin, diclofenac, sulindac, oxaprozin, flurbiprofen, etodolac, and nabumetone. This is not to say that this class of drugs is without side effects. The benefits of NSAIDs in the treatment of pain must be balanced against the risk of cardiovascular complications, including the potential for increased blood pressure, increased risk of heart attack, gastrointestinal irritation including the potential for stomach bleeding, decreased kidney function, and platelet inhibition, which can result in increased bleeding and even stroke. In most pain practices, NSAIDs are given out for the first 1–2 months to reduce acute pain and inflammation of muscles and joints. It is usually stopped or greatly reduced in dose because research data demonstrates that gastrointestinal bleeds occur after two consecutive months of taking NSAIDs, and most of these people unfortunately will not demonstrate any symptoms of gastrointestinal bleeding as it is happening. As a result, many people die each year from taking this class of drugs long term, and it is recommended that an NSAID be limited to the first 1–2 months for these reasons. Because it has been shown that heart failure is often worsened with the concurrent use of NSAIDs, they are not usually recommended in patients with this condition. It should be noted that some of these are sold over the counter and can pose risks if the patient is unaware of some of these very real side effects.

Some doctors try to reduce the amount of opioids they prescribe for a patient by prescribing NSAIDs. NSAIDs vary greatly in their side effects, half-life (see above), and strength. No specific NSAID is clearly superior for pain relief. Some doctors will try several different NSAIDs in an effort to find one that gives the best pain relief and/or the fewest side effects for a specific patient. A newer class of NSAIDs, described as "COX-2 selective agents," was developed over a decade ago to reduce gastrointestinal irritation such as stomach ulcers; however, these drugs have had other, highly publicized negative side effects, and many of them have been removed from the market.

The newer COX-2 selective drugs are equivalent anti-inflammatory agents compared with the NSAIDs and include: celecoxib (Celebrex), and the discontinued agents rofexcoxib (Vioxx) and valdecoxib (Bextra). The drug meloxicam (Mobic), which is considered an NSAID similar to the COX-2 selective drugs, has been reported to provide extended duration of pain relief with potentially fewer gastrointestinal side effects.

Topical (applied to the aching surface) NSAIDs such as diclofenac gel (Voltaren), diclofenac sodium topical solution (Pennsaid), and (Flector) patches are all newer treatment options available for patients with localized pain (for example, muscle, ankle, or knee pain). These newer products all provide effective pain relief, but precaution needs to be taken for long-term use due to the potential for gastrointestinal complications, as these are all formulations of NSAIDs. Even liver problems can arise in some patients.

The use of oral or injectable (into a vein or muscle) ketorolac (Toradol), an NSAID introduced over a decade ago, was believed to provide a very high level of pain relief. Due to fear of toxicity with extended duration of use, it is seldom used but for a few days of treatment and then stopped.

OPIATE (NARCOTIC) PAIN MEDICATIONS

Opiates have been used for pain control for several thousands of years, dating back to the times of the ancient Sumerians. The Sumerians documented poppy in their pharmacopoeia and called it, "HU GIL," the plant of joy. In the third century BCE, Theophrastus had the first documented reference to poppy juice. The word opium is derived from the Greek name for juice obtained from the poppy, *Papaver*, and the Latin name for sleep-inducing, *somniferium*. Arab traders brought opium to the Orient, where it was used to treat the symptoms of dysentery. Opium contains approximately 20 distinct, naturally occurring alkaloids, called opiates, such as morphine or codeine. In 1805, a German pharmacist, Sertüner, isolated a pure substance in opium and called it morphine. Morphine is named after Morpheus, the Greek god of dreams. After this initial discovery, many more opium alkaloids were discovered. Robiquet isolated codeine in 1832, and Merck isolated papaverine in 1848. In 1898, Bayer pharmaceuticals launched an alternative to opium and morphine, diacetylmorphine or heroin, from the German word for hero. By the middle of the 19th century, pure opium alkaloids, rather than basic opium preparations, spread throughout the medical community. Until the early 20th century, opioid abuse in the United States increased because of unrestricted availability of opium along with a massive influx of opium-smoking immigrants from the Orient. In fact, Thomas Jefferson grew opium poppies at Monticello. In 1942, the Opium Poppy Control Act banned opium production in the United States. It is important to differentiate "opioids," which are substances that act on the opiate receptor, and the term "narcotic," which is a substance that produces narcosis and can be abused, such as cocaine, cannabis, and barbiturates. Narcotics are derived from the Greek word for stupor. Narcotics were initially used for sleeping-aid medications rather than for opiates. Narcotic is now a legal term for drugs that are abused. In 2007, 93 percent of the opiates on the world market originated in Afghanistan. This amounts to an annual export value of about $64 billion.

In current medical practice, opiates are employed to provide pain relief from both acute and chronic conditions. Acutely, opioids are most commonly used to treat pain following injury, surgery, or labor and delivery. They are also used to treat discomfort arising from exacerbations of medical disorders. In addition, opiates have been used in lower doses to treat cough, and they can also be effective in causing constipation or treating diarrhea. It is important to remember, however, that opiates merely treat these symptoms; the underlying disease remains.

Opioid therapy involves the use of either weak or strong opiates, and often both are prescribed in conjunction to adequately control acute pain. Weak opiates typically come in oral (by mouth) preparations and are combined with other everyday medications in varying formulations to augment the response. These combinations often include acetaminophen (Tylenol), aspirin, or ibuprofen. All of these drugs have ceiling doses related to the non-opioid ingredient. Acetaminophen is included in a multitude of opioid formulations; its popularity is due to its property of not irritating the stomach. The limitations of these preparations come from the potential side effects of larger doses of the second drug along with the dose-dependent side effects of the opiate. Therefore, a larger dose of a drug combination with aspirin or ibuprofen over a long period of time can result in gastrointestinal issues, including bleeding. Another important example is acetaminophen poisoning, as it is one of the common causes of acute liver failure in the United States, and oftentimes, these patients are on acetaminophen-containing opiates.

Doctors and patients often look for "midrange" products that provide moderate pain relief without "major" risk of dependency or addiction. Some of these products include hydrocodone (Vicodin, Norco) and codeine (Tylenol with Codeine). These products are very effective for acute injuries, but the duration of pain relief is often brief.

Propoxyphene (Darvocet, Darvon) is structurally similar to methadone. Nausea, upset stomach, and constipation are often minimal compared to other opioids, but so is the degree of analgesia. Propoxyphene is reported to provide less than half the degree of analgesia as codeine or hydrocodone along with potential side effects that include heart damage, delusions, and convulsions. Propoxyphene when given in combination with aspirin or acetaminophen is thought to provide less analgesia than the aspirin or acetaminophen themselves. For these many reasons, the FDA recently banned propoxyphene use in the United States.

Hydrocodone is the most prescribed medication in the United States. It is available in many different concentrations formulated with a second drug, including acetaminophen (Lortab, Vicodin), aspirin (Lortab ASA), and ibuprofen (Vicoprofen, Ibudone). There are many different products sold under different trade names, including Hydrococet, Symtan, Anexsia, Damason-P, Dicodid, Hycodan (or generically Hydromet), Hycomine, Hycet, Lorcet, Novahistex, Hydrovo, Duodin, Kolikodol, Orthoxycol, Panacet, Zydone, Mercodinone, Synkonin, Norgan, Xodol, Hydrokon, and Norco. All of these products are routinely prescribed for acute and chronic pain. Ratios of hydrocodone to acetaminophen range from 2.5 mg/500 mg, 5 mg/325 mg, 5 mg/500 mg, 10 mg/325 mg, to a high of 10 mg/750 mg. Due to the lack of a controlled-release product on the market at the present time, dosing of every 4–6 hours is usually needed to maintain effective pain relief, and proper monitoring is required to prevent potential liver injury from large doses or chronic use of acetaminophen. Patients should not attempt to increase doses beyond the prescribed amount without first consulting their physician.

Unfortunately, because many patients do not get full relief from their pain, they ultimately require larger doses to try to control escalating pain. Because of toxicity in larger doses of these products, doctors usually attempt to utilize other secondary medications in an effort to prevent severe complications. Also, over a period of time, your body can develop what is termed "tolerance" to the same drug that was once effective. Larger and larger doses of the same drug are required to achieve the same effect. As larger doses are given by your physician, the risks of potential side effects and toxicity increase as well.

The "big guns" used in the treatment of severe pain include the use of even stronger opioid medications. Because of the risk of abuse, potential for side effects, and confusion about dependency, these more potent medicines should be used only in the setting of the most severe pain syndromes.

Morphine is the most studied opioid pain reliever and has been available in various formulations including immediate-release tablets, oral liquid, sustained release tablets, suppositories, and parenteral (injectable) formulations. MS-Contin and Oramorph SR (Morphine Sulfate Controlled-Release) provide 12 hours of relief in most patients, but lack a quick onset of action. Kadian is a newer morphine product formulated in sustained-release pellets that provides prolonged pain relief for up to 24 hours in selected patients. Morphine is also available in a bead-formulation (Avinza) consisting of immediate-release and extended-release "beads" that offer continuous opioid pain relief for an extended period of time. This product would not be particularly effective for immediate or as-needed (for breakthrough pain) use and requires proper patient education.

Some other medications are 100 or more times as potent as morphine. An example of one such very potent pain medicine is fentanyl. Fentanyl is available in a myriad of dosage formulations, including buccal soluble film (Onsolis), buccal tabs (Fentora), transdermal patches (Duragesic), lollipop (Actiq), and parenteral formulations (Sublimaze, Sufenta).

Oxycodone (Oxyir, Oxycontin) has a reputation of being overtly dangerous due to the many reported overdoses with its use. The numerous reports in the lay press stem from its incredible popularity with young adults, high-school kids, and celebrities. This formulation allows patients powerful, effective, and prolonged pain relief. Dosing of every 12 hours for the extended-release formulation and every few hours for the immediate-release formulation offer multiple prescribing options for physicians. Immediate-release liquid is also available for patients unable or unwilling to swallow tablets or capsules. Like many of the opioids, while tolerance to the sedation develops rapidly within days or weeks, constipation is a long-term complication. Chronic use of laxatives is often necessary with either polyethylene glycol-electrolyte solution (MiraLAX) or stimulant laxatives such as senna glycosides or sennosides, available with or without the popular stool softener docusate sodium (Senokot, Senokot-S, Colace, DSS, Surfak).

Methadone is an inexpensive opioid that is often given once a day because of its extended duration of action. It is effective for both chronic pain relief and to help patients who are suffering from opioid withdrawal symptoms in physically dependent individuals. Because of tolerance and possible accumulation of the drug in your system, treatment has to be adjusted often to provide optimal pain relief.

Percocet and Percodan offer dosage formulation that include either aspirin or acetaminophen combined with oxycodone in immediate-release tablets. Liver damage potential exists with Percocet due to its concentration of acetaminophen in concentrations of 325–650 mg per tablet, and it has attracted the attention of the FDA.

Meperidine (Demerol) is a very effective pain reliever with a fast onset of action after parenteral administration. High addiction potential and toxicity from its metabolite limit its chronic use. Oral tablets are available but seldom used for anything but acute pain.

Hydromorphone (Dilaudid) is a very effective analgesic that has been formulated in the past in an extended-release formulation (Palladone). Palladone was removed from the U.S. market due to concerns by the FDA of dose "dumping" or substantial release from its controlled release formulation in patients that used it with alcoholic beverages. A new formulation without this complication has recently been introduced in an extended-release formulation (Exalgo). This once-daily pain medication for opioid tolerant patients promises around-the-clock opioid analgesia for an extended period of time.

Oxymorphone (Opana, Opana ER) was first developed around 1914 in Europe and recently reintroduced in this country. It is reported to differ from many other opioids in that it generates less euphoria, sedation, and itching than other analgesics.

Another opioid product that is commercially available but seldom used is levorphanol (Levo-Dromoran). The product is considered similar to morphine, but with a longer duration (12−16 hours) of action and less associated nausea and vomiting.

Tramadol (Ultram) and tramadol with acetaminophen (Ultracet) are non-opioid dual-action analgesics that produce many of the same benefits and potential side effects of opioids with a reported reduction in the risk of dependency or addiction. Interactions with other medicines or history of seizures may increase seizure risk with chronic use and with specific medications including some antidepressants. Tapentadol (Nucynta) is a newer and similar type of product that produces powerful pain relief with less severe toxicity, even in higher doses.

In patients who have exhibited the potential to misuse or "tamper" with their medications, various formulations have been developed, including Embeda (morphine + naltrexone), Suboxone (buprenorphine and naloxone), and Talwin-NX (pentazocine + naloxone). Recently, Oxycontin has been reformulated to "prevent the opioid medication from being cut, broken, chewed, crushed or dissolved to release more medication." The new formulation involves the addition of "Remoxy," a substance that causes the tablet to be sticky and difficult to crush and prevents it from being able to be snorted or injected.

General Prescribing Principles

The type and the amount of opiate medication your doctor prescribes for your new-onset pain are based on a variety of factors. However, it is imperative to understand that no standard therapy exists. Opioid doses should be titrated to a response. Some patients may require considerably more than the average dose of a drug to experience part or complete relief from pain, while others may require a dose at more frequent intervals. Treatment often depends on a multitude of factors, and can be heavily influenced by your prior experience with opiates and other adjuvant (non-opioid) drugs. If you have never taken opiates, you are likely to require minimal amounts due to a lack of tolerance (see above) and the possibility of being more sensitive to an overdose. On the other hand, patients who have had previous opiate treatment or have substance abuse problems often require stronger and more frequent therapy. Lastly, patients receiving opiates on an intermittent or chronic basis often require maximum recommended doses. Many communities have pain specialists available to help manage these more challenging situations.

There is wide variability of responsiveness to opioid medications both in terms of pain relief achieved and side effects and complications that can occur. For some people, the biology of one's body may limit the effectiveness of certain classes of analgesic agents. For example, some patients are poor metabolizers of opiates. It is now understood that people who are poor metabolizers of a key enzyme in the opiate medications codeine and dihydrocodeine may not have success in achieving good pain relief. Likewise, a very long constellation of signs and symptoms, including increased heart rate and blood pressure, can be seen with opiate withdrawal. Still, doctors are taught not to automatically assume abuse if you report pain despite receiving medication. In fact, a lack of understanding of opioids by some practitioners and concerns regarding governmental retaliation for prescribing opioids can result in many practitioners under-dosing pain patients, which can often lead to treatment failure.

Doctors and the rest of the medical and research community continue to monitor the introduction of new pain medications that have the potential to provide safer and more effective treatment of pain conditions. You should not expect complete pain relief and must understand that safety and reduced suffering is the primary concern. Many doctors observe that unrealistic expectations by patients are often associated with requests for escalating doses of pain relievers (analgesics) that can contribute to more severe side effects and risks of complications and organ damage. Doctors need to assure patients of the need to remain on prescribed doses of medications consistent with their safe use, and not to escalate or increase doses of opioid medications on their own. As your doctor will explain to you, optimizing pain relief requires safe trials of medications until a specific combination (regimen) is determined with the most effective level of pain relief and least side effects.

In summary, a prudent physician will consider the benefits and the risks of taking these types of analgesic medicines, depending on the details of your pain state. The careful use of opioids by patients is crucial to prevent serious and even fatal complications, including progressive respiratory and central nervous system compromise. The concepts of your specific response to a given medication, duration of the medicine, and onset of pain relief are exceedingly important in efforts to find the best combination of opioid medications for you.

8

"ALTERNATIVE" METHODS TO MANAGING PAIN

Damien Tavares, MD, and Danielle Perret, MD

INTRODUCTION

An increasing number of Americans, both patients and physicians, are interested in complementary and alternative approaches to the management of pain. The utility of these techniques should not be underestimated. Good evidence shows that any treatment plan to successfully manage pain should be both comprehensive and multimodal. Pain pills and pain injections alone, without other therapies, will typically have limited efficacy, especially in the treatment of chronic pain conditions. Traditional approaches to pain medicine may include pain medications (both nerve pain medications and other analgesics), interventional procedures, and physical rehabilitation therapies. More and more pain physicians have found greater patient satisfaction when these techniques are coupled with a variety of complementary treatments, including: the use of manual medicine and manipulation; traction; massage techniques; heat, cold, and electrical therapies; orthotics (therapeutic braces); acupuncture; and the use of herbal medications and naturopathic foods (foods that have inherent medicinal value). Eastern exercise therapies are also reviewed in this chapter. Finally, one should not underestimate the power of pain psychology. Depending on patient preference, these alternative approaches can take the place of more traditional approaches; in the authors' experience in an academic pain practice, however, traditional and alternative approaches complement each other beautifully and can be used concomitantly. At the minimum, patients should be aware of the myriad of resources and techniques available to reduce pain and suffering.

MANUAL MEDICINE

Manual medicine is utilized by chiropractors, osteopathic physicians, and some physical therapists; all of these providers have specialized training in this modality. The function of manual medicine is to restore spinal mobility, flexibility, symmetry, and posture. After a thorough biomechanical evaluation, areas of restricted motion are identified. Various techniques are applied directly or indirectly to the restricted area. Both mobilization (using non-forceful movement of tissue within the range of motion of the joint) and manipulation (using high-velocity thrusts beyond the range of motion of the joint, resulting in the cracking sound that is associated with chiropractic adjustments) may be employed. Manual medicine is primarily indicated for neck and low back pain. Contraindications include spine fracture, cancer, and infection as well as spinal cord impingement or myelopathy (pressure on the spinal cord nerves), disc herniation, rheumatoid arthritis, and severe osteoporosis. To complement, extend, or substitute for traditional pain treatments, or when traditional pain treatments cannot be used (such as when a pregnant woman cannot receive a corticosteroid sacroiliac joint injection but has ongoing pelvic and buttock pain), manual medicine can provide great pain relief.

TRACTION

Traction is the process of applying a constant or intermittent force to separate the bony segments of the neck and low back. Its proposed pain-relieving effects include reduction of herniated disc material, muscle relaxation, and relieving pressure on nerves by widening the spaces where they exit and enter the spine. Traction is accomplished through various devices for both office and home use. An inversion table, commonly advertised on television, is a form of low back traction utilizing one's weight as a counterforce. Indications include neck and low back pain with or without nerve impingement. Contraindications to traction include spine fracture, cancer, and infection. Due to the forces applied to the spine, spinal cord impingement (pressure on the spinal cord nerves), severe osteoporosis, spinal ligament laxity (looseness), and artery injury or vascular disease in the neck should be ruled out before initiating traction.

MASSAGE

Massage is a broad term used to describe various soft tissue (tissue between skin and bone) manipulation techniques, primarily involving the use of a practitioner's hands, to produce physiologic effects. The effects of massage include muscle relaxation, improved circulation, and improved flexibility of scarred tissue. Massage is also utilized as an adjunct to enhance the effectiveness of other therapies including therapeutic exercise and manual medicine. Massage enhances the body's release of internally produced feel-good pain-relieving chemicals (endogenous opioids) and increases blood vessel diameter; the latter results in increased blood flow and increased oxygen supply to the tissue. Massage also has mechanical effects including the softening of scar tissue, the relaxing of tight muscles, and the increasing of blood and tissue fluid return to the heart; this reduces swelling. Massage can be beneficial for many conditions, including anxiety, stress, chronic pain conditions, arthritis, headache, and swelling. General precautions include the presence of infection, cancer, and recent tissue trauma or bleeding. Tables 8.1 and 8.2 describe various Western and Eastern massage techniques, respectively.

THE PHYSICAL MODALITIES

Cold and heat are both ancient therapies that have pain-relieving properties. Cold decreases inflammation and slows down the speed that pain travels; pain is, after all, an electrical signal that travels from our skin or muscle or bone through our spinal cord to our brain, where we perceive pain as a feeling. Cold

Table 8.1
Western Massage Techniques

	Description	Goal
Effleurage	Superficial gliding movement over skin, stroking-type of massage.	Muscle relaxation; to decrease swelling and improve circulation
Petrissage (kneading massage)	Compression of tissue between fingers and thumbs; alternating rolling motion type of massage.	To decrease swelling and improve circulation; to prevent or treat scar tissue formation; to treat sprains or tendonitis
Tapotement (percussion massage)	Rhythmic, with rapid strokes of various pressure.	To improve circulation; to aid with secretion clearance in those with pulmonary and sinus disease
Friction	Pressure applied by thumbs and fingers to site of injury. May result in bruising.	To prevent or treat scar tissue formation; to treat sprains or tendonitis
Myofascial Release	Prolonged light pressure applied to stretch connective tissue.	To reduce contractures; to improve joint range of movement
Rolfing	Combination of superficial types and deep types of massage.	To achieve improved posture and symmetric movements

Table 8.2
Eastern Massage Techniques

	Description	Goal
Acupressure	Pressure applied by thumbs and fingers over areas typically treated by acupuncture needles.	To restore energy flow or Qi
Shiatsu	Japanese version of acupressure.	To restore energy flow or Qi
Reflexology	Deep pressure applied to designated areas of the feet, which represent various parts of the body.	To treat high blood pressure, stress, digestive complaints, and fatigue

is an important therapy for acute or new injuries, especially for burn injuries and sports injuries, and cold therapy can limit the accumulation of swelling and reduce inflammation.

Heat therapy causes relaxation and feels soothing. In addition, heat therapy allows collagen, a fiber that composes connective tissue, to stretch. This ability means that tight joints can be stretched. In scleroderma, contractures, and even in rheumatoid arthritis, joint extensibility (flexibility and movement) can be increased.

Heat therapies may include heating pads, paraffin, ultrasound application, whirlpool baths, and others. Heat increases blood flow and may therefore decrease chronic (lasting more than about three months) inflammation. Heat, however, should not be used on a new (acute) injury as swelling and inflammation may increase.

Ice massage, ice packs, whirlpool baths, and vapo-coolant sprays are examples of cold therapies. These decrease acute inflammation and are invaluable in limiting the pain of new (acute) injury. Cold therapy can also temporarily reduce muscle spasticity.

Modalities are agents used to produce a physiologic response over the applied body area or part. Therapists commonly employ them as an adjunct to a prescribed physical or occupational therapy program. With proper training, many modalities can be safely self-administered by the patient to treat his or her pain. Common modalities are reviewed below and include the use of surface (or superficial) heat, deep heat, cold therapies, and electrical stimulation. Cold or heat sensitivity, blood vessel disease, or neuropathy (nerve injury) that impairs sensation is a contraindication to these therapies.

Caution should be taken when using heat or cold near open wounds or on patients with cancer. Cautions for the use of electrical stimulation include implanted electrical devices such as pacemakers. Heat and cold therapies should only be applied for 15–20 minutes at a sitting. This timing will minimize any skin irritation or injury. Properties of the various physical modalities, such as heat, cold, and electrical stimulation, are described in Table 8.3.

Table 8.3
Properties of the Physical Modalities

	Modality	Physiologic Effects	Indication
Superficial Heat	Hot packs Paraffin baths Whirlpool Fluidotherapy Electric heating pad Chemical packs Heating lamp	• Pain relief • Increase blood flow to affected area, which increases healing • Increased tissue metabolism to remove toxins from tissues	Chronic inflammation Tendonosis Arthritis
Deep Heat	Ultrasound Shortwave diathermy	• Pain relief • Increase blood flow to affected area, which increases healing • Increased tissue metabolism to remove toxins from tissues	Adhesive capsulitis Contractures
Cold	Ice packs Ice massage Chemical gel packs Cold hydrocollator packs Cold water immersion Vapo-coolant spray	• Pain relief • Decrease swelling • Decrease bruising • Decrease muscle spasm • Decrease inflammation	Acute injury Swelling/bruising Bursitis Tendonitis Minor burns Spasticity Fibromyalgia
Electrical Stimulation	Transcutaneous Electrical Nerve Stimulation (TENS) Interferential Current Therapy (ICT) Electrical Acupuncture	• Pain relief	Acute and chronic pain conditions Nerve (neuropathic) pain conditions

NATUROPATHIC HERBS AND FOODS

Certain spices and foods may help enhance health and wellness and may help treat pain. Antioxidants can guard the body from the damaging effects of free radicals, which cause damage to our cells. Free radicals are by-products of normal metabolism, and may also come from alcohol, smoking, fried foods, and pollution, and from toxins in the environment.

One teaspoon of cinnamon contains as many antioxidants as half a cup of blueberries; ginger contains an amazing anti-inflammatory ingredient called gingerol, which may work like aspirin and ibuprofen to inhibit an enzyme that causes inflammation. Ginger may help relieve the pain of arthritis and migraines and has recently been shown to relieve muscle pain following vigorous exercise.

Oregano has one of the highest antioxidant levels of any dried herb. One teaspoon of oregano has as many antioxidants as three ounces of almonds and one-half cup of chopped asparagus.

Red peppers have "heat" because of capsaicin. The hotter the pepper means that more capsaicin (and antioxidants) is on board. Cayenne, or ground red pepper, contains the most antioxidants; all red peppers, including paprika, are rich in antioxidants, however. Research shows that capsaicin promotes a feeling of fullness and may help curb appetite (people that add cayenne pepper to their meal eat fewer calories at that meal and at the next meal). Capsaicin (applied topically) is commonly used to treat painful conditions as it inhibits an important chemical involving in pain processing.

Other herbs and foods also have anti-inflammatory properties. Rosemary is highly antioxidant and aromatic. The antioxidant power of thyme comes from flavonoids, which are anti-inflammatory compounds. Research suggests that thyme may boost brain power (cognitive function) and cardiovascular health. Turmeric's active ingredient is yellow curcumin. Research suggests that this anti-inflammatory ingredient may inhibit cancer growth and protect the brain (preliminary studies show it helps prevent the growth of destructive brain plaques) and it is being studied to protect against Alzheimer's disease.

Using seasonings, herbs, and spices to substitute for mayonnaise, cream, or cheese will also cut a lot of calories; avoiding mayonnaise, cream, or cheeses will save a person from the harmful effects of those foods and will add antioxidant power to protect from inflammation and illness. This means there are triple benefits of adding spices to one's diet: (1) avoiding harmful foods; (2) boosting antioxidant power; and (3) cutting calories.

Some foods also have special properties. Chocolate, for example, contains substances phenylethylamine and serotonin, which can boost one's mood. Tables 8.4 shows special properties of the various herbs and foods.

Table 8.4
Properties of Naturopathic Herbs and Foods

Ingredient	Use/Properties	Notes
Allspice	• Anti-inflammatory • Muscle relaxant	
Anise	• Anti-inflammatory	High levels of antioxidants.
Caraway	• Pain relief • Anti-spasmodic	Used for rheumatoid arthritis, dental pain, and eye infection pain.
Cardamom	• Pain relief Anti-spasmodic	

(Continued)

Table 8.4 (Continued)

Ingredient	Use/Properties	Notes
Chamomile	• Anti-inflammatory • Sedative	Constituents include salicylic derivates (similar to aspirin). Used in anxiety disorders, nausea, and infantile colic.
Cinnamon	• Anti-inflammatory	
Clove	• Pain relief	Contains eugenol, which is useful for treating neuropathic pain (i.e., painful diabetic neuropathy). Also useful for earache, arthritis pain, and dental pain.
Coriander	• Anti-inflammatory • Muscle relaxant	Beneficial for headaches, muscle pain, and arthritis. Seeds can be used as a paste for mouth ulceration.
Epsom Salt	• Muscle relaxant • May be anti-inflammatory	Ingested or absorbed through skin. May be beneficial for fibromyalgia.
Fennel	• Anti-inflammatory	High levels of antioxidants.
Ginger	• Anti-inflammatory • Aids in stomach digestion	Used in traditional Chinese, Indian, and Arabic medicine.
Hops	• Anti-inflammatory	Used to treat insomnia. COX-2 inhibitor activity (similar to Celebrix).
Lavender	• Anti-inflammatory • Muscle relaxant	Beneficial for headaches and fibromyalgia.
Lemongrass	• Anti-inflammatory	
Marjoram	• Pain relief • Sedative	Used for external application for bruises and sprains.
Nutmeg	• Pain relief • Muscle relaxant	Active ingredient in commercial topical analgesic creams and ointments.
Peppermint	• Pain relief • Antispasmodic	Contains menthol which is used in topical analgesic in creams and ointments; contains azulene which is anti-inflammatory. Soothes stomach pain and colic.
Red Chile	• Pain relief	Contains capsaicin, an important pain reducer that reduces substance P, a key pain chemical. Initial topical application of capsaicin may cause a burning sensation for 3–4 days but will remit; excellent analgesia can be the end result.

Table 8.4 (Continued)

Ingredient	Use/Properties	Notes
Rosemary	• Anti-inflammatory	Contains four anti-inflammatory substances (camosol, oleanolic acid, rosmarinic, and ursolic); used in traditional Mexican and native Southwest Indian medicine.
Sage	• Pain relief	Used for sore throat.
Spearmint	• Anti-inflammatory	
Thyme	• Pain relief • Antispasmodic	
Turmeric	• Anti-inflammatory	COX-2 inhibitor activity (similar to Celebrex).

A variety of naturopathic medications are also available and can be found over the counter (without a prescription) in traditional pharmacies or in health food and naturopathic medicine suppliers; some can be prescribed at integrative medicine centers. Glucosamine-chondroitin, DL-Phenylalanine (DLPA), and Wobenzym N have particular efficacy in reducing pain. *Always consult a physician before initiating treatment with a naturopathic medication*; some can adversely change the metabolism of other medications, changing the efficacy of antibiotics, birth control pills, blood-thinning pills, and others. To cite just one example from the over 29,000 herbals available worldwide, garlic, a commonly used herbal that has been shown to lower blood pressure, can also cause nausea, thin your blood, cause uterine contractions, and produce other potentially unwanted side effects.

THERAPEUTIC EXERCISE AND AQUATIC THERAPY

Therapeutic exercise is a broad term used to describe the primary method by which physical and occupational therapists modify a patient's function. Physical therapists tend to focus on the legs, the lower trunk, the torso, and the back and neck. Occupational therapists, in contrast, tend to address shoulder, arm, and wrist and hand impairments. Goals typically include improving range of motion/stretching, strengthening, endurance, and balance training. Abnormal range of motion around a joint can lead to joint dysfunction that results in muscle imbalance and pain. Without adequate flexibility, available strength is less useful and may lead to muscle wasting and a vicious cycle of worsening muscle imbalance. The usual progression in strengthening involves utilizing one's own body weight with gravity eliminated, then training against gravity and finally adding resistance, including the use of weights. Abnormal balance due to neurologic impairment (i.e., stroke, Parkinson's disease) or abnormal joint function can result in falls (with sustained injury) and sudden muscle strains as a person tries to prevent a fall. Therapists can provide balance training and fall prevention techniques. Endurance training can improve heart and lung function resulting in improved blood flow and tissue oxygenation. Endurance training enhances well-being, decreases depression, and has been shown to improve pain in patients with fibromyalgia and multiple sclerosis.

Aquatic therapy is a form of therapeutic exercise that has several added benefits compared to traditional forms of exercise. The viscosity of the water provides resistance training. The buoyancy of the water decreases weight bearing and is ideal for patients with severe arthritis of the hips, knees, and legs; it is also helpful for very obese patients. The hydrostatic (compressive) forces of the water can reduce leg, ankle, and foot swelling. Centers of aquatic therapy have special classes with heated pool temperatures (where a patient can usually wear his or her own clothes and where no bathing suit may be required); these have been shown to reduce pain in patients with fibromyalgia. Open wounds are a contraindication for this type of pool therapy due to a risk of wound contamination. In addition, patients with multiple sclerosis should avoid warm pools because heat may exacerbate their symptoms.

EASTERN MOVEMENT THERAPIES: TAI CHI AND YOGA

Tai chi is an ancient Chinese martial art that utilizes controlled, graceful movements to enhance energy flow, or Qi, throughout the body. It is useful in treating pain secondary to knee arthritis and can reduce the risk of falls in the elderly by simultaneously improving balance. It has been shown to provide pain relief and improve well-being in patients with chronic pain conditions, such as fibromyalgia, as well as provide spinal flexibility in patients with ankylosing spondylitis (disease of the spinal joints). A recent study shows that tai chi reduces pain and improves the functional capacity of those with knee osteoarthritis. Another study shows that tai chi is effective in treating tension-type (muscle spasm) headaches by reducing stress.

Yoga is an ancient Indian movement art that focuses on stretching, controlled breathing, and distinctive postures. It has been found to have multiple physical and physiologic benefits such as improved balance, flexibility, and decreased blood pressure. It can alter an individual's pain experience by reducing stress and by decreasing depression and anxiety. There are many forms of yoga practiced throughout the world. Viniyoga is a therapeutically oriented type of yoga practiced to treat and prevent pain. "Energy" yoga is another form, which is thought to reduce labor pain and the need for analgesic medication through the use of special breathing techniques. Caution must be taken when initiating a yoga program due to its rigorous physical nature. However, overall, there are many exciting studies that demonstrate the efficacy of tai chi and yoga in the treatment of chronic pain.

MIND–BODY THERAPY: THE ROLE OF PAIN PSYCHOLOGY

In the culture of traditional American medicine, the mind and the body are thought of as separate entities. By the inherent nature of pain, however, pain is a combined mind-body experience because pain is multifactorial (with contributions from the nervous system both outside and inside the brain). The role of emotional, cognitive, and behavioral factors also equally contribute to the pain experience. In some chronic pain states, these factors may be the primary movers governing the pain experience when tissue damage is negligible. The rational to applying mind-body therapies to pain management is that learning or applying cognitive and behavior responses to pain and stress can provide an individual with a sense of control over his or her pain. This can reduce anxiety, depression, and many maladaptive behaviors that are often associated with chronic pain. Many distraction techniques provide a great source of relief for many chronic pain patients. Mind-body therapies are often used as an adjunct to a comprehensive, multidisciplinary pain management program; they may also be used as a stand-alone therapy. Available methods include hypnotherapy, biofeedback, and cognitive behavioral therapy.

Hypnotherapy involves the use of imagery; its goal is to produce a state of focused consciousness and body relaxation. It has been used preemptively (to provide pain treatment before the pain begins) and to treat acute pain secondary to an interventional procedure or surgery or anticipated pain such as that which occurs during childbirth. It has also been used to treat chronic pain states such as fibromyalgia (full-body tenderness) and myofascial (localized muscle tenderness) pain syndromes. With proper training, some individuals can be taught to perform self-hypnosis.

Biofeedback is another available technique in pain psychology. This involves the process of using specialized monitoring devices that detect and amplify various physiologic functions such as muscle tension, blood pressure, breathing rate, heart rate, and skin temperature. These parameters are typically under unconscious control. Biofeedback converts these responses into information that can be accessed consciously. This allows a patient, for instance, to visually (or through auditory feedback) "see" tension in the body and to correct or relax certain overcompensated muscles (the correction can also be "seen" by monitoring the physiologic parameters after the conscious effort to relax). The net effect of this technique is to train the body to reduce the pain from many conditions that are related to stress, posture, or muscle tightness or tension. Biofeedback has been used, for example, to treat tension and migraine headaches, fibromyalgia, and temporomandibular joint (TMJ) disorder.

Cognitive behavioral therapy (CBT) is typically performed by a clinical psychologist. The goal of CBT is to identify positive and negative consequences associated with the pain experience in order to reduce or eliminate them. An individual is taught self-coping and problem-solving techniques to treat his or her pain. CBT is commonly used to treat chronic pain, headaches, and fibromyalgia.

ORTHOTICS

Orthotics is a broad category that describes braces/splints that are used to promote function, provide stability, and reduce pain. They are used to immobilize affected structures to facilitate healing and to prevent deformity such as painful contractures. Acutely inflamed joints or tendons are provided rest during immobilization with an orthotic, which reduces pain and inflammation. Leg orthotics can also unload painful joints by shifting weight bearing to areas that can better accommodate the force or simply correct biomechanical alterations. By relieving pressure on painful areas of the body, orthotics can play an important role in reducing pain. In the authors' own experience treating many patients who have sustained a spinal compression fracture secondary to osteoporosis, spinal braces, which restore posture (and height), can relieve 50 percent or more of the pain. Tables 8.5, 8.6, and 8.7 show orthotic choices for selected arm, spine, and leg conditions, respectively.

Table 8.5
Selected Arm Conditions and Orthotic Choice

Condition	Orthotic	Objective
Elbow sprain	Sleeve brace	Joint support
Lateral epicondylitis (Tennis elbow)	Tennis elbow orthosis	Shortens origin of the wrist extensors
Cubital tunnel syndrome	Elbow pad	Minimize pressure over cubital tunnel
Carpal tunnel syndrome	Wrist splint	Minimize wrist flexion
Wrist sprain	Wrist splint with wrist placed in slight extension	Joint support
Carpal metacarpal (thumb) arthritis	Thumb splica splint	Immobilize joint
Stenosing tenosynovitis (de Quervain's)	Thumb splica splint	Immobilize wrist, CMC joint, and MCP joint of the thumb
Ulnar collateral ligamentious injury of first CMC (thumb)	Hand-based thumb spica splint	Immobilize wrist
Trigger finger	Trigger finger splint	Decrease excursion through first annular pulley at base of MCP joint
Digital sprains	Finger extension splint	immobilize PIP joint in extension but allow flexion of the DIP joint
Mallet finger	DIP extension spint	Allow healing of DIP

CMC = carpal metacarpal joint; PIP = proximal interphalageal joint; DIP = distal interphalageal joint.

Table 8.6
Selected Spine Conditions and Orthotic Choice

Condition	Orthotic	Objective
Whiplash Cervical ligament injury Stable cervical fractures	Depending on severity of injury, soft versus hard cervical collars	Pain relief, allow healing
High thoracic scoliosis (>T9)	Cervico-thoracic-sacral orthosis (CTLSO), a.k.a. Milwaukee brace	Arrest scoliosis progression
Low thoracic scoliosis (≤T9) Lumbar scoliosis	Thoraco-lumbo-sacral orthosis (TLSO)	Arrest scoliosis progression
Cervical (neck) fracture	Depending on location and severity, Halo device, Minerva body jack, 4-poster brace, Yale cervicothoracic brace	Immobilize fracture to allow healing
Thoracic compression fracture	TLSO: including Taylor brace, Knight-Taylor brace, Jewett brace, and cruciform anterior spinal hyperexten-sion (CASH) brace	Minimize forward flexion/ posture, maximize healing, and pain relief
Back injury prevention	Lumbar corset	Controversial, sensory feedback to individual, which acts as a reminder to maintain proper body mechanics; prolonged use may weaken back muscles
Sacroilliitis	Sacroiliac belt	Decrease motion at SI joint

INTERVENTIONAL PROCEDURES: ACUPUNCTURE AND OTHERS

Acupuncture is a form of traditional Chinese medicine, which is a common adjunct in contemporary Eastern and Western medicine. It involves the insertion of very fine needles into distinct anatomic locations to facilitate energy flow, which is also called Qi. Electro-acupuncture, which has excellent literature supporting its use to provide pain relief, is a variation commonly practiced in the West. A generator delivers electrical current via probes directly to the inserted needles; this is thought to enhance the effects of acupuncture. Acupuncture has been used to treat nausea and many chronic pain conditions including fibromyalgia and myofascial pain syndrome. Acupuncture probably has a variety of explanations to account for its pain-relieving properties. At least partially,

Table 8.7
Selected Leg Conditions and Orthotic Choice

Condition	Orthotic	Objective
Patellofemoral pain syndrome	Knee sleeve brace with patella cutout or buttress	Minimize patella tracking
Knee osteoarthritis, medial component	Medial unloader brace	Provide medial knee support, correct knee biomechanics, minimize further degenerative joint disease
Knee osteoarthritis, lateral compartment	Lateral unloader brace	Provide lateral knee support, correct knee biomechanics, minimize further degenerative joint disease
Internal derangement (meniscal/collateral ligament tear)	Hinge brace	Provide medial and lateral support
Leg length discrepancy	Heel lift	Correct discrepancy
Metatarsalgia	Rocker bar Metatarsal bar	Relieve pressure over metatarsals
Plantar faciitis	Ankle dorsiflexion night splints	Allow plantar fascia to heel in stretch position
Achilles tendonitis	Heel lift	Pressure relief
Heel spur without associated plantar fasciitis	Heel cushion	Pressure relief
Heel spur due to plantar fasciitis (from high arch/hyperpronation)	Thomas heel University of California Berkeley Laboratory (UCBL) orthotic	Arch support

acupuncture may treat pain by increasing the body's own production of natural pain-relieving compounds (endogenous opioids). Studies show that acupuncture also has beneficial effects on the cardiovascular system and is useful in the treatment of nausea.

Cupping is a form of traditional medicine commonly practiced throughout Asia and the Middle East. Cupping utilizes a glass or bamboo cup to create suction over a painful area or acupuncture site. The inside of the cup is first heated to remove oxygen, creating a vacuum. Negative pressure inside the cup creates a suction effect on the skin, increasing blood flow to the area. Some forms of cupping utilize an external pump rather than heat. There are two forms of cupping, namely, dry and wet. In dry cupping, the skin is intact. Wet cupping, in contrast, requires that a small laceration is made over the area where the cup will be applied. The negative pressure causes blood to flow into the cup, which is thought to enhance energy flow of Qi. Both forms of cupping have been used for many chronic pain conditions including, arthritis, back pain, cancer pain, and migraine headaches. Cupping should not be used over open sores, over frail/thin skin, or when allergic skin conditions are present. Application to the face or the abdomen and/or low back of pregnant women should be avoided. Wet cupping has rarely been associated with transient reflex unconsciousness (vasovagal response or fainting).

Trigger point injection therapy involves the use of a needle, with or without local anesthetic, to treat hyperirritable muscle nodules known as taut bands. The taut bands are found over tender areas known as trigger points, which, upon palpation, often result in a typical pain radiation pattern. Persons that have asymmetric or altered posture or that spend many hours daily overusing certain muscle groups (such as computer programmers, administrative assistants, readers, quilters, etc.) may be prone to this regional muscle pain syndrome. A needle is directed into the taut band of the muscle, and vigorous repeated probing of the needle is performed. The patient may feel an involuntary twitch that is felt as a needle "catch" by the practitioner. After needling, the area is treated with soft tissue massage or a vapo-coolant spray followed by muscle stretching. The goal of therapy is to relax the contacted muscle.

Viscosupplementation is the administration of a hyaluronate-containing solution into a joint. It is a proven therapy to relieve pain and improve function with current FDA approval for the treatment of knee osteoarthritis. It has also been reported to be beneficial for shoulder and hip osteoarthritis. It is typically given in a series of three injections. Individuals with an egg allergy should avoid this therapy.

Prolotherapy is a form of "regenerative" therapy thought to strengthen ligaments, tendons, and joint capsules. It involves the use of injecting a sclerosing solution such as concentrated dextrose (sugar water) into injured tissue in order to initiate a local inflammatory reaction. The goal is to promote or accelerate the body's natural response to tissue injury. It is a potential option for patients who have failed conservative management and are considered nonsurgical candidates. Treatment may be painful, and the patient should abstain from using anti-inflammatory medications, which can counteract the effects of prolotherapy. There is limited evidence for pain relief from this therapy, although many physicians offer this treatment and a growing number of patients report treatment success.

Platelet-rich plasma (PRP) therapy is a newer form of "regenerative" therapy. It involves the use of the patient's own blood, which is processed to isolate very high concentrations of important growth factors. Current literature supports its effectiveness for chronic non-healing tendon injuries including lateral epicondylitis (tennis elbow) and plantar fasciitis (pain of the foot). Similar to prolotherapy, a patient may be a candidate for PRP therapy if he or she has failed conservative management and is not a surgical candidate. Treatment may be painful, and the patient should abstain from using anti-inflammatory medications. For the most part, prolotherapy and PRP therapies are still considered experimental (from an insurance coverage point of view), but may hold future promise as important treatment modalities.

Botulinum toxin therapy involves the injection of a potent neurotoxin from the bacterium *Clostridium botulinum*. It inhibits muscle contraction with initial effects in three days, with peak action in three weeks, and with a duration of approximately three to four months. It is FDA (Food and Drug Administration) approved to treat dystonia (an abnormal muscle positioning), but has also been found effective for spasticity, contractures, myofascial (regional muscle) pain, and refractory tension headaches. It may also possess inherent analgesic properties independent of its muscle paralysis affects, and it has also been recently used to treat knee osteoarthritis.

Additional Resources

National Center for Complementary and Alternative Medicine: http://nccam.nih.gov/
WebMD: Complementary Medicine: http://www.webmd.com/balance/tc/complementary
    -medicine-topic-overview

9

ADDICTION TO PAIN MEDICATIONS AND PAIN MANAGEMENT CHALLENGES

Kathryn Nixdorf, MD, and Grace Chen, MD

INTRODUCTION

Prescription medications play a vital role in clinical medicine. But unfortunately, addiction to prescription medications has become an increasingly alarming problem in the United States. Pain medications, specifically opioids (narcotics), are amongst the classes of medications most highly abused.

Examples of opioid medications that have been abused, according to the American College of Family Physicians, include:

- Opium
- Codeine
- Fentanyl
- Heroin
- Hydrocodone
- Hydromorphone
- Methadone
- Morphine
- Oxycodone
- Oxymorphone
- Paregoric
- Sufentanil
- Tramadol

As prescription medications are being misused or used for nonmedical purposes, the effects on public health are increasing, leading to an increasing number of accidental deaths, emergency room visits, and the emergence of associated health problems. Public awareness of this problem is spreading, with several recent high-profile celebrity deaths attributed to prescription medication abuse or misuse. This chapter will serve to discuss the unique issues of addiction in pain management, including the challenges facing both patients and physicians.

Prior to discussing the role of pain medications in addiction, we must first define and discuss the vocabulary used when discussing addiction and effects that medications have on the body. This is especially important in regard to pain management, as many patients have a fear of some pain medications because of feared stigma of "addiction."

DEFINITIONS

Addiction

The medical definition for the term "addiction" has been the topic of robust discussion. In 2001, several organizations dedicated to the treatment of pain, including the American Pain Society, American Academy of Pain Medicine, and the American Society of Addiction Medicine came to a consensus definition of addiction. This definition stated, "Addiction is a primary, chronic, neurobiologic disease, with genetic, psychosocial, and environmental factors influencing its development and manifestations. It is characterized by behaviors that include one or more of the following: impaired control over drug use, compulsive use, continued use despite harm, and craving." In short, this includes compulsive use of a drug despite harmful consequences, including at work, socially, or within the family. As stated in the definition, addiction is considered to be a disease, with relapses occurring.

Abuse

Abuse includes the use of a prescription medication without medical supervision for the intentional purpose of getting high, or for a reason other than what the medication was intended. This can include taking a medication by a different route than how it was intended. For example, if a delayed-release medication is crushed, this can result in significantly higher blood levels than was intended by the prescription. As expected, this can lead to adverse events or even death due to the elevated blood levels.

Misuse

Drug misuse and drug abuse are commonly interchanged terms. In this chapter, we will use the term "misuse" as incorrect use of medications, different from how it was prescribed. Examples include missing dosages, taking the medication with other medications or substances that may interact with it, or not taking the medication with food as recommended. The concern with medication misuse is unintentional side effects or adverse events.

Physical Dependence

Physical dependence is a state of adaptation that occurs with chronic use of a drug, when the body develops tolerance and has withdrawal symptoms (as defined below). Physical dependence can occur with several types of medications, including opioid pain medications, heart medications, antidepressants, and antianxiety medications. Gradual tapering of these medications is typically required, as rapid discontinuation can lead to withdrawal symptoms.

Tolerance

Drug tolerance is the body's reaction to drug decreases, requiring higher amounts of that drug to get the same desired effect. Tolerance to a drug can also develop in some cases as the body builds resistance after repeated doses. Research on opioids, such as morphine, has revealed several changes that explain why opioid tolerance occurs, including changes in the opioid receptors.

Withdrawal

Withdrawal symptoms are symptoms that the body experiences after decreasing or stopping a medication. These symptoms can be physical or mental. In order to experience a withdrawal from a medication, your body must first develop a physical dependence on a medication. Having withdrawal symptoms is not unique to pain medications. For example, people who stop smoking tobacco "cold turkey" will often develop withdrawal symptoms such as anxiety, hunger, and headaches. These symptoms can vary amongst individuals, but in general, medications and illicit drugs have common symptoms that are associated with their withdrawal.

ADDICTION TO PAIN MEDICATIONS

Pain medications are used by people experiencing chronic and acute (new onset) pain, and are helpful for decreasing suffering associated with pain and increasing ability to participate in activities of daily life. When taken responsibly, they play an important role in a comprehensive pain management plan. The National Institute on Drug Abuse, which is part of the U.S. Department of Health and Human Services, has evaluated the trend of addiction to prescription medications. Opioids, which are pain-relieving medications, are amongst the most abused prescription medications in the United States, along with CNS depressants and stimulants.

Between 1999 and 2005, admissions for the treatment of prescription pain medication abuse increased by more than 300 percent. The Center for Disease Control (CDC) reported that unintentional poisoning deaths involving narcotics and hallucinogens grew 55 percent from 1999 to 2004.

WHY DO PEOPLE BECOME ADDICTED TO MEDICATIONS?

Drugs of abuse (both prescription and illicit) exhibit their affect by altering chemicals within the brain. One such chemical is dopamine, which is present in areas of the brain involved with emotion, cognition, pleasure, motivation, and movement. Dopamine acts as a messenger within the brain. When our body completes a behavior or task that is life sustaining (such as eating), dopamine is released, leading to a sense of well-being or euphoria. These circuits in the brain are in place to teach us to repeat these behaviors. When some drugs are used, they can release 2–10 times the amount of dopamine than natural rewards do. Some of these effects are also much quicker or longer-lasting than the body's own natural reward system. The powerful effects these drugs have on the reward circuitry of the brain teach the body to repeat the behavior, making it a habit.

The body responds to these higher amounts of neurotransmitters by decreasing their natural production as well as decreasing the receptors available to activate these circuits. This leads to tolerance, or an increased amount of drug needed to obtain a desired effect.

When a drug of abuse is stopped, there is a sudden decrease in these chemicals, which results in decreased stimulation of the pleasure centers and resulting depression, apathy, and decreased ability to experience pleasure. At this point, people will start to take these drugs in order to feel "normal" again, rather than for the indication for which they were prescribed.

Other neurotransmitters, locations, and circuits of the brain are affected by drug abuse as well. Imaging of the brain has been done in people with addictions, showing that addiction alters the areas of the brain involved with memory, learning, decision making, and behavior control. These changes can persist long after the drug has been stopped. Areas of the brain involved with habit forming are altered as well, leading to association of drug use with environmental cues, which is called "conditioning." Factors such as location, smells, specific individuals, psychiatric illness, and medical conditions can trigger a craving, even years after the drug has been stopped. Drug abuse can lead to changes in cognition and impulse control, leading to poor self-control in order to obtain these drugs.

Specific risk factors for developing addiction have been identified. These include a medical condition requiring use of a medication typically associated with addiction, such as pain medications, antianxiety medications, or stimulants; family history of addiction; excessive alcohol consumption; fatigue or overwork; poverty; depression; and obesity. Prescription drug abuse is typically the same between men and women, except among 12- to 17-year-olds, where a report by the National Institute on Drug Abuse found that females are more likely to use psychotherapeutic drugs for nonmedical purposes.

ADDICTION IN TEENS

Addiction and abuse of prescription medications is growing at alarming rates amongst teenagers. Concern over this growing problem has led to several studies to determine the extent of the problem. The Office of National Drug Control Policy, acting by directive of the Executive Office of the president of the United States, created a report entitled "Prescription for Danger: A Report on the Troubling Trend of Prescription and Over-the-Counter Drug Abuse Among the Nation's Teens."

The report found that drug abuse starts early, and peaks during the teen years. The prescription medications most commonly abused by teenagers are pain medications, antianxiety medications, sleeping aids, and stimulants such as Ritalin (NSDUH; see Additional Resources at the end of this chapter). With the exception of marijuana, prescription drugs are abused more in teens than any illicit drug (NSDUH). In addition, a growing number of teens are abusing over-the-counter medications and cold remedies for the purpose of getting "high" (SAMHSA; see Additional Resources). Part of this increasing trend has been attributed to the role of peer pressure.

In 2006, 2.1 million teens admitted to abuse of prescription drugs (NSDUH). The majority of these teens (64%) stated they used prescription drugs because they were able to get these drugs easily and for free, primarily from friends and relatives. Many teens stated they abused prescription drugs because they felt that because they were prescription, rather than illicit drugs, they would provide a "safe" high. In one study it was found that nearly half (49%) of teens who have abused prescription pain medications have also used two or more other drugs, most commonly alcohol and marijuana. They also found that among teens, 13 is the mean age of first nonprescribed used of sedatives and stimulants, and 60 percent of teens (age 12–17) who have abused pain medications tried them before age 15, and 18 percent used them at least weekly in the past year.

Each year, a survey called "Monitoring the Future" (MTF) is completed by 8th, 10th, and 12th graders nationwide. The purpose of this study is to evaluate the use of prescription drugs, including Vicodin and Oxycontin, for non-medical purposes. In 2008, 15.4 percent of these students had reported use of Vicodin or Oxycontin in the preceding year. The number of people having used in the preceding year increased with age, including 9.7 percent of 12th graders versus 2.9 percent of 8th graders having used Vicodin, and 4.7 percent of 12th graders versus 2.1 percent of 8th graders having used Oxycontin in the preceding year.

Symptoms and Diagnosis

Recognizing the signs of addiction is the first step in identifying someone at risk for addiction or those who are in need of receiving appropriate treatment and counseling. If a patient is prescribed a medication, it is expected that they are taking this medication appropriately per the directions provided. Those with addictive behaviors begin using their medication differently than prescribed, such as more frequent use of the medication. A person may lose control over their medication use and request early refills as they have used all of their medication before it is due. If they are not able to receive these medications from their primary physician, they may begin to visit other doctors or emergency rooms in order to obtain more medication. Some say they must take the medication in order to "feel themselves," not because they are in pain, but because the medication has an effect on their mood. The extreme of this is use of the medication for purely nonmedical use, such as for the purpose of getting high. Abusers may take a medication that is provided to another person.

Treatment

There are multiple treatments available for the treatment of addiction, and the key to successful treatment is adapting the treatment plan to be individualized. Placing someone into an addiction treatment program without addressing their unique situation places them at a higher risk of relapse. The patient, health care providers, and families must understand that addiction is a chronic lifelong disease with risk for relapse, even after long periods of being abstinent. As a person ages, their situation may change, requiring adjustments in their treatment management. Recognizing this chronic disease requires lifelong attention.

Detoxification from a drug in the acute setting is often inadequate to fully address the needs of someone with an addiction. A comprehensive treatment plan must address not only the drug abuse, but also medical, psychological, social, work-related, and legal problems that affect the individual. There is a strong association between drug abuse and mental health disorders, and therefore people with addictions should be carefully evaluated for a possible coexisting mental health disorder. Treatment plans also need to reflect personal characteristics of the individual, including age, gender, culture, and ethnicity.

As previously mentioned, drug abuse can lead to conditioning, which means that specific environmental triggers can set off cravings for a drug. An individual addiction treatment plan needs to identify those triggers, which can be difficult as they are not always apparent. Avoiding these triggers, or creating an alternative and acceptable behavior, is a key part of a successful treatment plan. Biologic changes within the brain cause this conditioning, and it is a difficult behavior to unlearn.

Several medications are available, in a monitored system, to help individuals with addiction to opioid drugs. Much of the information regarding treatment of opioid addiction is available from treatment of heroin addiction. Methadone is a synthetic opioid that decreases withdrawal symptoms and cravings and can block effects of other opioids and heroin, such as euphoria. Buprenorphine, found in Suboxone, is a medication that controls withdrawal symptoms and blocks dopamine receptors in the brain. This causes a block in the effect of these drugs of abuse to cause a "high" feeling. Suboxone can be prescribed only by a physician who has completed a certification and is licensed to prescribe the drug. Naltrexone is an opioid receptor blocker that can cause severe withdrawal symptoms in a person who takes an opioid, thus deterring the use of the medication. Naloxone is a short-acting medication that also blocks opioid receptors and can be used in the case of opioid overdose.

It should be noted that preferably in intensive-care settings, Ultra Rapid Detoxification (UROD) procedures are performed by a few super specialized experts in the United States and elsewhere for opioid dependence. In these UROD procedures, patients are withdrawn under general anesthesia over a two- to eight-hour period after being given a cocktail of medicines to minimize changes in heart rate or blood pressure. These patients are then seen by counselors post procedure and given naltrexone for a period of time. The advantage of this procedure is that patients essentially are asleep for most of the withdrawal and are no longer on pain medications such as methadone or suboxone.

Counseling is the cornerstone of drug abuse treatment. There are several different types of therapies available, which can be done in an individual setting, with a group, or both. The benefit of individual therapy is the ability to work on unique problems and identify specific factors leading to a person's addiction. Group therapy allows for a person to feel a sense of commonality and social reinforcement; in other words, group therapy helps someone to understand that they are not alone in their struggles. Group therapy helps build a community, which can help them through the treatment process and help to hold them accountable.

Different types of therapies include cognitive behavior therapy, motivational interviewing, motivational therapy, and group therapy. Some of the goals of therapy include providing a motivation for change, providing motivation or incentives for stopping the drug, recognizing and replacing risky behaviors, and providing problem-solving skills to deal with the struggles of becoming abstinent.

The obvious question in patients with chronic pain and addiction to pain medication is that if they abstain from opioids, what else would they use to treat their chronic pain?

Surprisingly, there are many medication and non-medication choices for treatment of pain in a person who wishes to abstain from opioid medications. Medication treatment of chronic pain that does not involve opioids includes anti-inflammatory medications such as ibuprofen or naproxen, antiseizure medications such as gabapentin or pregabalin, antidepressants such as duloxetine and vanlafaxine, and muscle relaxants such as tizanidine and cyclobenzaprine.

Some non-medication treatments of pain include physical therapy, pain psychology, heat, ice, massage, chiropractic care, surgeries, and spinal cord stimulators. Your doctor would be best to advise you as to which type of care is best suited for you.

PSEUDOADDICTION

Pseudoaddiction is a term that is more frequently used in the field of pain management. This term applies to a patient whose pain is inadequately treated, and who begins to display behaviors similar to those with an addiction. Possible behaviors include becoming mentally focused on their pain and obtaining pain medications, watching the clock in order to take the next dose, outward display of painful behaviors (such as moaning or grimacing) in order to obtain more pain relief, and frustration with health care providers. These behaviors, also seen in addicted individuals, can further perpetuate the problem, as health care providers are reluctant to give more medications for fear of exacerbating the problem. This can even lead to illegal behaviors such as obtaining medications on the street or taking other people's prescribed medications.

Underlying these behaviors is a person with inadequately controlled pain. Factors contributing to pseudoaddiction include prescribing medications that are not appropriate, inadequate doses of medications, prescribing dosing intervals that do not accurately reflect the duration of action, and use of medications "as needed" rather than on a scheduled basis. Correction of these problems and adequate treatment of the pain stop these behaviors, which distinguishes it from addiction where the behaviors will persist.

It is very difficult for a health care provider to distinguish between addiction and pseudoaddiction, as those with addiction will claim their pain is untreated in order to obtain medications, even when that may not be the case. Pain is a subjective complaint, which means we cannot complete a test or study to prove that someone is experiencing pain. Therefore, a health care provider must continue to reassess a medical situation and a treatment plan to distinguish between the two. This reassessment may include changing doses, changing medications, psychological evaluations and drug testing.

PROGNOSIS

According to research papers and eMedicine, opioid treatment relapse rates vary from 25 to 97 percent. Cigarette smokers have higher rates of relapse than nonsmokers. How well people do with opioid addiction treatment varies widely according to the type of agent abused, medical care received, patient's employment, legal situation, family, and psychological difficulties. Statistically, the success rate is much better in people who abuse opioids and are professionals than in individuals with a poor education level and low job prospects. However, it is hard to translate this to individual patients, as there are many complicated factors that may change the course of addiction in each individual.

ADDITIONAL RESOURCES

Betty Ford Center at http://www.bettyfordcenter.org

Drugs, Brains, and Behavior: The Science of Addiction. 2010. National Institute on Drug Abuse. http://www.nida.nih.gov/scienceofaddiction/

Hazelden at http://www.hazelden.org

Monitoring the Future (MTF). 2007. National Institute on Drug Abuse (NIDA)

Narcotics Anonymous at http://www.na.org

National Survey on Drug Use and Health (NSDUH). 2007. Substance Abuse and Mental Health Services and Adminstration (SAMHSA)

Prescription for Danger: A Report on the Troubling Trend of Prescription and Over-the-Counter Drug Abuse among the Nation's Teens. 2008. Office of National Drug Control Policy, Executive Office of the President.

Substance Abuse and Mental Health Services Administration at http://www.samhsa.gov

Wu, Pilowsky, & Patkar. 2007. "Non-prescribed Use of Pain Relievers among Adolescents in the United States." Drug and Alcohol Dependence.

10

How to Apply for Disability Benefits

Ruth Van Vleet, MS, CRC, CDMS, and
Kathleen McAlpine, CRC, CDMS

If you have been in pain for a number of years, and you have been unable to work due to the pain, you may apply for disability benefits. Some individuals, through their employer, either funded by their employer or themselves, may have long-term disability insurance policies. If you have this benefit, you may discuss the terms of your policy with your Human Resource or Benefits Department to determine if you qualify for such benefits and to find out how to apply. Long-term disability benefits assist in meeting financial obligations and are often time limited. In addition, you should contact the insurance company to discuss your plan and obtain a copy of your policy. If you have a copy of the plan, it will allow you to familiarize yourself with the process.

Another source is Social Security Disability benefits. To begin this process, it is recommended that you coordinate with the Social Security office in your area by telephone or in person. The Social Security Administration can provide information about benefits you may qualify for based on your disability. Benefits are based on your inability to work due to a medical condition that is expected to last at least one year. In order to qualify for Social Security Disability benefits, you must have been employed and paid Social Security taxes. You must also meet the definition of being medically disabled. If you have worked, you must not have earned beyond what is considered SGA (Substantial Gainful Activity). Please refer to the Social Security website, and Figure 10.1.

One may also qualify for Social Security Insurance (SSI). To qualify for this benefit, you must have limited income and be considered disabled with a medical condition that would be expected to last at least one year or longer and not be working or earning an income.

Just because your doctor tells you that you are disabled does not mean that the Social Security Administration will consider you disabled. You can be disabled and not be able to perform your previous employment requirements, but may be able to perform other jobs available in the national or local economy. To qualify for benefits, Social Security does not take into consideration your locale, and it often evaluates you on positions available within the entire United States. Should you wish to pursue Social Security benefits, you

Figure 10.1
Outline of the process of applying for disability.

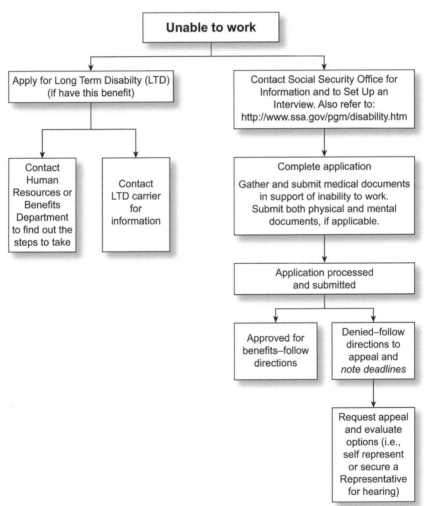

will need to complete a Social Security application and provide documents of your medical records from your physicians, hospitals, treatment centers such as social service agencies and psychiatrists, and pharmacies. The Social Security application process is a long process that can take several months after the application is submitted to receive a decision. After the application is evaluated, you will receive a response. If the response is not favorable, you need to respond within the time frame outlined in the correspondence you receive.

In evaluating options available to you, it is recommended that you review the U.S. Social Security website, http://www.socialsecurity.gov, or call 1-800-772-1213. You may also want to consult an attorney or representative to review your records to see if you meet the Social Security requirements for disability. An organization such as the National Organization of Social Security Claimant's Representatives at http://www.nosscr.org can provide you with a list of Social Security claimants' representatives in your area. The NOSSCR website will also have a list of frequently asked questions defining what disability is under Social Security, types of Social Security Disability benefits, and how to apply. You may also want to contact your local bar association or social service agencies to inquire of Social Security representatives in your locale. They may be able to assist you in navigating the Social Security process as well as in compiling data needed to apply for Social Security Disability or to appeal your case if you have been denied. Figure 10.1 outlines steps you should follow to assist you in your application for disability benefits should you become unable to work.

PART II

SPECIFIC PAINFUL CONDITIONS AND TREATMENT OPTIONS

11

HEADACHE

C. Obi Onyewu, MD, Frank J. E. Falco, MD, Sareta Coubarous, DO, and Rajesh Jari, MD

INTRODUCTION

More than 30 million people in the United States suffer from headaches that are associated with losses in the billions of dollars in terms of missed workdays, reduced work productivity, and medical costs. There are many pain sensitive structures in your head, including the scalp, nerves, brain, blood vessels, and muscles. Some structures in your face may also refer pain and present as headaches.

Headaches can be divided into two categories, primary or secondary. A primary headache is one in which there is no identifiable cause and includes tension, migraine, and cluster headaches. A secondary headache is caused by an identifiable disease such as infections, tumors, trauma, and medication side effects. The treatments for headaches have improved dramatically over the last few years, and many patients have benefited with improved outcomes.

PRIMARY HEADACHES

1. *Tension Headaches:* This is the most common type of headache, often involving a squeezing type pain that feels like a band around your head. Usually the pain is not aggravated by physical activity, although light or noise can have an adverse effect. Nausea and vomiting are rarely associated with this type of headache. If headache frequency is more than 15 episodes per month, then it is defined as chronic. Tension headaches can last from 30 minutes up to 7 days.

2. *Migraine Headaches:* This is the second most common type of headache. There are two common patterns for migraines, those that occur with or without an aura (aura refers to feelings and symptoms noticed shortly before the migraine begins). There are visual auras (most common) which include flashing lights, zigzag lines, spots in the visual field, and blurred vision. Sensory auras include pins and needle sensation, and numbness in the arms, hands, and face. Other aura symptoms include arm or leg weakness, an unpleasant taste and/or smell, and difficulty remembering words. These aura symptoms precede the migraine headache, start over a 5- to 10-minute timeline, and reverse within an hour. When a headache occurs without an aura, it is usually described as throbbing on one side of your head that often involves your forehead.

Sensitivity to light and sound and experiences of nausea and vomiting are often present. Migraine pain can be aggravated by any kind of physical activity, and retreating to a dark and quiet room during the headache is advise. Although migraines occur more often in women, men can have them too.

Chronic migraine headaches are defined by more than 15 headache days per month, of which at least 8 are migraine headaches that have persisted for three months. In addition, there are many conditions that become worse in the presence of a migraine, including depression, sleep disturbances, anxiety, bipolar disorder, fibromyalgia, epilepsy, and stroke.

3. *Cluster Headaches:* The term "cluster" is derived from the characteristic number of headaches that frequently occur close together up to eight times a day, and all are grouped over a period of time lasting several weeks or months. Cluster headaches are often tied to a seasonal time table, occurring at roughly the same time and season each year. These headaches are much less frequent than migraine or tension headaches and affect less than 1 percent of the population. They occur five times more often in men than women. They typically present as multiple daily attacks on a regular schedule. Often cluster headaches occur during asleep and may provoke wakefulness at the same time each night.

The pain usually occurs on one side of the head, lasting from 15 minutes up to 3 hours, and can be deep and searing, similar to a "red hot poker." Classic symptoms including teariness, bloodshot eyes, stuffy nose with dripping, pinpoint pupils, eyelid swelling, and droopy eyes. Cluster headaches, in contrast to migraines, do not have a throbbing quality. All are associated with physical activity, such as rocking or changing posture.

SECONDARY HEADACHES

1. *Cervicogenic Headaches:* These headaches are triggered by muscles or bones in your neck that refer pain into your head. The pain is usually on one side and made worse upon neck movement to one side or the other. The pain is generally not very severe and does not shift from one side of the head to the other. There may be decreased range of motion in your neck, shoulders, or arms.

2. *Occipital Neuralgia:* This is a common cause for acute and chronic headaches. This pain is commonly located in the upper neck and the back of your head. The condition is caused by injury or inflammation to the nerves. It can be caused from trauma to these nerves, neck arthritis, or in rare cases from a tumor. The

headaches are typically chronic on a daily basis and are often associated with muscle spasms. Your doctor can diagnose these headaches based on physical findings such as nerve tenderness and muscle spasms.

3. *Headaches and Brain Tumors:* A headache is a common complaint in patients with a brain tumor; however, brain tumors rarely cause headaches. There are natural concerns that a brain tumor may be the cause of headache, but there are usually other symptoms occur before headaches, including weakness, seizures, and changes in mental faculties such as memory loss.

4. *Headaches associated with Meningitis:* Meningitis is an inflammation of the protective covering of your brain and spinal cord that is caused by an infection. Patients with meningitis often complain of a severe headache, neck stiffness, fever, confusion, vomiting, and an inability to tolerate loud noises or light. Meningitis can be life threatening and requires prompt attention and treatment.

5. *Headaches associated with Subarachnoid Hemorrhages:* A subarachnoid hemorrhage is bleeding in the area between the brain and its covering. It is a form of a stroke with bleeding due to a rupture of one of the blood vessels in your brain. The bleeding causes an irritation of your brain covering that causes a "thunderclap" headache described as your worse headache ever. You often will experience vomiting and decreased alertness, which can progress to a coma. This condition can be life threatening and is considered a medical emergency requiring immediate medical treatment.

6. *Medication Overuse Headaches:* This form of headache is also known as a rebound headache and frequently occurs concomitant with a migraine or a tension headache that transitions over time to a chronic daily headache. This often results in an overuse of headache medications that ultimately cause severe "rebound" headaches for several days to weeks upon discontinuing medication.

Other Causes of Headaches—Facial Pain

Facial pain can often worsen or trigger your headaches. Facial pain can be caused by any disease that affects any part or parts of the face. The following disorders of the face are common causes of referred headaches.

1. *Sinusitis:* Over 37 million people suffer from headaches and facial pain resulting from sinusitis, which is an inflammation of sinuses found around your face and head. Any sinuses can become enlarged and inflamed after an infection, leading to severe pain. Some symptoms can include early morning headaches, pain with head movement, and pain when pressing on any of the affected sinuses. Other symptoms along with sinusitis include frontal headaches, pain and swelling around the eyes, cheekbone pain, fever, weakness, cough, nasal congestion, rhinitis, sore throat, painful swallowing, and a constant nasal drip. Your doctor may need to get a CAT scan of your head in order to confirm the diagnosis of sinusitis. Occasionally, your sinusitis may worsen and become chronic resulting in chronic head and facial pain. Sinusitis can become worse if your immune system is compromised, such as in cancer, after an organ transplant, or with HIV.

2. *Trigeminal Neuralgia:* This is a painful condition of the trigeminal nerve, which provides sensation to your face. The pain is severe and described as a stabbing pain involving one side of the face lancinating (stabbing) pain in the distribution of one or more of the branches of the fifth cranial nerve. The pain is often triggered by the slightest stimulation, such as touching your face or brushing your teeth. The pain is described as sudden in onset, intense, sharp, stabbing and/or burning that lasts only for a few seconds to as long as a few minutes.

3. *Temporal Mandibular Joint (TMJ) Syndrome:* The temporo-mandibular joint is the joint of your jaw that allows you to open and close your mouth. Common symptoms include joint spasms and localized jaw pain that is made worse with chewing. Difficulty opening your mouth as well as clicking or popping of your jaw may occur. Other symptoms may include an earache and headache.

4. *Temporal Tendonitis:* Temporal tendonitis is the "tennis elbow" of your jaw where the tendon of the muscle most responsible for closing your jaw becomes inflamed and painful from overuse. The symptoms are similar to a migraine headache, particularly in its location, which is along either side of the forehead. Other symptoms include TMJ pain, ear pain and/or pressure, cheek pain, tooth sensitivity, neck pain, and/or shoulder pain.

DIAGNOSIS

Diagnosing the type of headache that you have is very important so that you can have the best possible outcome. Your doctor will ask you to give a complete history, which may include any of the following information.

- Headache history?
- How long and how frequent?
- Pain location?
- Pain intensity and quality (e.g., severity and adjectives such as throbbing, burning)?
- Pain fluctuations (e.g., on waking up, or in bright light)?
- Relieving factors?
- Aggravating factors?
- Medication history and allergy history?
- Associated factors (e.g., visual problems, teariness, and/or weakness)?

Physical examination may include:

- Vital signs—blood pressure, heart rate, temperature
- Mental status including speech, memory, alertness, and orientation to time and place
- Eye examination
- Neurological examination of the nerves, sensations, muscle strength, and reflexes
- Neck motion, muscle tenderness, muscle spasms

Diagnostic tests that the physician may order include:

- Radiological: x-rays, CT (CAT) scan, MRI, or Ultrasound
- Lumbar puncture: spinal fluid is obtained and assessed
- Blood studies

MANAGEMENT

Successful treatment of your headache is dependent upon an appropriate evaluation leading to the correct diagnosis. Treatment should always be tailored to your condition. An accurate diagnosis is important in developing the appropriate treatment plan for you.

1. *Migraine Headaches:* The treatment goals for migraines are to prevent or abort your headache symptoms. Preventative treatment involves avoiding the things that trigger your headache. Different medications can be prescribed by your doctor for prevention, to reduce the number of your headaches, and to stop your migraine shortly after the early symptoms. Depending on the frequency of your symptoms, your doctor will choose the appropriate treatment.

    The first-line medications for acute attacks are generally over-the-counter drugs such as Tylenol and ibuprofen, which are used for mild to moderate migraines. If these are ineffective, then prescription medications such as triptans, ergotamines with or without caffeine, corticosteroids, and opiates are used to stop your migraine headache. Some of these medications can be administered by nasal spray, under your tongue, by injection under your skin and/or by mouth. The advantages of the different ways of taking these medications include a quick onset of pain relief with the nasal, tongue, and injectable forms, which also are beneficial if you are experiencing nausea and vomiting. Your doctor should be informed if you are pregnant or suffer from heart, kidney or liver disease since these medications may be harmful if used under these conditions.

    Opiates are another type of medication that can be helpful in stopping a migraine headache. Opiates are narcotic pain medications that are used as a last resort when you cannot tolerate the other medications or the other medications fail to provide you pain relief. They can be habit forming and should be prescribed with extreme care.

    Corticosteroid medications might be useful over a limited period of time and under strict supervision as they have significant side effects when used for a prolonged period of time. However, in most cases they can be used alone or in combination with other medications for difficult migraines.

    Medications given to treat the symptoms of migraines can be used alone or in combinations. They can reduce your pain, nausea, and emotional distress. Medications in this group include those for the treatment of nausea, insomnia, anxiety, depression and inflammation.

    Once the diagnosis of chronic migraine headaches is made, your doctor will plan treatment to include preventative drugs that can decrease the frequency and severity of migraines. These medications are usually taken daily or on a schedule when a particular trigger can be predicted such as the menstrual cycle. These medications include seizure, blood pressure, and depression drugs that have a preemptive effect for migraines.

Other complementary approaches that have been shown to be effective in the treatment of your migraine headaches include nutritional interventions and lifestyle changes. Your doctor may recommend limiting your caffeine intake or even eliminating caffeine altogether. You may also need to avoid tyramine-containing foods including chocolate, aged cheese, yogurt, sour cream, soy sauce, avocado, chicken liver, nuts, yeast extracts, tap beer, cured meats, and wine. Tyramine is derived from the amino acid tyrosoine and stimulates the release of adrenaline that has an adverse effect on migraine headaches. Other foods and products to avoid include nitrates that dilate your blood vessels such as processed meats, as well as products containing monosodium glutamate and nutrasweet preparations all of which can trigger your headaches.

2. *Tension Headaches:* Management of tension headaches is similar to that for migraines. Conservative treatment includes relaxation techniques such as meditation, sleep hygiene, and a regular exercise program including stretching. The use of over-the-counter pain medications such as aspirin, acetaminophen, and ibuprofen can also be effective in treating your tension headaches. Your doctor may also use prescription muscle relaxants and even opiates when more conservative treatments do not work. You must take care not to overuse your pain medications, as these can cause rebound headaches. Your doctor may use preventative medications similar to those used for migraines to treat tension headaches that become chronic.

3. *Cluster Headaches:* There is no known cure for cluster headaches at this time. The goal of treatment is to prevent and shorten the duration of your headaches and decrease the severity of your pain. The use of 100 percent oxygen inhaled through a face mask can be very effective in treating these headaches. The use of injectable or nasal inhalation triptans is often effective in stopping your cluster headache. Ergotamine tablets or suppositories may be prescribed by your doctor if the triptans do not work. Short courses of oral corticosteroids have been shown to help stop a cluster headache cycle. Again, preventative treatments can be started by your doctor when your cluster headaches are chronic. First-line preventative medications include the use of blood pressure and psychiatric drugs such as lithium that have been effective in preventing chronic cluster headaches.

4. *Temporo Mandibular Joint Syndrome:* Treatment options for temporo mandibular joint (TMJ) syndrome focus on ways to relax the jaw and facial muscles. This may be accomplished through lifestyle changes, oral splints, medications, bite adjustment, orthodontics, or dental surgery. The treatment for TMJ syndrome is often directed either at the joint itself, or at the fatigue of the temporalis muscles.

Your doctor or dentist may recommend an over-the-counter pain medication or prescribe stronger pain medication. If oral medications alone are not helpful, a corticosteroid injection into your TMJ joint can provide TMJ and headache pain relief. The corticosteroids help to ease your pain by reducing joint inflammation. Radiofrequency is a procedure that destroys the nerves that provide sensation and pain for your TMJ in order to provide you with prolonged pain relief. This procedure is performed after corticosteroid injections have been performed, providing only temporary relief.

Botulinum toxin or Botox injections are another treatment option available than can provide you with pain relief from your TMJ disorder. This is injected into the temporalis muscle that is used for chewing to reduce muscle spasms and pain.

There are several forms of noninvasive therapies that can help you with your TMJ pain. The most common is the use of a bite guard. Grinding or clenching your teeth in your sleep causes TMJ pain and headaches in the morning. Wearing a soft or firm bite guard device inserted over your teeth prevents the teeth from compressing together and therefore can prevent your pain. The bite guard can be custom made by your dentist or purchased over the counter. Another noninvasive therapy is cognitive behavioral therapy (CBT). The symptoms of TMJ disorder may be made worse by poorly managed stress or anxiety. A psychotherapist with experience in CBT can teach you how to be aware of your stress or anxiety. Once you are aware of any stress and/or anxiety, you can learn how to change your behavior, and relaxation techniques that can help you manage your stress.

There are orthodontic surgical and other invasive procedures that attempt to improve TMJ symptoms that cause headaches. These procedures are performed by dentist and they include corrective dental treatment to improve the bite by balancing the biting surfaces of your teeth, replacing missing teeth, or replacing fillings or crowns. However, these types of treatments don't always improve pain. Arthrocentesis is a procedure which involves inserting a needle into the joint and irrigating it with fluid to remove debris and inflammatory byproducts. Surgery is always the last resort, and your doctor or dentist may suggest surgery to repair or replace the joint.

5. *Trigeminal Neuralgia:* Trigeminal neuralgia is a difficult and complex pain disorder to treat. Medications are used initially as a conservative way to reduce or block the pain; these typically begin with an antiseizure and/or an antispascticity drug. The less commonly used medications to treat trigeminal neuralgia include the antidepressant drugs. Complementary and alternative treatments for trigeminal neuralgia include acupuncture, biofeedback, vitamin therapy, nutritional therapy, and electrical stimulation of the nerves.

Surgical microvascular decompression and gamma knife radiation are two procedures that have been shown to provide relief in some cases. Radiofrequency is another common procedure used for the treatment of trigeminal neuralgia.

6. *Medication Overuse Headaches:* Treatment for headaches due to medication overuse starts with weaning yourself off of the medication of overuse. If the medication happens to be a short-acting analgesic, then you may have a more difficult time weaning off of it. Issues complicating treatment for these types of headache include physical and psychological dependency, which makes it difficult to wean off of any opioid analgesics. Your doctor will have to gradually decrease the medication to avoid precipitating any rebound headaches and to also avoid withdrawal symptoms. Once off the medication, your doctor will avoid restarting the medications again if the medication is a narcotic. If it is a non-narcotic, your

doctor may reintroduce the medication with very close supervision after three months. Psychological treatment may be necessary for you in order to successfully remain off the analgesic drugs responsible for your rebound headaches.

7. *Occipital Neuralgia:* Occipital neuralgia can be a challenging diagnosis to make especially if it is associated with neck pain and the neck pain is your main complaint. Appropriate treatment can begin after the diagnosis of occipital neuralgia has been confirmed by your doctor. Occipital neuralgia can be treated in several ways. These include occipital nerve blocks, peripheral nerve stimulation, oral steroids, radiofrequency or chemical rhizotomy, cryoneurolysis, and medications for neuropathic pain. Less commonly, a microdecompression or surgical neurolysis of the occipital nerves can provide relief if more conservative treatment and interventional procedures fail to resolve or improve your symptoms.

Conclusion

Treatment of headaches is a challenging process. Making the correct diagnosis is paramount for successful treatment of your headaches. In order to make the correct diagnosis your doctor will require details of events that surround the occurrence of your headache. Your doctor will often require a headache diary be kept. Great challenges in treating headaches exist, even though there have been significant advances in medical technology and the medications used in treating headaches. Lifestyle changes are often helpful, including smoking cessation, sleep hygiene, stress reduction, and avoiding known triggers. Alternative and nontraditional therapies can also be helpful. These would include acupuncture, meditation, massage therapy, and chiropractic manipulation.

Additional Resources

National Headache Foundation: http://www.headaches.org
WebMD: http://www.webmd.com

12

PAIN IN THE EAR, EYE, AND FACE

Christopher Annis, MD, and
Magdalena Anitescu, MD, PhD

The human head is a complex structure containing more than just the brain. Each of us, for the most part, is born with two eyes, two ears, a nose, and a mouth. Unlike headaches, which affect nearly everyone at some point in time, painful conditions affecting the ears, eyes, and face are somewhat less prevalent. This chapter provides the reader with a basic overview of the many facets of ear, eye, and facial pain. Some terms are described in detail; the reader is encouraged to look up other words that are not clear. Understanding where to find information and understanding one's condition are as important, if not more important, than understanding the treatment. One must take responsibility for his or her disease, as only then will true healing begin.

Ear pain, for which the medical term is *otalgia*, can be caused by conditions in the ear itself (known as *primary otalgia*), or be referred from other locations within the head and neck (known as *referred otalgia*). In fact, almost 50 percent of adult patients with ear pain seen by primary care physicians have referred otalgia. In dealing with any type of pain related to the ear, one must first understand the underlying anatomy. The exact minutia of the ear's anatomy is far greater than the scope of this text; however, the ear is essentially broken down into three areas; the external, middle, and inner ear. Each has its own distinct anatomical landmarks, blood and nerve supplies, and pain generators. The same nerves that supply the ear actually go on to supply some of the sensation to the face, tongue, and skin around the head and neck.

As there are many parts that make up the ear, there are many possible causes of pain in the ear. Some of the more commonly seen causes of primary otalgia include trauma, environmental insults (i.e., frostbite, sunburns, etc.), infection (both bacterial and viral), and cancers. Each has its own set of symptoms, means of diagnosis, and treatment. Referred otalgia also has multiple etiologies, many more than primary otalgia. Some of the more common causes of referred otalgia include temporomandibular joint disorder (TMJ disorder), gastroesophageal reflux disease (GERD), cancer, neuralgias, and a condition known as Eagle's Syndrome when recurrent otalgia is due to an excessively elongated styloid process (a structure found behind the ear) in conflict with adjacent structures.

Depending on the origin of otalgia, a myriad of associated symptoms can be found. Sometimes patients can experience hearing loss, drainage from the ear (known as *otorrhea*), ringing in the ear (known as *tinnitus*), itching of the ear (known as *pruritis*), or aural fullness. For instance, patients with Meniere's disease sometimes describe ear pain as aural fullness, or a sensation as if wearing ear muffs. Patients with chronic myringitis have symptoms of otorrhea, hearing loss, aural fullness, tinnitus, and pruritis. Patients with otalgia caused by bacteria or viruses (termed *otitis media* or *otitis externa* depending upon location) can experience facial palsy or weakness, a rash of the outer ear, external auditory canal, and occasionally the tympanic membrane. In fact, some patients develop a condition called Ramsay Hunt Syndrome stemming from the same virus that causes chicken pox. This pain is known as neuropathic pain and tends to be sharp, short lived, and intermittent in nature.

Diagnosis begins with determining whether or not the pain sensed is coming from the ear itself, or if it is referred pain. This is accomplished first by doing a simple ear exam and obtaining a detailed history. The doctor, whether it is the primary care physician, otolaryngologist (ENT physician), or pain medicine physician, will examine the external ear first. The doctor will look for any obvious deformities, lesions, or rashes. The exam may involve pulling on the ear or parts of the ear in an attempt to elicit the pain, followed by the examination of the external auditory canal and tympanic membrane (or eardrum). Using a special tool known as an otoscope, the doctor will add light and magnification to aid in the examination. This part of the exam will reveal any possible inflammation of the canal, buildup of waxy substances (known as cerumen), and issues with the eardrum itself. Next, the doctor will turn his attention to the middle ear. This part of the ear contains the bones that help relay sound as well as the eustachian tube (that part of the ear that causes it to "pop" while on a plane or diving). Finally, the doctor will possibly evaluate the inner ear and assess one's hearing and response to rotational changes.

Following the examination of the ear, the doctor will turn his attention to the head, neck, and neurological examinations. This part of the overall examination will help narrow down the possibilities for what can be the cause of the ear pain. Sometimes the doctor will need imaging studies such as MRI or CT scans to help make the diagnosis.

As with most things in medicine, treatment of any ailment depends on the cause. Antibiotic therapy in both topical and oral forms is typically employed for otitis media and externa. Keeping one's ear dry and avoiding movement of the ear itself, in conjunction with intermittent use of topical antibiotics and cleansing preparations, is the usual treatment for chronic myringitis. Surgical debridement (clearing away of dead tissue and debris) is the treatment for malignant otitis externa and mastoiditis, which are two infectious conditions that affect not only the ear but also the bony structure behind the ear. Otic (ear) drops, oral antibiotics, corticosteroids, and topical analgesia are used for a condition known as bullous myringitis. Neuralgia, or nerve pain, is difficult to treat but possibly requires no intervention at all. More severe cases of otalgia related to neuralgia can be treated with medications such as carbamazepine or phenytoin. Sometimes though, the above treatment options will take care of the cause of the pain, but not the pain itself. When that occurs the doctor may perform more interventional or nontraditional techniques. One recommendation may be nerve blocks which act as a form of "roadblock" of the transmission of the painful stimuli. If this treatment works, the interventional pain physician can then burn, or ablate, the nerve. With the appropriate treatment, otalgia can be managed quite easily. However, as stated above, there are instances where the pain does not present itself until after the condition resolves.

In identifying the most common sources of eye pain, the same general diagnostic and treatment principles apply. The first step is to determine whether the pain is coming from the eye itself or if it is referred from an area elsewhere. Eye pain can even be caused by systemic (whole-body) conditions such as multiple sclerosis or ankylosing spondylitis (a condition that makes the spine very stiff but is also associated with eye pathology), or by conditions localized to the eye itself. One must be familiar with the anatomy of the eye, for it is made up of many little parts, each with its own nerve and blood supply. To simplify things, only issues affecting some of the major structures are discussed. These include: the sclera, uvea, and the most commonly affected, cornea.

One of the most common eye conditions leading to pain in patients between the ages of 40 and 50 is glaucoma. The eye has fluid that is constantly produced and reabsorbed. When that fluid cannot be reabsorbed, pressure builds up in the eye, a condition known as glaucoma. When this happens suddenly, it is called *acute angle closure glaucoma* and is a medical emergency. Patients have an acutely painful red eye along with blurred vision and halos surrounding sources of light. One might also have a headache, be nauseated, vomit, or even have abdominal pain. Headache may also be associated with a condition known as *scleritis*. In this rather uncommon condition that affects the white part of the eye, one may experience a severe "boring" pain that is made worse with eye movement. Unlike acute angle closure glaucoma, the pain that comes with scleritis comes on over the course of weeks. Oftentimes in scleritis, there is blurred vision, tearing, redness of the eye and pain when the globe (the main part of the eye) is touched. *Anterior uveitis (iritis)* is another relatively uncommon inflammatory process involving the iris (the colored part of the eye) and/or the ciliary muscles (the muscles around the pupil). Similar to scleritis and glaucoma, there is pain, redness of the eye, blurred vision, tearing, and an aversion to light (called photophobia). This condition usually occurs between the ages of 20 and 50. While most cases of uveitis have no identifiable cause, systemic conditions caused by the genetic condition called HLA-B27 may be the culprit. HLA-B27-associated uveitis can present in two different time courses, depending on the underlying systemic disease. While the onset can be varied, recovery occurs within two to four months. Other causes of uveitis that are not HLA-B27-related include trauma, infection, and inflammatory conditions such as sarcoidosis and rheumatoid arthritis.

Pain arising from the outermost portion of the eye, the cornea, can be severe if the cornea is inflamed, as is the case in *keratitis*. This painful condition also has two different possible causes: infectious and noninfectious. Keratitis, regardless of the cause, produces a sensation as if one has an eyelash stuck in the eye. Photophobia, tearing, and redness are also present. Infectious agents causing keratitis include bacteria, viruses, and fungi. Some of the more common noninfectious causes include UV keratitis (from welding or light exposure), dry eye syndrome, agitation from rubbing the eye, chemical injury, and contact lens use. Corneal abrasion (a scratch on the eye) can also lead to eye pain. The presenting symptoms are similar to keratitis in that one experiences eye pain, tearing, redness, and a foreign body sensation.

The evaluation of a patient with eye pain is similar to that of ear pain. A detailed history is obtained including duration, quality, and severity of the pain, alleviating and exacerbating factors, and associated symptoms that may indicate more of a whole-body process. Next, the evaluating practitioner will examine the eye itself. First, the outer surface of the main part of the eye (the globe) along with the eye lid and structures around the eye will be examined. A visual acuity test will assess for vision loss. Next, using a tool called an ophthalmoscope, the examiner will look *in* the eye. The ophthalmoscope will reveal any problems with the posterior (back) part of the eye known as the retina. In this part of the eye, one finds the blood vessels as well as the insertion point of the optic nerve, the main nerve of the eye that allows each of us to see. After evaluation of the main part of the inside and outside of the eye, the practitioner will evaluate the surface of the globe. This is done to look for scratches, ulcerations, irregularities, and infections. A substance known as *fluorosceine* will be administered topically to the eye. The eye will then be examined underneath a special light known as a *Wood's lamp*. The fluorosceine will glow under the Wood's lamp, similar to a white shirt under a black light. It will reveal any areas of corneal abrasion or ulceration. Another tool, known as a *Slit lamp*, will also be used. This microscope-like tool allows the practitioner to take a closer look at the *anterior chamber*, checking for uveitis.

The treatment for eye pain is as varied as the causes; however, the thing to remember is that to treat the pain, one must treat the underlying cause. In some instances, emergent evaluation by an ophthalmologist is required. Most forms of treatment of eye pain involve topical medications. Eye lubricants, analgesics, antimicrobials, beta blockers, and pilocarpine are all administered via drops. Oral medications such as steroids, nonsteroidal anti-inflammatory drugs (or NSAIDs), and immunosuppressive agents are also employed. In the case of acute angle glaucoma, medications that decrease the overall fluid content in the eye (as well as the body) are used. Besides evaluation from an ophthalmologist, one may also need to see a rheumatologist as there may be a systemic (e.g., whole body) component as discussed earlier.

Depending on the cause, healing can take anywhere from days to weeks. However, the pain associated with the various conditions may also become chronic, lasting well beyond the time to heal from the underlying cause. When that occurs, it is important to remember that the goal of therapy shifts from complete relief to that of tolerance. A pain medicine specialist may use multiple oral and topical medications in conjunction with one another and may refer a patient to a pain psychologist. This person is someone who is skilled in helping patients adjust their lives and create positive coping strategies when dealing with their pain. This multidisciplinary/multimodal approach holds true for all types of chronic pain, whether in the eye, ear, or as we will find, the face.

Within the face are hundreds of different muscles, blood vessels, nerves, and other tiny structures. While we will not be discussing headache in this chapter (please see Chapter 11), it behooves one to know that headache and facial pain affect roughly 300 million people a year and cost over $1 billion for medication and close to $13 billion if one takes into account lost work/reduced productivity. There are many ways to classify and describe face pain. One method involves location; either central or peripheral, with peripheral comprising the majority of cases. Most of the time, this pain originates from the mouth or adjacent structures, such as the teeth or the hinge of the jaw (henceforth referred to as TMJ, which stands for temporomandibular joint). For instance, peripheral facial pain can be caused by dental disease, infections, or ulcerations of the lining of the mouth or even the sinuses. Central facial pain, on the other hand, is caused by other factors such as tumors, vascular issues, and sometimes unknown sources that make up or come from the structural components of the face. Facial pain can also be classified by symptomatic classes, each with its own set of diagnoses. These broad categories include those pertaining to the muscles and bones (musculoskeletal), alterations in the blood vessels and nerves together (neurovascular), and abnormalities to the nerves themselves (neuropathic). Breaking from the format we have tried to keep during the prior portion of this chapter, we will now describe some common causes, symptoms, and diagnostic features related to face pain, each pertaining to a single etiology.

Up to 12 percent of the population can be affected by *temporomandibular disorder*, a broad classification that describes pain involving the muscles used to chew and the joints involving the jaw. One will typically experience "clicking" when opening the jaw, tenderness overlying the muscles near the jaw, pain near the ear or temple, and sometimes referred pain to the area above the eye or into the teeth. Sometimes patients will experience fullness of the ear, dizziness, and neck soreness. The cause of pain in the temporomandibular joint is usually due to displacement of a disc found in the joint itself. Other causes include degeneration and/or inflammation of the joint such as in arthritis. This condition tends to be more common on one side but can be bilateral. When being evaluated for TMJ dysfunction or disorder, the evaluating physician will first do a detailed history and physical exam. They will look for one's jaw to move to the affected side when opened fully. Mouth opening tends to be reduced as well. They will feel the joint itself, attempting to feel the disc slipping out of place. Imaging studies such as MRI or CT will also aid in revealing more serious possibilities such as tumors.

As mentioned above, the topic of headache is covered in Chapter 11; however, we will briefly touch on the subject of migraines, as they can present with facial pain referred to areas such as the ear and above the eye. Fear of light or of sounds (photophobia and phonophobia, respectively) are common, as is nausea. Again, evaluation starts with a history and physical and frequently involves the imaging studies mentioned above.

Similar to, but different from migraines and headaches, *neurovascular orofacial pain* is a condition that produces pain in the mouth and areas around the mouth. This location of pain is what separates neurovascular orofacial pain from other forms of face pain. It may also be present below the eyes and around the ears, but is usually a throbbing pain that sometimes wakes a patient from sleep. Some patients also experience a feeling of swelling in the cheeks, excessive sweating, a stuffy nose, sensitivity to cold drinks, and the above-described phono- and photophobias. Evaluation involves a history, physical, and imaging.

In terms of neuropathic facial pain, two of the most common causes include *trigeminal neuralgia* and *burning mouth syndrome*. Trigeminal neuralgia, once called *tic douloureux*, is a short-lasting, excruciating, usually one-sided facial pain that has multiple causes such as tumors, cysts, viruses, trauma, and systemic diseases such as multiple sclerosis (MS). The pain is often described as an extremely sharp, or lancinating, electric-like pain that lasts typically for only a few seconds. Despite the attacks only lasting for seconds to minutes, repeated attacks can lead to facial pain that lingers continuously. Unfortunately, evaluating one for this condition can be problematic. Light touch, eating, talking, yawning, even a light breeze can lead to an attack. It has been proposed that one of the causes of trigeminal neuralgia involves compression of the nerve that bears the syndrome's name. This is usually from a vascular structure, be it a main vessel or one much smaller (micro compression). *Glossopharyngeal neuralgia* is a pain syndrome similar to trigeminal neuralgia, however much less common. It has similar inciting factors such as yawning, chewing, laughing, and talking; however, the location of the pain is in the distribution of the named nerve. Neither condition demonstrates abnormalities that can easily be seen on physical exam, nor is there a typical etiology in most cases. Regardless, a detailed history and physical exam should be obtained in each patient. Again, MRI and CT scans are obtained to rule out conditions such as tumor or other forms of microvascular compression.

Burning mouth syndrome, one of the most difficult to manage and get rid of problems causing facial pain, is a syndrome typically seen in postmenopausal women. There are multiple causes. Sometimes it can be spontaneous without any known cause (*idiopathic*), and at other times allergies, local infections, hormonal changes, vitamin deficiencies, diabetes, and autoimmune disorders can be the culprit. Patients experience a "burning" sensation in their mouths, typically the front portion of the tongue, top of the mouth, lips, and gums. It usually gets worse by the end of the day, and some patients have described altered taste (many times metallic). Unfortunately, the pain from this condition can last from months to several years. Diagnosis relies upon history and physical, ruling out treatable infectious causes or other reversible systemic conditions.

Another common area that causes referred facial pain is the nose. Pain associated with this location can be described as aching, diffuse, and nonpulsatile. Patients who have pain referred from the nose (*sino-nasal pain*) can experience it in various locations depending on which part of the nose is affected. The teeth, eye, temple, and forehead can all be possible destinations for the referred pain from the nose. During the evaluation of sino-nasal pain, the evaluating physician may use a tool called a speculum to inspect the inside of the nose. Sometimes, an otoscope (a device used to look into the ears) is used. In either case, the mucous membranes of the nose are evaluated for infection, inflammation, and possible tumor. Imaging studies may be ordered.

Ophthalmic zoster (*herpes zoster ophthalmicus*), a common cause of facial pain due to reactivation of hibernating chickenpox, should be suspected in elderly individuals or immunocompromised patients (difficulty fighting off infections). Pain develops on one side of the forehead as a stabbing, "knife-like" sensation followed by the formation of little raised blister-like lesions (vesicles). The skin overlying the affected area may become red and swollen. Aside from the history and physical, the evaluating practitioner may also take scrapings of the skin to send for analysis by a lab.

Treatment for many of the above conditions takes a somewhat similar approach. If the underlying cause is known, treat that first. For conditions like ophthalmic zoster, one will likely be prescribed an antiviral medication. Infectious causes of sino-nasal pain will be treated with antibiotics. For conditions that have a less defined cause for the pain, the treatment changes. In patients who develop postherpetic neuralgia, which can occur following the treatment for ophthalmic zoster, medications like amitryptyline or gabapentin may be used. While these medications were originally used for other disorders (i.e., amitryptyline is an antidepressant), they have been found over time to be helpful for these pain conditions. Patients that have one of the neuralgias (trigeminal or glossopharyngeal) may be treated with the antiseizure medication carbamazepine. Other medications that may be tried are phenytoin or valproic acid, both antiseizure medications. The muscle relaxant baclofen may be useful. A class of medications called benzodiazepines showed efficacy in certain conditions. With prescription drugs becoming the number one drug of abuse, it is prudent to start analgesic therapy (or pain control therapy) with non-opioid medications like NSAIDs, Tylenol, or a medication called Tramadol. In fact, recent evidence has revealed that combining acetaminophen (Tylenol) and NSAIDs like ibuprofen works better than either alone.

If conservative treatment is ineffective, more aggressive modes of treatment can be employed. For instance, the doctor may refer you to a pain medicine specialist who can offer treatments such as radiofrequency (RF) thermocoagulation or ablation. This treatment involves using x-ray to guide a very small needle next to the nerve that is suspected of causing the pain. Medication is injected to numb that nerve. Then, a small amount of heat is used to make a lesion in the nerve which can block transmission for six months, sometimes up to a year. RF ablation has been found to be effective in 95 percent of patients, especially when diagnostic blocks are performed beforehand. No lesion is made through those procedures, but rather the nerve is bathed in local anesthetic solutions in order to specifically identify the culprit. Similar to RF thermoablation, regional anesthetic techniques can be used to temporarily ease the pain caused by some of these syndromes. Various injection techniques, many performed under x-ray, can be used to not only help confirm a diagnosis, but also help treat it. Individual branches of the trigeminal nerve can be blocked to help localize facial pain. Sometimes other approaches need to be taken. For instance, in refractory trigeminal neuralgia, a neurosurgeon may be asked to perform procedures such as posterior fossa microvascular decompression, or stereotactic radiosurgery with a gamma knife. These techniques involve more specialized equipment, combining CT scanning and either general anesthesia or conscious sedation.

The outcome for facial pain is varied. In most cases, the pain subsides anywhere from one to four weeks after its onset. Some of the conditions mentioned above, like postherpetic neuralgia, burning mouth syndrome, glossopharyngeal, and trigeminal neuralgia, can exist for months to years. However, with proper treatment, many patients can begin to manage their pain on a daily basis. An understanding of how physicians go about diagnosing these conditions can help a patient help themselves.

Appendix A
Ear Pain

Condition	Symptoms	Evaluation	Treatment
TMJ disorder (R)	• Pain in the jaw, near the ear • Pain in the ear itself • "Clicking" sound when opening the mouth • Fullness of the ear • Dizziness • Neck soreness	– History and physical – MRI/CT	• NSAIDs • Bite-blocks
GERD (R)	• Sour taste in the mouth • Sore throat • Dull ear pain • Chronic cough • Chest pain • Trouble swallowing	– History and physical – Esophageal pH monitoring	• Lifestyle modifications • PPIs • H2-blockers
Eagle's Syndrome (R)	• One-sided sore throat • Trouble swallowing • Ringing in the ears • Neck pain • Ear pain	– History and physical – CT	• Surgery
Meniere's disease (P/R)	• Dizziness/vertigo • Nausea • Vomiting • Sweating • "Drop attacks"— sudden attack causing the individual to fall down • Jerky eye movements (nystagmus)	– History and physical – Audiometry – MRI	• Antihistamines (Benadryl) • Steroids • Diuretics (water pills) • Anti-nausea meds • Meclizine (anti-vertigo)
Chronic myringitis (P)	• Otorrhea • Aural fullness • Hearing loss	– History and physical – Otologic exam – CT/MRI	• Topical analgesics • +/– antibiotics • +/– surgery (for perforated eardrums)
Otitis media/ externa (P)	• Otorrhea • Aural fullness • Rash on outer ear, canal, or eardrum	– History and physical – Otologic exam	• Topical analgesics • +/– antibiotics • Maintaining dry ears • Surgical debridement for severe cases

*P = primary otalgia; R = referred otalgia.

Appendix B
Eye Pain

Condition	Symptoms	Evaluation	Treatment
Acute angle closure glaucoma	• Acutely painful eye • Red eye • Blurred vision • +/− halos surrounding light • +/− headache • +/− nausea and vomiting	− History and physical − Tonometry − Ophthalmoscope − Slit-lamp	• Topical Beta-blockers • Topical steroids • Diuretics
Scleritis	• Severe "boring" pain worse with eye movement over the course of weeks • Headache • Blurred vision • Tearing • Red eye	− History and physical − Blood work − Ophthalmoscope − Florosceine/ Wood's lamp	• Oral NSAIDs • Oral steroids • +/− Oral • Immunosuppressive drugs
Anterior uveitis (iritis)	• Painful eye • Red eye • Blurred vision • Tearing • Photophobia	− History and physical − Blood work − Ophthalmoscope − Tonometry − Slit-lamp	• Topical steroids • Oral steroids • Oral immunosuppressive drugs • Topical drugs to dilate the pupil • Topical antivirals/ antibiotics
Keratitis	• Painful eye • Red eye • Foreign-body sensation (like an eyelash) • Photophobia • Tearing	− History and physical − Ophthalmoscope − Slit-lamp − Fluorosceine/ Wood's lamp	• Topical eye lubricant • +/− Topical steroids • Oral analgesics • Oral antihistamines • +/− topical antibiotic/ antimicrobial
Corneal Abrasions	• Painful eye • Red eye • Foreign-body sensation (like an eyelash) • Photophobia • Tearing	− History and physical − Ophthalmoscope − Slit-lamp − Fluorosceine/ Wood's lamp	• Topical NSAIDs • +/− Oral analgesics • Topical Antibiotic

Appendix C
Face Pain

Condition	Symptoms	Evaluation	Treatment
Temporomandibular disorders	• Pain in the jaw, near the ear • Pain in the ear itself • "clicking" sound when opening the jaw • Fullness of the ear • Dizziness • Neck soreness	– History and physical – MRI/CT	• NSAIDs • Bite-blocks
Neurovascular orofacial pain	• Pain in the mouth and areas around the mouth • Pain below the eyes and around the ears • Throbbing pain that wakes one from sleep • Sensation of swelling in the cheeks • Excessive sweating • Stuffy nose • Sensitivity to cold drinks • Phono- and photophobia	– History and physical – MRI/CT	• Gabapentin • Amitryptyline • Carbamazepine • Analgesics/NSAIDs • Microvascular decompression • Nerve blocks • Radiofrequency ablation
Trigeminal Neuralgia	• Lancinating, electric-like pain in the distribution of the trigeminal nerve that last for seconds • Pain is exacerbated by light touch, talking, eating, yawning	– History and physical – MRI/CT	• Gabapentin • Amitryptyline • Carbamazepine • Analgesics/NSAIDs • Microvascular decompression • Nerve blocks • Radiofrequency ablation
Glossopharyngeal neuralgia	• Lancinating, electric-like pain in the back of the mouth, near the ear, and back of the tongue • Pain is exacerbated by light touch, talking, eating, yawning	– History and physical – MRI/CT	• Gabapentin • Amitryptyline • Carbamazepine • Analgesics/NSAIDs • Nerve blocks • Radiofrequency ablation

(*Continued*)

Appendix C (continued)

Condition	Symptoms	Evaluation	Treatment
Burning mouth syndrome	• "Burning" sensation in the mouth, typically near the front portion of the tongue, top of the mouth, lips, and gums • Pain becomes worse by the end of the day • +/− altered taste	− History and physical − MRI/CT − +/− blood work	• Gabapentin • Amitryptyline • Carbamazepine • Analgesics/ NSAIDs • Nerve blocks
Sinonasal pain	• Diffuse, aching, nonpulsatile pain near the eye, temple, forehead, and teeth	− History and physical − MRI/CT	• Antibiotics/ Antivirals • Analgesics/ NSAIDs
Ophthalmic zoster	• Pain on one side of forehead with blisters • Stabbing, "knife-like" pain of the skin overlying the affected area	− History and physical − MRI/CT	• Antivirals • Analgesics/ NSAIDs • Nerve blocks • Radiofrequency ablation

Appendix D
Treatment Modalities in Ear, Eye, and Facial Pain

Conservative Treatment	Interventional Treatment
Ear • Topical and oral medication • Bite blocks • Keeping the ear dry	Ear • Occipital nerve block
Eye • Topical and oral medication • Eye lubricants	Face • Gasserian nerve block • Glossopharyngeal block • Microvascular decompression
Face • Oral medication	

For more information on various medications used in the treatment of ear, eye, and face pain, please first consult your physician. Websites like WebMD, while helpful, may lead to unnecessary worry and possible misdiagnosis by the patient. However, if one is looking for more information online, http://www.rxlist.com has easily indexed sections on common dosages, indications, side effects, and contraindications. Appendix E provides a list of the commonly prescribed medications.

Appendix E
Commonly Prescribed Medications

Tylenol	Carbamazepine
Ibuprofen	Cyclobenzaprine (Flexeril)
Gabapentin (Neurontin)	Baclofen
Pregabalin (Lyrica)	Phenytoin
Tramadol (Ultram)	Amitryptyline (Elavil)
Hydrocodone/APAP (Vicodin)	Timolol eye drops
Oxycodone/APAP (Percocet)	Pilocarpine eye drops
Morphine	Acyclovir
Lidocaine patch/cream	Capsaicin

ADDITIONAL RESOURCES

American Academy of Otolaryngology: http://www.entnet.org
WebMD: http://www.webmd.com

13

NECK AND SHOULDER PAIN

John C. Pan, MD, Pamela Law, MD, and David E. Fish, MD, MPH

INTRODUCTION

Neck and shoulder pain are often related. If you experience pain in the shoulder, the source of the problem may be in your neck, and vice versa. That is why doctors frequently examine both in order to find out the cause of your pain. Neck and shoulder pain is very common, affecting 10–20 percent of the population. One out of three people can recall at least one episode of significant pain in the neck in their lifetime.

The key to successful management of neck and shoulder pain is to identify the source of pain. Since there are multiple interconnecting structures in the neck and shoulder that may cause pain, knowing the anatomy can help you better understand your pain.

ANATOMY OF THE NECK

Cervical spine refers to the portion of the spine in your neck. It supports the head and allows the head to move through these motions: rotation, flexion (forward bending), extension (backward bending), and side bending.

Vertebrae are the bones of the spine. There are seven cervical vertebrae, designated as C1 through C7 from top to bottom, which form a column to protect the spinal cord.

Intervertebral disks provide cushion between the vertebrae and allow flexibility. Each intervertebral disk is named by the level of vertebrae above and below. For example, the disk between the C5 vertebra and the C6 vertebra is the C5-6 disk.

Muscles help to protect, stabilize, and move the neck.

Ligaments refer to the tissues connecting bone to bone. They provide structural stability of the spine. A *sprain* is an injury to a ligament caused by stretching it too far from its normal position. The ligament can have a partial tear or be completely torn.

Facet joints are small joints in the neck connecting each vertebra to the level above and below. These joints have surrounding capsules and allow movements of the spine.

Cervical spinal cord is the portion of the spinal cord in the neck. It is located in the spinal canal formed by the vertebrae.

Nerve roots arise from the spinal cord. A left and a right nerve root exit the cervical spinal canal at each vertebral level through openings known as *intervertebral foramen (pl. foramina)*. The cervical nerve roots are designated as C1 through C8, according to the level at which they exit the spine. Upon exiting the spine, cervical nerve roots combine around the shoulder and form the nerves going into the arm. The nerve supply of the shoulder, arm, and hand entirely originates in the neck.

All of the structures listed above can be sources of pain if injury, irritation, or inflammation occurs.

ANATOMY OF THE SHOULDER

The shoulder is a combination of joints and associated muscles, tendons, and bones where the top part of the arm bone (humerus) forms a joint with the shoulder blade (scapula). The muscles, tendons, and ligaments hold the shoulder in place and maintain a balance between motion and stability. The shoulder joint provides a wide range of motion to the arm, allowing you to scratch your back or throw a ball.

The *rotator cuff* is a structure surrounding the "ball" of the shoulder (head of the humerus) consisting of the supraspinatus, infraspinatus, subscapularis, and teres minor muscles and their tendons. These tendons and muscles cover and hold the head of the humerus into the scapula as well as lift and rotate the arm.

The *acromion* is a bony structure forming the front edge of the shoulder blade. It sits over and in front of the head of the humerus.

Tendons are cords that connect muscle to bone.

Bursae (sing. bursa) are small, fluid-filled pads that act as cushions among your bones and the tendons and muscles near your joints.

SYMPTOMS

The most common causes of neck and shoulder pain are injuries to the muscles, tendons, and ligaments. Other common causes include nerve root impingement and joint or disk trauma. In rare instances, neck or shoulder pain can be caused by an infection or tumor. If the pain is accompanied by fevers or unexplained weight loss, it is important to see your doctor immediately.

Neck and shoulder pain does not always require medical attention. However, you should notify your doctor if you experience:

- Pain radiating to the shoulder, arm, or hand
- Numbness, tingling, or abnormal sensation in the arm or hand
- Weakness or loss of strength in the arm or hand
- Loss of coordination or ability to do simple tasks such as holding a fork or buttoning a shirt
- Difficulty with walking and stiffness in the arms or legs
- Loss of control of urination or bowel movement

Cervical Strain and Sprain

A cervical strain is an injury of the muscles or tendons produced by excessive forces on the cervical spine. A cervical sprain is the overstretching or tearing of the ligaments of the cervical spine. Cervical strains and sprains are the most common injuries after motor vehicle accidents and sports injuries.

Cervical Radiculopathy

Cervical radiculopathy refers to injury, irritation, or inflammation of a cervical nerve root. It is most commonly due to disk herniations and arthritic changes of the spine. Arthritis of the spine causes thickening of the ligaments, overgrowth of the bone, enlargement of the facet joints, and flattening of the disks. The combined effect is a narrowing of the exit space for the nerve roots, which can cause impingement and inflammation of these roots.

Symptoms of cervical radiculopathy are often described as sharp pain shooting from the neck into the arm or hand. Frequently, there is also numbness and a tingling sensation along the course of the radiating pain. If the injury is severe, the arm and hand can lose strength and become weak. The symptoms may be worse with turning or bending the neck toward the painful side and extending the neck backwards.

Cervical Facet Joint Pain

Cervical facet joints, the small joints between the vertebrae in the neck, are a common source of chronic neck pain. As arthritic changes and inflammation of the joints occur, the nerves to the facet joints can convey severe pain. Unlike cervical radiculopathy, cervical facet pain does not follow a nerve root pattern. Instead, the pain can run diffusely over the neck and upper back, known as "referred" pain, as the brain has trouble localizing these internal structures. Cervical facet joint pain is usually caused by arthritis or trauma such as auto accidents or a fall. It is usually worsened by sudden movements or staying in poor postures for a prolonged period. Examples of these are kneeling in the garden, bending forward to lift, straining to read a book, or working for a long time in front of a computer. Often there is associated spasm of the muscles in the neck, making it difficult to differentiate from muscle pain.

Cervical Myelopathy

In the late stages of spinal arthritic changes, bone spurs and thickened ligaments begin to narrow the spinal canal, through which the spinal cord runs. This condition is called *spinal stenosis*. When spinal canal narrowing becomes severe, the whole spinal cord can be compressed, resulting in a serious condition called cervical myelopathy. This is different from cervical radiculopathy, in which only the exit spaces of cervical nerve roots are narrowed, and legs are not affected. Cervical myelopathy can affect both the arms and the legs, causing pain, weakness, and spasticity in the limbs. Spasticity refers to a loss of control and stiffness of a limb. You may experience difficulty walking due to loss of control of where you place your feet. You may have numbness and tingling sensation of both arms and legs. You may lose the sensation that allows you to tell where your arms and legs are when your eyes are closed.

Whiplash Syndrome

Whiplash injury occurs with sudden excessive flexion and extension injury of the neck. Typically, it happens to occupants of a vehicle struck from behind by another vehicle, but can occur with any type of direction of force. During the impact, the head and neck do not suffer a direct blow, but undergo forceful passive movements that cause injuries to facet joints, disks, ligaments, supporting structures and muscles. The most common symptoms can be neck pain and headache, followed by shoulder pain, dizziness, visual disturbances, and arm tingling.

Shoulder Separation and Acromioclavicular (AC) Joint Sprains

A shoulder separation involves the acromioclavicular (AC) joint. The AC joint is where the collarbone (clavicle) meets the acromion, both of which are attached by the acromioclavicular (AC) ligament. The most common cause for an AC ligament sprain or separation of the AC joint is a fall directly onto the shoulder. Shoulder separations can be mild or severe, depending on whether the injury tears the AC ligament or its neighboring coracoclavicular (CC) ligament, putting the collarbone out of alignment. The most severe shoulder separation tears both the AC and CC ligaments and causes the "separation" of the collarbone and scapula. The scapula moves downward creating a bulge above the shoulder.

Nonsurgical treatments, such as a sling, cold packs, and medications, can often help manage the pain. Most people return to near full function even if a deformity remains, but it is also possible to have continued pain even with only a mild deformity. Surgery can be considered if pain persists or the deformity is severe.

Impingement Syndrome and Rotator Cuff Tendonitis

Because the shoulder is a highly mobile joint, the rotator cuff can become compressed by surrounding structures, like bone. Tendons of the rotator cuff muscles can become trapped under the acromion. This can cause shoulder pain called *impingement syndrome*. The pain may be due to compression, irritation, or tearing of any part of the shoulder, including muscle, tendon, or bursa. Compression and irritation of the rotator cuff tendons can lead to inflammation, or *rotator cuff tendonitis*. Impingement syndrome and rotator cuff tendonitis can occur after general wear and tear as you get older, from activity that requires constant use of the shoulder like baseball pitching, or from an injury.

Rotator Cuff Tear

While the rotator cuff can be torn from a single injury, such as during a shoulder fracture or dislocation, rotator cuff tears are usually the result of overuse of the shoulder over a period of years. The most common symptom is shoulder pain, often for several months. Other symptoms include pain when lifting the arm, pain when lowering the arm from a fully raised position and weakness when lifting or rotating the arm. Some symptoms of a rotator cuff tear may develop right away after an injury; when the tear occurs, there may be sudden pain, a snapping sensation, or immediate weakness of the arm. Alternatively, initial symptoms may be less dramatic and only present with overhead activities such as reaching or lifting. Lying on the affected shoulder also can be painful. Over time, the pain may become more noticeable with less activity.

Biceps Tendonitis

Biceps tendonitis is the inflammation of the biceps tendon and a common cause of shoulder pain due to its position on the front of the shoulder joint. Because the biceps tendon is physically located between two rotator cuff tendons (subscapularis and supraspinatus), it can share inflammatory processes involving the rotator cuff. Consequently, biceps tendonitis is frequently diagnosed in association with rotator cuff disease. Typically, biceps tendonitis causes aching pain in the front of the shoulder, exacerbated by lifting or pushing motions. Biceps tendonitis frequently occurs from overuse syndromes of the shoulder, which are fairly common in overhead-activity athletes such as baseball pitchers and tennis players.

Shoulder Dislocation and Glenohumeral Instability

The shoulder is an easy joint to dislocate because of its mobility. Dislocation means the head of the humerus dislodges from its usual position within the glenoid socket. A partial dislocation, also called a subluxation, means the head of the humerus is only partially and transiently out of the glenoid socket, while complete dislocation means it is all the way out. Both partial and complete dislocations cause pain and unsteadiness in the shoulder. Symptoms to look for include swelling, numbness, weakness, and bruising. Sometimes a dislocation may tear ligaments or tendons or damage nerves. Shoulder dislocation often recurs, which can lead to repeated dislocations and glenohumeral instability, which is excessive mobility of the humeral head in its socket. Patients with glenohumeral instability experience pain and unsteadiness in the shoulder joint. Initial treatment is conservative, focusing on strengthening the muscles of the shoulder. If conservative treatment fails, surgery may be undertaken to stabilize the shoulder.

Adhesive Capsulitis or Frozen Shoulder

Pain due to *adhesive capsulitis* (also known as *frozen shoulder*) is usually dull or aching and worsened with attempted motion. The pain is usually located over the outer shoulder area and sometimes in the upper arm. The hallmark of the condition is restricted motion and stiffness in the shoulder. The causes of adhesive capsulitis are not fully understood, but the process involves thickening and contracture of the connective tissue surrounding the shoulder joint. Adhesive capsulitis can develop after a time when you have been less active because of another injury, such as a rotator cuff injury or arm fracture, or after recovering from shoulder surgery.

Symptoms of adhesive capsulitis typically occur in three stages. During the first *stage*, your shoulder may ache and feel stiff, progressively becoming more painful. This stage may last about 3–8 months. During the second stage, you may experience less pain, but your shoulder becomes stiffer. This stage usually lasts about 4–6 months. The third and final stage, which usually lasts about 1–3 months, is not very painful. It becomes very hard to move your shoulder. After a while, the stiffness improves and you regain some shoulder mobility. Although full movement may not return, you should be able to do more activities.

For more than 90 percent of people with adhesive capsulitis, the pain and stiffness improve with simple treatment. However, recovery can take several years. Treatment is aimed at pain control with anti-inflammatory medication and the restoration of motion with stretching and therapy.

Glenoid Labrum Tear

The glenoid labrum is a soft fibrous tissue rim that surrounds and deepens the glenoid socket to help stabilize the head of the humerus in the shoulder.

Injuries to the labrum can occur from an acute injury, such as falling, or repetitive shoulder motion. Throwing athletes and weightlifters can experience glenoid labrum tears. Symptoms include pain, especially with overhead activities; locking, popping, or grinding sensations; a sense of instability in the shoulder, and decreased strength and range of motion.

Thoracic Outlet Syndrome

Thoracic outlet syndrome occurs when the blood vessels or nerves in the thoracic outlet—the space behind your collarbone (clavicle)—become compressed. This can happen after trauma from a car accident or after repetitive injuries from work or sports-related activities. Even an injury that happened long ago may lead to thoracic outlet syndrome in the present. The most common symptoms of thoracic outlet syndrome are pain in your shoulder, arm, and neck and numbness and tingling in your fingers. Depending on the extent of nerve and blood vessel compression, other symptoms include aching in your arm or hand, weakened grip, a bluish discoloration or paleness of your hand, arm swelling, and a throbbing lump near your collarbone.

DIAGNOSIS

Shoulder and neck pain is generally diagnosed using a three-part process:

First, you will be interviewed for your *medical history*. It is important to tell your doctor about any injuries or conditions that might be causing the pain, in addition to your general medical conditions. Be prepared to answer some of these important questions your doctor may ask:

- How long have you been feeling pain?
- Did your pain start suddenly or gradually?
- Is the pain dull, sharp, or shooting?
- Do any particular neck or arm movements make the pain improve or worsen?
- Are you experiencing numbness or weakness in any part of your body?
- Does the pain radiate to other parts of your body?
- Have you injured your neck, shoulder, or arm recently?
- What medications and supplements are you taking?

The doctor will then perform a *physical examination*, during which he or she will examine your neck and shoulder to feel for injury and to observe the range of movement, the location of pain, and the stability of the joint.

Lastly, the doctor will order any relevant *tests*. He or she may order one or more of the following to make a diagnosis:

- *Standard X-ray:* In this common procedure, a low level of radiation is passed through the body to produce a picture of your bones. This is useful for diagnosing fractures or other problems of the bones. However, soft tissues, such as muscles and tendons, do not show up on x-rays.

- *Arthrogram:* This diagnostic exam involves a series of images, often x-rays, taken after injecting contrast fluid into the shoulder joint. The injection is normally done under a local anesthetic to minimize pain. The contrast fluid enhances images by outlining soft tissue structures of the shoulder, and can be used to study tears of the rotator cuff and abnormalities of the glenoid labrum. Computerized tomography (CT) scans or MRI scans can be used as an alternative to x-rays, depending on the part of the shoulder that needs to be imaged.

- *Ultrasound:* A noninvasive procedure, this imaging technique involves a small, handheld scanner, which is placed on the skin of the shoulder. Ultrasound waves are reflected off internal structures of the neck and shoulder to form images. The accuracy of ultrasound for the rotator cuff is particularly high.

- *MRI (Magnetic Resonance Imaging):* Another imaging test, MRI is a procedure in which a machine with a strong magnet produces a series of cross-sectional images. No radiation is involved, and images are of a high quality, especially for soft tissues like muscles, tendons, and ligaments. Structures such as nerve roots, spinal cord, intervertebral disks, and rotator cuff are readily seen, making MRI a valuable test for many neck and shoulder conditions.

- *Electrodiagnostic Studies:* Nerve conduction study and electromyography (EMG) are two types of electrodiagnostic studies that are usually performed together when your pain may be related to a pinched or damaged nerve. Nerve conduction study involves attaching small electrodes to the skin over the hands and arms. Mild electrical currents are delivered through your nerves to assess the speed of the conduction and the health of the nerves. Some patients find this test uncomfortable and compare it to receiving a shock similar to static electricity. However, each stimulation only lasts less than a second. Electromyography (EMG) involves inserting a very fine needle through your skin into muscles to determine whether nerves are functioning properly.

Treatment Options

Medications

Acetaminophen and nonsteroidal anti-inflammatory drugs are frequently used to relieve neck and shoulder pain. Nonsteroidal anti-inflammatory drugs (NSAIDs; examples include ibuprofen and naproxen) provide analgesic effect at low doses and anti-inflammatory effect at high doses. Muscle relaxants are occasionally used in conjunction with NSAIDs for muscle spasm. If an injured nerve is the primary source of pain, low-dose antidepressant or antiseizure medication such as gabapentin may be used.

Physical Therapy

Physical therapy for neck and shoulder pain can provide symptom relief and prevent pain in the future. A typical course of physical therapy includes twice-a-week sessions and a home exercise program. The goals are to increase strength, regain mobility, and learn about postures and methods to prevent injury. Therapy sessions may incorporate heat, ice, ultrasound, transcutaneous electrical nerve stimulation (TENS), massage, and neck traction. The duration of therapy depends on how your symptoms respond to therapy. It is important to note that physical therapy works the best when you actively participate and perform home exercises as directed.

Cervical Collar

Soft cervical collars provide comfort mainly by reminding you to maintain proper neck and head positions. They can be used in the first two weeks of your pain, but should not be used for longer than a few weeks, because they can cause weak neck muscles.

Corticosteroid Injection

Corticosteroids are medications with strong anti-inflammatory properties, and inflammation is a common problem in patients with shoulder and neck pain. For shoulder pain, injection of a combination of local anesthetic and corticosteroid into the joint spaces or bursae can relieve pain, both in the short-term and long-term periods. Pain caused by common shoulder conditions, like rotator cuff tendonitis and adhesive capsulitis, may be alleviated by a corticosteroid injection. Ultimately, the effects of the corticosteroid may last from a few weeks to a few months.

Nonsurgical Interventional Procedures

A variety of nonsurgical techniques are available to treat and diagnose neck and shoulder pain. Often, these are performed with the guidance of fluoroscopic x-ray.

Cervical Epidural Steroid Injection

Epidural steroid injection relieves pain by delivering corticosteroid to the epidural space of the spine, where the medication can flow along compressed nerve roots and decrease inflammation. This may start the process of nerve root healing by decreasing pain while the intervertebral disk pathology is naturally healing. The effects may last a few weeks, and sometimes up to a few months. More than one injection may be required to achieve sustained relief of your pain. Judicious use of cervical epidural steroid injection is important, because rare but severe complications have been reported. Your doctor may consider this procedure if the pain does not improve with other more conservative treatments. It is important to find an interventional pain specialist who regularly performs these procedures so that a good result will occur, and to minimize the potential for complications. Do not assume that every pain specialist is automatically the right person to perform a cervical epidural steroid injection.

Facet Joint Medial Branch Block

Medial branches are small nerves that provide sensations to the facet joints. Local anesthetic medication can be injected into the facet joints or on the corresponding medial branches to block painful sensation from the facet joints. This is usually done for diagnostic purposes and should not relieve long-term pain. If the injection alleviates your pain significantly for a few hours to weeks, then facet joints are likely to be the source of pain. At that point, another procedure known as *radiofrequency ablation* (RFA) is often done to use heat to block the medial branches and provide more prolonged pain relief. Successful radiofrequency ablation of the medial branches can achieve four to six months of pain relief. Unfortunately, this procedure has diminishing returns and may become less effective over time, but the natural healing of the joint may have occurred by then. The RFA procedure may be used for 1 to 3 years as a pain management option for the typical patient.

Surgery

Surgeries for cervical herniated disks or arthritis-related cervical radiculopathy can be considered when there is intractable pain, severe or worsening weakness, or progression to myelopathy. For cervical radiculopathy, surgery can sometimes achieve quicker improvement three months post surgery than nonsurgical treatments, but unless there is neurological decline, conservative options should be considered as a first line treatment. At one year after surgery, people with conservative treatments may do as well as people who had surgeries, and therefore conservative options may continue to be a reasonable alternative to surgery. For cervical myelopathy, surgical decompression may be needed for severe cases or worsening neurological symptoms despite conservative treatments. People with severe cervical disk pain may also be surgical candidates to remove parts of the pathological disks and fuse the spine at the involved levels.

PROGNOSIS

Because neck and shoulder pain is most commonly caused by sprains and strains, you can usually expect to feel much better or even have full recovery in three months or less. If pain persists for longer than six months, it is unclear at times what the extent of the injury is to the ligaments, disks, joints, or nerves. Beyond sprains and strains, the extent of relief from other causes of neck and shoulder pain varies. Some conditions can be recurrent or persistent, such as arthritic facet joint neck pain or shoulder instability. Some conditions require surgical repair, physical therapy, or other treatment measures for maximal recovery. In general, a longer duration of symptoms, gradual onset of pain, litigation, and higher pain severity are associated with more persistent symptoms.

With time and conservative therapy, most neck and shoulder pathology will recover, and only a few patients will end up going to surgery for persistent symptoms. It is important to follow through with the plan recommended by the healthcare practitioner.

ADDITIONAL RESOURCES

"Neck Pain." American Academy of Orthopaedic Surgeons: http://orthoinfo.aaos.org/topic.cfm?topic=A00231

"Neck Pain." MayoClinic.com: http://www.mayoclinic.com/health/neck-pain/DS00542

"Neck Pain." Medline Plus: A Service of the U.S. National Library of Medicine, National Institutes of Health: http://www.nlm.nih.gov/medlineplus/ency/article/003025.htm

"Shoulder Injuries and Disorders." Medline Plus: A Service of the U.S. National Library of Medicine, National Institutes of Health: http://www.nlm.nih.gov/medlineplus/shoulderinjuriesanddisorders.html

"Shoulder Pain." American Academy of Orthopaedic Surgeons: http://orthoinfo.aaos.org/topic.cfm?topic=a00065

"Shoulder Pain." FamilyDoctor.org: http://familydoctor.org/online/famdocen/home/healthy/physical/injuries/268.html

"Shoulder Pain." MayoClinic.com: http://www.mayoclinic.com/health/shoulder-pain/MY00189

"Shoulder Pain." Medline Plus: A Service of the U.S. National Library of Medicine, National Institutes of Health: http://www.nlm.nih.gov/medlineplus/ency/article/003171.htm

"Shoulder Problems: Questions and Answers about Shoulder Problems." National Institute of Arthritis and Musculoskeletal and Skin Diseases, National Institutes of Health, Department of Health and Human Services: http://www.niams.nih.gov/Health_Info/Shoulder_Problems/default.asp

"Shoulder Problems: What Are Shoulder Problems? Fast Facts: An Easy-to-Read Series of Publications for the Public." National Institute of Arthritis and Musculoskeletal and Skin Diseases, National Institutes of Health, Department of Health and Human Services: http://www.niams.nih.gov/Health_Info/Shoulder_Problems/shoulder_problems_ff.asp

14

ABDOMINAL (BELLY) PAIN

Frank J. E. Falco, MD, Renato Vesga, MD,
Syed A. Husain, DO, and Jignyasa L. Desai, DO

BACKGROUND

Abdominal (belly) pain is located from the breast bone to the hips and spans from one side of the rib cage to the other. Abdominal pain generally results from a problem related to the organs within the abdominal area. It can also be referred by an organ outside of the abdominal cavity, such as a bladder infection. Abdominal pain can also be caused by a disease process such as diabetes. Diagnostic tests, laboratory analysis, and radiologic imaging such as x-rays or an MRI (magnetic resonance imaging) scan can help to establish the source of the abdominal pain. Treatment options depend on the diagnosis. This chapter reviews the most common causes and treatment options for abdominal pain.

SIGNS AND SYMPTOMS

Your doctor will ask many of the following questions to help differentiate amongst the vast diagnoses of abdominal pain. It is important to be honest with your doctor and not to leave anything out when explaining your pain and symptoms. You never know what piece of information will be important in establishing a diagnosis. Symptoms to discuss with your physician include nausea, vomiting, bloating, gas, jaundice (yellow coloring of the skin or eye), reflux, appetite loss, dark stool, vomiting blood, weight loss, constipation, diarrhea, and mucus or blood in the stools. You should also mention any food intolerances, especially lactose and wheat. Any prior history of abdominal surgeries, colonoscopies, endoscopies, test or blood results, and previous treatment are important to review with your doctor.

Abdominal pain may be the only presenting symptom you have in a number of serious conditions. You should take any form of abdominal pain seriously. A sudden onset of severe abdominal pain with signs of vomiting, muscle stiffness, abdominal distention, dizziness, or loss of consciousness signifies a serious problem that requires you to receive immediate treatment. Severe abdominal pain can be caused by a number of different problems, including an acute appendicitis, peptic ulcer disease with perforation, acute pancreatitis, cholcystitis, bowel obstruction, a vascular problem, or a serious infection, all of which need urgent medical attention. These conditions should be treated immediately at a hospital and may require surgical treatment.

COMMON ACUTE ABDOMINAL CONDITIONS

Acute appendicitis is caused by a bacterial infection of your appendix, which is a fingerlike pouch of the intestine that sometimes can become obstructed by stool, which then develops into an infection. In severe cases, the appendix can swell and rupture, spilling the infection into the abdominal cavity, which is a surgical emergency. You might experience indigestion a few days before developing appendicitis. Children can have either diarrhea or constipation before a case of appendicitis. The location of the pain is epigastric (above the belly button) or periumbilical (around the belly button) in location, which then localizes to the right lower abdomen. Other symptoms such as nausea, vomiting, and fever may occur. There is local tenderness, rigidity, and distention of the abdomen to touch. A perforation (rupture) may result in a high fever, intense tenderness, an elevated white blood cell count, nausea, and/or vomiting. During the physical examination, there is right lower abdominal pain on touching or pushing. The diagnosis of appendicitis is confirmed by a CT (computer tomography) scan and blood work. The blood work is analyzed for an increased white blood cell count and inflammatory markers. Treatment is based on severity of the case, but oftentimes it is surgical, which is either by laparoscopy (small incision) of the abdomen, or an open surgical removal (laparotomy) of the appendix. Intravenous fluids, antibiotics and pain medications are also part of the treatment plan.

Peptic ulcer disease is caused by *Helicobacter pylori* (a bacteria) in 90 percent of cases. Other causes include overuse of steroids, cigarette smoking, and rapid gastric emptying of the stomach. Perforation of a gastric or duodenal ulcer is a surgical emergency that can lead quickly to death if not treated immediately. Usually, there is a sudden, sharp, severe pain that can be generalized. The pain will be so severe that patients can be found in a fetal position, and any movement exacerbates the pain. On examination, there is generalized tenderness, guarding (preventing touching of the painful area), and rigidity (stiffness of the abdominal muscles). In severe cases, there is so-called shock that consists of a reduced body temperature (95°F), cold extremities, pale face, low blood pressure, and rapid heart rate. A routine diagnostic study of the abdomen includes x-rays or a CT scan of the abdomen after swallowed barium (a liquid x-ray contrast). A barium swallow is an upper intestinal study that will show leakage of the barium contrast if there is a perforation of the stomach or intestines. Nonperforated ulcers can be treated with medical management using antibiotics and medications that protects the stomach lining from the gastric (stomach) acid. Perforated ulcers are treated with surgery.

Acute pancreatitis is the sudden inflammation of the pancreas, the gland organ that produces digestive enzymes and insulin in the digestive and endocrine systems. Abdominal pain can also be related to chronic pancreatitis. Acute pancreatitis can lead to death without immediate treatment. Pain from acute pancreatitis is excruciating and located in the epigastric (above the belly button) area. Pain often radiates to the left shoulder and left upper abdomen. The diagnosis is made with a CT scan and/or an MRI scan, and blood work. Mild cases are often successfully treated with simply stopping food intake and intravenous fluids for hydration. Surgery is indicated for necrosis (premature death of cells and living tissue) of the pancreas in the setting of acute pancreatitis. The most common cause of death in acute pancreatitis is infection. Antibiotics are an important aspect for the treatment of pancreatitis. Pain management includes the use of strong opioids (narcotics) in moderate to severe cases such as morphine.

Gallbladder disease may include biliary colic, cholecystitis, choledocholithiasis, and cholangitis (these conditions are described below). Biliary cholic is caused by gallstones that directly block the cystic duct. Cholecystitis is an inflammation of the gallbladder due to obstruction of the cystic duct, most commonly a result of a gallstone. Choledocholithiasis is an obstruction of the common bile duct by a stone from the gallbladder. Cholangitis is inflammation of the entire bile tract, with associated infection that can be life threatening without immediate treatment. There is pain associated with biliary colic. It is a steady pain that can refer to the right shoulder or right lower back. In severe cases, the gallbladder can rupture spilling contents of bacteria and infection into the abdominal cavity, which is a surgical emergency. Sometimes a continuous low-level inflammatory state develops in the gallbladder that is a source of chronic pain. Pain is generally located in the right upper abdomen. Other symptoms include vomiting, jaundice, fever, tenderness, and rigidity. Other diseases that can cause right upper abdominal pain include hepatitis, pleurisy (inflammation of the lining of your lungs), heart attack, and inflamed duodenal (small bowel) ulcer. The diagnosis is made through a HIDA (nuclear study of your gallbladder) scan, or a CT scan. Treatment is generally a cholecystectomy (surgical removal of the gallbladder).

Acute (sudden onset) intestinal obstruction can present with a number of different symptoms based on location and type. Intestinal obstruction can be the result of several different problems including volvulus (an abnormal twisting of the bowel onto itself), diverticulitis of the colon, strangulated hernia, abdominal tumors, intussusceptions (telescoping of one portion of the bowel in the other) and malrotation. The severity is based on whether the mesentery (supporting soft tissue structures) and blood vessels are affected in the obstruction. Pain may be mild to severe and referred to the epigastric and umbilical regions. The pain is typically episodic, colicky (comes in waves of intensity), and results from intestinal peristalsis (contractile propulsions) attempting to overcome the obstructed segment. Vomiting, constipation, abdominal distention, and tenderness are other symptoms that may occur. The diagnosis may be made by a barium enema or CT scan of the abdomen. Treatment is based upon the cause of the obstruction and can range from a simple decompression of the abdomen with a nasogastric tube (a tube placed through the nose down into your stomach) attached to suction to surgical resection.

Peritonitis is inflammation of the tissues that line the abdomen and cover the organs in your abdomen. This is a very serious diagnosis, since peritonitis is the single most common cause of death. The infection in the peritoneum can develop from an abdominal wound or spread from blood, organs, or the lymphatic system. Common causes are from a rupture of organs, such as the appendix, duodenal ulcer, diverticulum, gallbladder, or biliary ducts. Pain is constant and generally over the abdomen. The initial pain is at the site of rupture and then spreads along the peritoneum. The symptoms experienced include abdominal distention, fever, fluid in the abdomen, and low urine output. The toxic symptoms of peritonitis and shock present later in the course of the infection and indicate the severity of the diagnosis. This must be addressed immediately, and surgery is a must to treat the cause of peritonitis.

An acute-onset of abdominal pain might be due to an *infectious etiology,* especially if there has been recent travel to a tropical region. Malaria, sickle-cell anemia with associated crisis, amebiasis (a microscopic parasite), and infestation with parasites such as worms, giardia (a microscopic protozoa), and tropical sprue (malabsorption disease of unknown cause found in the tropics) are just a few of the potential infectious etiologies. This is a condition that is often misdiagnosed and is dependent upon the history provided to the physician. The history is typically one of recent travel, including camping or traveling overseas. Symptoms typically include dysentery (inflammatory disorder of the intestine), colicky pain, fevers, vomiting, and leukocytosis (a raised white blood cell count above the normal range in the blood). The pain is diffuse and located in all four regions of the abdomen. Severe gas pain can occur secondary to bacterial overgrowth in the small intestine and presents as severe spasms. The diagnosis is based primarily on blood work and imaging to rule out other conditions. The mainstay of treatment consists of antibiotics and intravenous fluid replacement. In the case of malabsorption, it is important to receive replenishment of vitamins such as vitamin B and vitamin D as well as iron.

Gastroparesis is a chronic condition characterized by abnormal gastric motility, where the stomach is not emptying solid foods in a normal fashion. The hallmark symptoms experienced are nausea, vomiting, and abdominal pain. This is often a disabling disorder marked by chronic pain, depression, anxiety, frequent hospitalization, poor social functioning, nutritional deficiencies, and unemployment. Gastroparesis can usually be diagnosed by ingesting a radioactive tracer (typically in the form of a sandwich) and determining whether your gastric emptying rate of the tracer is normal or abnormal. Unfortunately, the diagnosis of gastroparesis is easier to establish than identifying the actual cause. In the majority of cases, a specific cause for gastroparesis is never found, adding to the frustration surrounding this condition. The most common identifiable cause of gastroparesis is diabetes followed by abdominal surgery. Other causes include eating disorders, adverse effect of certain medications, and gastrointestinal diseases such as gastroesophageal reflux, peptic ulcer disease, chronic pancreatitis, and celiac disease (an autoimmune disease leading to small intestine damage from eating gluten and other proteins found in wheat and other grains).

There are multiple factors involved in treatment of gastroparesis which consist of education, diet adjustments, treating identifiable causes, and symptom management. Liquid supplementation with vitamins and other nutrients as well as pureed food are the foundation of diet, since liquids are unaffected by gastroparesis. The diet should not include high-fiber fatty foods that delay gastric emptying. Drugs that improve gastric emptying such as metoclopramide (Reglan), tegaserod (Zelnorm), domperidone (Motilium), and erythromycin can be part of the treatment plan but need more clinical investigation to determine their effectiveness. Electrical stimulation of certain gastric pacing cells by implanting a neurostimulator can enhance gastric emptying. Neurostimulation can also be used as a means of controlling chronic abdominal pain associated with gastroparesis.

CHRONIC ABDOMINAL PAIN

Chronic abdominal pain is abdominal pain that persists for a minimum of three months. This may be continuous or intermittent. There are many causes of chronic abdominal pain, and these are related to many of the above acute pain syndromes.

Treatment Options

Chronic abdominal pain affects up to 20 percent of Americans. Many treatments for abdominal pain exist. After the initial evaluation and treatment for chronic pain states there is often residual discomfort. This abdominal pain can be treated in many different ways just as in other areas of the body that can be pain generators, including oral medications and interventional procedures. Interventional procedures can be used to identify a cause for abdominal pain as well as for treatment. Interventional procedures can often be a better choice than oral pain medications, which can produce side effects that can even worsen symptoms. There are several interventional pain management options available, including diagnostic and therapeutic injections to help identify and treat the cause of your abdominal pain.

The first step in treating abdominal pain is to identify the cause. There are two categories of abdominal pain: either pain that is originating from internal organs or pain from the abdominal wall. A proper workup for your abdominal pain includes a thorough history and physical exam, laboratory testing, and imaging. There are times when it can be difficult to make a diagnosis even with these evaluations. It is important to start looking at exactly where the pain is originating from. Dividing the abdomen into the upper, middle, and lower regions helps to group potential structures that could be causing the pain.

Certain nerves correlate with different areas in the abdomen. Blocking (numbing) the nerve that supplies a particular structure that is sending the painful impulse to the brain can narrow down which structure is causing pain. In this way, blocking certain nerves that innervate the upper, middle, and lower abdomen as well as the pelvis can localize the source of pain. Once the pain is identified, the same nerve can be injected with a neurolytic agent such as alcohol (neurolysis) to provide long-term relief. These types of injections are performed in a sterile environment using x-ray (fluoroscopic) guidance and sedation to maintain comfort during the injection.

The celiac plexus is a group of nerves that supply many upper and mid-abdominal structures. Mid-abdominal pain can be diagnosed and treated with a celiac plexus block which can help if there is pain in the liver, pancreas, gallbladder, stomach, spleen, kidneys, intestines, and adrenal glands. This block is particularly helpful for pancreatic cancer pain. Lower abdominal pain including pelvic pain can be diagnosed and treated using a hypogastric block. The hypogastric block can be particularly useful if there is interstitial cystitis or cancer involving the testicles, prostate, or rectum.

Abdominal pain can also be coming from the abdominal wall. Nerves in the abdominal wall can be injured from trauma or after surgery. The abdominal nerves include the ilioinguinal, iliohypogastric, and genitofemoral nerves. These nerves can be blocked in the same diagnostic fashion and, if pain relief is adequate with the local anesthetic, a neurolytic injection can provide long-term relief.

There are other treatment options if these blocks do not provide long-term relief. One of these treatments, if there is visceral (abdominal organ) pain, is a spinal cord stimulator, a device that is implanted in your body. It functions by sending electrical impulses to the spinal cord and blocking pain signals from reaching the brain. By blocking the pain signals, the brain does not perceive the pain. The spinal cord stimulator offers a much more permanent solution for abdominal pain than the neurolytic blocks.

ALTERNATIVE TREATMENTS

Sometimes interventional procedures are not the best option. In these instances there are other methods for providing relief of abdominal pain. In certain circumstances, osteopathic manipulation can help alleviate abdominal pain. The body can be seen as a complex machine with each structure providing a certain function. This relationship between structure and function is important for performing daily functions at an optimal level. As with any portion of the body, the abdomen has certain nerves and structures that function together in balance to perform jobs like digestion. Your "balance" between certain nerves in the body can be thrown off. The goal of these treatments is to restore the balance. The advantage of the manipulation is that it is noninvasive. As with other treatment options, osteopathic manipulation may have to be performed multiple times to provide more permanent pain relief.

Another treatment option includes homeopathic medicine. Although not incorporated into mainstream medicine, one might consider homeopathy that relies on natural substances in the environment that have healing characteristics. Homeopathic medicine can be useful in treatment of acute abdominal pain with spasms, constipation, belching, bloating, heartburn, nausea, and vomiting. These natural remedies can be a part of initial treatment for abdominal pain. Some of the more common homeopathic substances used in the treatment of abdominal pain include Chamomilla, Chelidonium Majus, Colocynthis, Lycopodium, and Nux Vomica.

Abdominal pain is a complex diagnosis and includes many organs within the body cavity. Proper diagnosis and evaluation will help guide the decision for the specific type of treatments to be used. Multiple options exist in treating abdominal pain, and it is important to use all members of the medical staff to help create and execute the treatment plan. It is important to discuss in detail the expected outcomes and any potential complications that may arise. These discussions will help both you and your treating physician gain trust and help provide you with a more desirable outcome in the long term.

ADDITIONAL RESOURCES

Friedman, Scott. *Current Diagnosis and Treatment Gastroenterology.* McGraw Hill, 2003.
Silen, William. *Cope's Early Diagnosis of the Acute Abdomen.* Oxford University Press, 2005.

15

LOW BACK PAIN

Rinoo V. Shah, MD, MBA, and Alan D. Kaye, MD, PhD

INTRODUCTION

Low back pain is a common condition that affects millions of Americans. About 10 people out of 100 will experience low back pain in any given year. Over your lifespan, you may be just as likely to own a car as you are to get low back pain! A lot of money is spent on getting treatment for this pain; in 2007, more than $30 billion was spent on low back pain care. This figure doesn't calculate the personal cost and time lost due to disability. Low back pain doesn't discriminate. It likes all sexes, ages, income levels, marital statuses, athletic abilities, memetic preferences, and skin tones. Low back pain may express a preference, however, for smokers, machine operators, and commercial drivers. Those with anxiety, depression, obesity, jobs requiring heavy lifting, and poor job satisfaction may be vulnerable to low back pain as well.

SYMPTOMS

Low back typically refers to a region of the body at the level of the waist. The pain may extend up to below the rib cage, and down to the buttocks and legs. The pain can be described as aching, shooting, burning, stabbing, and/or tingling. The pain may get worse with sitting, standing, movement, twisting, and/or lifting. Patients often fidget while sitting or may have to use their hands to get out of a chair. The pain may linger for many years, and the details of what started the pain may get fuzzy. Unfortunately, the patient may fixate on a specific cause of the back pain. Patients sometimes blame themselves for a specific event—they do not understand that one will most likely get pain, no matter what they do. Patients should not blame themselves—this is not productive. Many patients develop a fear. This mini posttraumatic stress reaction following back pain is of major consequence. Our entire society is geared toward healthy mobility. If one is scared of developing a severe back pain attack, they may not wish to go outside or interact with family and friends. They may become very nervous about going anywhere without painkillers. Returning to work may cause anxiety and apprehension about their pain returning. Back pain is unfortunately a pejorative disease—many patients are not proud of this disease. There may be many rallies for heart disease and cancer, but no "walks for back pain sufferers." Back pain patients are often not treated well by colleagues and medical professionals; this unfortunately leads to a sense of victimization, frustration, and anger.

Back pain is alarming, and one of the most common reasons to see a doctor. Fortunately, most episodes resolve. The back pain that does not resolve after three months is referred to as chronic low back pain. Patients that recover from back pain may have another episode in their lives.

DIAGNOSIS

Physicians use certain medical tools and skills to figure out what causes back pain. Many folks criticize doctors when they search for the source of low back pain. These tools and skills can be expensive, but they can be very reassuring to the patient. Fewer than 1 out of 100 patients have a disastrous cause of low back pain, such as cancer. These tools can guide treatment as well.

Low back pain is evaluated, first and foremost, by telling a story—the patient's story. The doctor may also use guided questions: "Where is your pain?" "What does it feel like—sharp, stabbing, shooting, twisting, burning?" "On a scale from 0 to 10, with 0 representing no pain and 10 representing the worst pain possible, what is your pain?" "Does the pain go anywhere, such as down to your buttock or leg?" "Is the pain worse with sitting, bending, or walking?" or "Do you have any numbness in your groin, leaking of urine, or soiling of your underwear?"

A doctor may look for red flags during the interview—these symptoms require heightened attention. These include major trauma, falls, motor vehicle accidents, and sudden changes in pain intensity or one's ability to do daily activities. Back pain in someone older than 50 or younger than 20 could be due to a severe illness. Chills, fevers, or an unexplained weight loss may alert a doctor to cancer or infection. Risk factors for a spinal infection include urinary tract infections, intravenous drug abuse, and a weakened immune system. Patients with spine cancer or infection could have severe rest and nighttime pain. An elderly or chronically ill patient that develops sudden back pain, following a mild activity, may have a fractured bone in the back.

During the examination, a physician may ask you to disrobe. You should consider asking for a chaperone. The doctor may first observe you and how you behave with back pain. The physician will observe your walking, sitting capacity, and facial expressions. You may be asked to twist forward, backward, and sideways. The doctor may feel your back muscles to look for muscle spasms or "trigger points." The curvature of your spine will be visualized. They will do a comprehensive exam not directly related to your back. For example, they may observe your pupils if you are on narcotics, your breathing rate, your sweating rate, or your blood pressure.

The back examination will focus on looking (inspection), touching (palpation), movement (range of motion), and aching (body tenderness). Light tapping (percussion) may elicit pain over a broken spine bone. Tenderness over a muscle may be present in a muscle spasm. Range of motion may be restricted in someone with arthritis. There are some specialized tests. Your doctor may ask you to lie flat and lift your leg; if you get shooting pains down the leg, you may have a pinched nerve. Your doctor may check the strength, sensation, and reflexes in your leg. This is a test to pinpoint nerve damage. The doctor may observe how you walk. If you bend forward to relieve pain, this may be a sign of crowding of the nerves (spinal stenosis). If you get leg cramps after walking a short distance, this may be a sign of either crowding of the nerves (spinal stenosis) or blockage of the blood vessels (vascular claudication). The doctor may put your leg in a figure-of-four position and push down. If you hurt in the buttock, this could be a buttock joint problem (sacroiliac joint). If the pain is in the groin, this could be a problem with the hip joint. The doctor may also perform a general exam to evaluate your overall health and look for a total body condition, manifesting in your back.

X-rays are used to look at the bones and the alignment. A fracture can be pinpointed with x-rays. Comparing x-rays can help identify if a fracture is recent and the cause of pain. Patients may have degeneration or "age-appropriate changes" of the spine; the spine ages, whether we like it or not. No one would call gray or white hair "degenerative hair disease." For some reason, we use these negative connotation words such as degeneration. This can lead to anxiety and doesn't inform the patient about how they compare with others. Degeneration simply is a comparison between a younger version of your spine and an older version of your spine. This is a natural process of aging. Degeneration occurs at many levels in the low back and is present in many patients without symptoms. In isolation, degeneration cannot pinpoint who has pain. X-rays are important for identifying bone cancers, bone thinning (osteoporosis), and prior surgery. A doctor can review your x-ray with you and should review this type of study when planning a procedure.

Bone scanning is useful in pinpointing an active process. A radioactive tracer is injected through a vein. The patient is placed in a detector at different times after the injection. The anatomic details are not as great as other studies, but a silhouette of the person's bones can be identified. The tracer goes to the area of greatest activity. Areas of greater activity can alert the doctor to an area where bone is being turned over. The bone scan can alert the physician to a cancer, infection, fracture, or autoimmune "attacking your own body" disease. The bone scan can be used even with metallic implants.

CT scanning is an advanced tool. Its main goal is to look at the bones and create a cross-sectional and 3D view. It can demonstrate the relationship between the bones and the nerve structures. CT scans can also look at bony alignment. The main problem is the radiation exposure. CT scanning can be useful in detecting bony changes missed by x-rays and with greater anatomic detail, as compared to a bone scan. It can be performed quickly and is well tolerated by patients who are claustrophobic (scared of tight spaces).

MRI is the main imaging tool of choice in this modern era. It is a very versatile tool, and its costs have come down in recent years. It is excellent for looking at different structures in the low back. It can give excellent detail in distinguishing different tissues in the low back: bone, discs, ligaments, nerves, spinal fluid sac, and spinal cord. It is the best test for looking at soft (non-bony) tissues. An MRI is extremely safe, but it can be a problem for patients scared of tight spaces. An MRI cannot be administered to patients with pacemakers. The best part for patients is that an MRI of the low back can be very educational. The patient's doctor can show the patient what is exactly wrong.

Electrodiagnostic studies are used to study the function of nerves. A specialist will evaluate your muscles and nerves to pinpoint a pinched nerve, compression, or nerve disease.

TREATMENT

Rest

Modified rest with a quick return to normal activity is a good approach to managing low back pain. One large trial overturned the conventional wisdom that seven days of bed rest is necessary; two days is more than sufficient. Return to normal activity as quickly as possible works for most cases of back pain. Clearly, cancer, fractures, infections, and other very severe and progressive causes of low back pain may require longer periods of rest. There may be no difference in the type of activity that is necessary.

Drugs

Pain management uses different classes of drugs to help with pain. A pain ladder is used to guide treatment. Higher levels of pain require climbing up the painkiller ladder. The variety of drugs one uses is just as important as an individual drug's potency. Imagine going to a buffet when you are hungry. You may get a balanced meal, with a drink, salad, appetizer, main dish, and dessert. If you are really hungry, then you will get more food. This approach is used, by analogy, in pain management. I like to call it diversify, balance, and ramp up the painkillers. The analogy, however, fails because some drugs have a ceiling effect—this means more of a drug doesn't give pain relief. There is one exception: opioids (narcotics). The World Health Organization advocates a balanced approach, with increased amounts depending on the pain severity.

Nonsteroidal anti-inflammatory drugs (NSAIDs) are the most commonly used drugs for back pain. They reduce inflammation, which is common in low back pain. Ibuprofen is a common, over-the-counter NSAID. NSAIDs can be given by mouth, by vein, or through the skin. Ketorolac is a potent NSAID that can be given by vein. There are many creams that contain an NSAID, such as methyl salicylate. Some recent innovations include an NSAID patch, which can be applied to a part of the body. NSAIDs have risks with long-term use: stomach ulcer disease, kidney problems, high blood pressure, and heart attacks.

Acetaminophen reduces pain, but not inflammation. This is a good alternative or supportive drug for pain control. Many drugs are paired with acetaminophen, and patients must be careful about the total daily dose. Patients should talk to their doctor about how much acetaminophen they can consume in a day. Too much acetaminophen can cause liver damage.

Muscle relaxants are another class of drugs. They are not similar, and different drugs have different types of action. Some work on the central brain and spine tissues and cause sedation. Doctors often prescribe methocarbamol, baclofen, and cyclobenzaprine. All of these drugs can cause sedation, constipation, dry mouth, and retention of urine. They should be used with caution and used for the short term. They may be dangerous with other sedatives and alcoholic drinks. Carisoprodol is a controversial drug, since this may cause dependency. Practitioners and law enforcement encounter the slang "hillbilly cocktail": carisoprodol, valium, and oxycodone.

Antiseizure drugs are used for nerve pain and, not typically, for muscle, bone, and back pain. One common drug is gabapentin. This drug can be used to help with burning pain and "touch-me-not pain" (allodynia). This drug may be helpful in managing patients who need higher and higher doses of potent narcotic painkillers.

Sedative drugs can be used for nerve pain disorders or muscle spasms. Clonazepam is used for pain radiating to the legs, especially when associated with an irresistible urge to move the legs. Diazepam is a very potent sedative with drug dependency concerns. This can be helpful in a back pain flare-up situation that is associated with anxiety.

Tramadol is a painkiller that mimics to a mild extent some of the properties of an antidepressant and a narcotic. This drug is often used to help with pain, prior to going onto a stronger narcotic pain killer. Caution should be used with the use of tramadol and certain muscle relaxants, such as cyclobenzaprine. There is a concern about seizures.

Opioids are commonly used for pain control. They are considered to be scalable, which means they do not have a ceiling effect. A variety of opioids are available. Some are short acting and some are long acting. They may be delivered by mouth, by vein, or by absorption through the skin. Chemists have formulated different versions of opioids, but they act in very similar ways. They are potent and are used very commonly in surgery. They can cause constipation, itching, sleepiness, confusion, and euphoria. The latter reason is why they are abused and sought by patients not in pain. They will cause physical and psychological dependence. Addiction is uncommon in appropriately selected patients. Recent evidence points to a paradoxical phenomenon. Historically, opioids have been known to cause tolerance—wherein the same drug dose leads to a reduced effect. These patients need a higher dose. The paradox is that opioids may worsen the pain state (hyperalgesia), and this heightened pain state requires more opioids. The use of high-dose opioids has been advocated by some. More recent research suggests that this may not improve function and pain. Many patients are known to hoard medications, and some may divert the medications. Since opioid abuse and diversion (selling the pills for profit) are major public health and law enforcement concerns, the prescribing of these drugs is heavily regulated.

The use of these opioid drugs for long-term pain control and functional improvement is mired in controversy. Since pain can only be measured by the patient's own report, a doctor has to rely on surrogate actions to determine if a patient is "legitimate." This may include urine drug screens, written agreements, use of one pharmacy, use of one physician, pill counts, and strict controls on when a patient can refill medications. Although there is literature supporting the role of opioids in chronic low back pain, there is literature contesting this. Recent research suggests that the benefit of long-term opioids for chronic low back pain remains questionable. The American Society of Interventional Pain Physicians published guidelines in 2008 regarding opioids for non-cancer pain. They concluded the evidence was limited. What about the day-to-day practice? Many physicians are reluctant to prescribe opioids and feel pressured by chronic pain patients to write them. A chronic low back pain patient may experience these challenges. Ultimately, the physician must work closely with the patient to set goals, monitor functional improvement, and set controls, such as a drug screen. The patient has responsibilities, as well, to safeguard these drugs and use them appropriately.

Physical Therapy

Physical therapy can be passive or active. Passive physical therapy uses heat, cold, massage, electrical stimulation, or ultrasound. This is passive because the patient doesn't have to do much. These therapies can provide temporary pain relief, but not long-term relief.

Active physical therapy typically includes exercise. Exercise for weight loss, or body core muscle strengthening, may be helpful. Physical therapy focuses on functional rehabilitation. Physical therapy attempts to get the patient back on track—this is an important paradigm shift. Many physicians are quick to advise rest and to allow a patient's pain to determine what that patient can do. Physical therapy focuses on promoting normal activity. Physical therapy focuses on muscle reconditioning, movement, range of motion, strengthening, and stretching. Other goals include improving posture, manipulation, traction, biofeedback, electrical stimulation, heat, cold, and return to work. Some physical therapists specialize in manual medicine and McKenzie exercises. They may set up a special program individualized to a patient's needs. If one has a herniated disc in the low back that is pinching the nerve, the McKenzie therapist may use certain "extension" exercises. The goal is to get the pain away from the leg and to centralize it to the back. These therapists envision that they are coaxing the disc to relocate itself—this is ultimately speculation, but McKenzie exercises can be helpful. In simplistic terms, the goal of acute low back pain physical therapy is to reduce pain, and the passive approach dominates. An active, exercise-based approach is rolled out after the pain subsides. Chronic low back pain focuses on active exercises and personal strategies to help the patient cope with pain. This therapy seeks to maintain function and improve pain coping.

Acupuncture

Acupuncture and dry needling play an important role in chronic low back pain. Although the studies have not been of the highest quality, acupuncture and dry needling may be helpful in the short term. Dry needling may be just as effective as acupuncture. The scientific "gate theory of pain" may be a better model than "holistic or ancient" theories to explain the pain relief with acupuncture, or for that matter, acupressure. The gate theory is a classic theory about why patients get pain relief. When non-painful (touch) or weakly painful (acupuncture needle) stimuli flood the nervous system, a "gate" is activated. This gate then blocks the pain signal. We invoke this "gate" instinctively. We drink lots of water after eating something very spicy; we dip our hands in cold water following a burn; and we lick paper cuts to reduce pain. There are a number of holistic theories about acupuncture, but no one really knows why this works. Small needles are placed over painful parts of the low back. Many licensed acupuncturists will place them in particular locations. Some will hook up the needles to an electric current to help with the pain. There are some risks associated with needling, and relief is short-lived. Many acupuncturists advocate repeated treatments. A patient should know if acupuncture helps within one or two treatments; it is not necessary to have multiple sessions to figure out if this treatment is right for you. If the treatment does work, then the relief may be short-lived. In this scenario, the patient may need multiple treatments. Like other therapies for chronic pain, acupuncture cannot cure the "pain"—if your pain is cured, then your body should get the credit!

Alternative Therapies

Spinal manipulation and chiropractic care play an important role in the management of low back pain. The purpose is to mobilize the spine to its maximal range of motion. Usually this is performed by a chiropractor or osteopath. The literature is controversial. Many studies have failed to demonstrate any improvement in pain, over conservative care. Spinal manipulation is helpful in an acute episode of low back pain. Chiropractors may be of benefit to some patients with chronic low back pain. In spite of the studies, we all instinctively "crack" or "snap" our backs.

Holistic approaches are numerous. They include acupuncture, nutritional counseling, stress management, yoga, meditation, chiropractic adjustment, vitamin therapy, and magnets. Many patients seek these treatments out due to their frustration with the poor outcomes of conventional medical care. Some specialists contend that this is just a placebo—but, this may not be reassuring to a patient who has undergone multiple, perhaps unnecessary surgery. Clearly, many patients are willing to seek these holistic providers. A physician should be sympathetic and help patients research these therapies. Patients should understand the safety, cost, and research associated with therapy. Patients should understand their expectations with holistic care.

One important consideration is that holistic care evolved outside of traditional medicine and traditional insurance markets. Patients clearly exercised a choice. They voluntarily spent their own money, their own time, and their trust to seek holistic care. Holistic care has been admonished by traditional medical providers and not financially supported by health insurers. In a sense, holistic care represents the original form of "consumer driven" health care. The longevity and robustness of holistic care in the USA suggest that these forms of therapy have survived due to patient satisfaction and some positive outcomes. The other reason is that patients are clearly frustrated with traditional medical care in the treatment of chronic low back pain. Hopefully, a competing scientific framework can be used to study this problem, instead of just traditional evidence-based medicine. Behavioral economics is an emerging field in economics that may impact medicine. This field may help physicians and patients make better informed decisions, by actually determining why patients make specific choices in health care. The rise of holistic care in chronic low back pain indicates that physicians must do a better job in delivering traditional health care and in improving outcomes. Providers of holistic care, likewise, have an ethical responsibility in providing informed consent, which discusses risks, benefits, and alternatives. Holistic providers must be willing to discuss the evidence for their treatments, as doctors are obligated to discuss the evidence for traditional medicine. A patient must seek this information.

Biofeedback

A special noninvasive technique, known as biofeedback, may help reduce pain. This requires special equipment and supervision. Patches are placed on your body, over the painful area. The muscle tension is measured. The patient must slowly work toward reducing the tension. They will look at an animation on a computer screen; this animation may be a game, with the goal of reducing muscle tension. The person wins the game by reducing muscle tension. This is a "mind-over-body" control method. Sensors are placed over the muscle of interest. Respiration and heart rate may be monitored. The patient is asked to concentrate on reducing the spasm, heart rate, and respiratory rate. Biofeedback has the added bonus of helping the patient concentrate on something besides their pain.

Patient Education

Patient education is important. Education about a home exercise program, proper ways of lifting objects, and improving self-confidence are goals. Patients are educated on maintaining their heart fitness, stopping smoking, eating right, and participating in their communities.

Interventional and Minimally Invasive Treatment Options

These are discussed in the next chapter.

Surgical Options

Surgery for low back pain has increased in utilization. There have been major improvements in the technology and surgical approaches. Surgery is becoming less invasive, and the focus is shifting toward preserving motion. Unfortunately, the outcomes are still mixed—particularly for chronic low back pain. Surgery often has good outcomes for well-defined pain syndromes, but these are rarer than nonspecific low back pain. These include fractures (broken backbone), ruptured or herniated discs (torn shock absorbers in the spine), advanced spinal stenosis (crowding of the soft nerves by hard bone spurs, ligaments, and discs). Even when the diagnosis is clear, the results may be questionable. There continues to be an epidemic of patients with failed back surgery syndrome. Many of these patients find themselves returning back to pain specialists. Surgeries can fail, even with perfect technique. Although pain treatment can fail as well, these treatments are reversible and the patient can walk away. The patient can pursue other treatments—they have not "burned bridges" with conservative care. Surgery, on the other hand, is irreversible. There is no doubt surgery has helped countless patients in pain and mobility, but there are many patients who didn't get better. The patient should carefully weigh the pluses and minuses about surgery. The patient should seek multiple opinions, if necessary.

Prognosis

Acute back pain episodes often resolve and are self-limited. Chronic low back pain usually does not go away. The lack of a cure is frustrating for patients and physicians alike. Many patients may undergo multiple therapies and take multiple medications. These patients may never fully recover. The lack of a cure is part of the reason many patients seek care from a pain management specialist. A pain management specialist recognizes that chronic pain is not curable and will require long-term treatment. There is a growing acknowledgement that chronic pain may not be a symptom, but a disease of the nervous system. There are many chronic diseases, such as diabetes, which are not curable and require long-term treatment. This chronic disease model is important in shifting the focus from cure to pain control. Patients may not want to hear this in the beginning, but over time, they will come to terms with this truth.

One of the most frustrating aspects of pain is the inability to answer "Why did I get chronic low back pain?" or "Why doesn't it go away?" In our opinion, the root cause of chronic pain may be answered by looking into our deep past. Evolutionary medicine is a nascent field that may help explain why pain occurs. Chronic pain is so common that it defies logic as a treatable disease. Chronic pain is incredibly complex and has many redundant pathways to keep the pain alive. I have always been amazed that a small quarter-inch tear in our discs (shock absorbers) could cause so much disability and pain. As we transitioned to an upright species, nature couldn't go back to the drawing board and create a new disc. We essentially have the same types of discs that our four-legged or horizontal ancestors had a long time ago. Upon becoming upright, the forces across the disc have increased compared to our "horizontal" ancestors. Industrialization of society (with constant repetitive motion and heavy lifting), reduced autonomy to self-regulate how hard you could work, prolonged life expectancy, smoking, and obesity may have contributed to the accelerated wear of our discs. Consequently, people feel pain and become progressively disabled. Chronic low back pain patients are apt to forget that we have the ability to stand upright and live long lives. Chronic low back pain is an unfortunate price to pay.

Another speculation is that our bodies have these chronic pain alarm systems to protect us. These protective mechanisms smother us, instead of helping. Imagine if the airport was on high security every day or if mandatory curfews were enacted. In chronic pain, these nerve pathways are on high alert and "want" to put your body on curfew. If you don't stop and slow down, the pain will get worse and harder to stop. This is speculation, but is a good model for patients to understand that they have some control of their pain.

ADDITIONAL RESOURCES

American Academy of Orthopaedic Surgeons: http://orthoinfo.aaos.org/topic.cfm
　　?topic=a00311
e-MedicineHealth: http://www.emedicinehealth.com/back_pain/article_em.htm
National Institute of Neurologic Disorders and Stroke: http://www.ninds.nih.gov/disorders/
　　backpain/detail_backpain.htm

16

Arm, Leg, and Phantom Limb Pain

Jung H. Kim, MD, and Tamer Elbaz, MD

In this chapter, the common injuries and disorders that cause pain in the arms and legs are presented, including phantom limb pain.

Arm Pain

Elbow

- *Tennis Elbow:* The medical term for tennis elbow is "lateral epicondylitis" (inflammation of the lateral epicondyle or the outer part of the arm bone). It is actually a misnomer because it is a degenerative process rather than an inflammatory one as the word epicondylitis indicates. Pain is caused by degenerative changes that occur in the tendons of the forearm muscles that extend to the wrist. Overuse of these muscles can cause very small tears in the tendons of these muscles at the outer side (away from the body) of the elbow.

  It is more commonly seen in males between the ages of 40 and 50 years, and caused by frequent use during activities that require wrist extension, such as the backhand stroke in tennis. The presence of this condition is not limited to tennis players; it is also commonly seen in housekeepers (repeated sweeping motion), assembly line workers, typewriters, and bowlers.

  Pain is the main presentation of this condition. The pain is located at the outer side of the elbow, but often spreads down to the forearm and rarely to the wrist. Pain could limit everyday physical activities from gripping, shaking hands, or even turning a doorknob. Results of x-rays are generally normal in this condition, and the diagnosis is made by a physician using medical history and physical examination.

Initial treatment includes anti-inflammatory medications such as ibuprofen and naproxen. It is very important to limit or, better yet, discontinue the activity that caused tennis elbow. If pain does not improve, steroid injection into the elbow can be helpful. These injections have the potential to weaken the tendons and cause them to rupture. If conservative treatment options fail, surgery to repair the damaged tendon may be considered.

- *Golfer's Elbow:* The medical term for golfer's elbow is "medial epicondylitis." Again, it is caused by degenerative changes such as micro (very small) tears of tendons located on the inner side of the elbow, not a true inflammatory reaction. Repeated motions of wrist flexion and internal rotation of the wrist may cause this painful condition, and the occurrence is three to seven times less frequent than tennis elbow.

Pain occurs gradually. Common symptoms include pain during flexing the wrist against resistance or making a tight fist, as well as handgrip weakness. X-rays are often normal, but unlike tennis elbow, calcium deposits can be seen on the inside of the elbow.

Treatment starts with discontinuation of aggravating activities. For pain control, anti-inflammatory medications are useful. If pain persists, corticosteroid injections can be used at a cost of further weakening the tendon and increasing the risk of rupture.

Wrist and Hand

- *De Quervain's Tenosynovitis:* It is named after the Swiss surgeon Fritz de Quervain, who first described the condition in 1895. Shear and micro trauma to the tendons of two muscles, abductor pollicis longus and extensor pollicis brevis are responsible for this degenerative process. These two muscles basically share the same function, which is to move the thumb away from the hand. Therefore, repetitive movements of the thumb in the above-mentioned direction or forceful cocking of the wrist could often cause this syndrome.

Pain is often subtle, and it is located over the outer half of the wrist on the thumb side. Pressure over this area can increase the pain; thus activities such as playing racket sports, golf, or fly fishing may aggravate the pain.

Treatments include anti-inflammatory medications or homemade remedies such as using an ice pack and giving the wrist a rest. A thumb splint is often required as well, but it must be removed several times a day to prevent stiffness and to give gentle rotation of the thumb. Almost always, corticosteroid injections into the area decrease the pain. However, it should be noted that repeated injections could weaken the tendons, which makes them easier to rupture.

- *Carpal Tunnel Syndrome:* Carpal tunnel is a well-defined space surrounded by hard surfaces. One of the hand bones, the scaphoid, forms the wall on the thumb side, while the hamate and the pisiform bones form the wall on the pinky side. The floor is made of carpal (hand) bones and ligaments, and the thick carpal ligament that goes side to side across the wrist forms the roof. This tunnel houses many tendons that control the movement of the fingers and a nerve that transmits movement and sensation to the first three and a half fingers, the median nerve. When this nerve gets compressed within this tight space, a painful condition known as carpal tunnel syndrome occurs. Any process that increases the volume of the carpal tunnel can result in this syndrome. But the most common cause is swelling of the tissue surrounding above-mentioned tendons.

Carpal tunnel syndrome is caused by entrapment of a nerve called the median nerve as it travels over the wrist. It is most commonly seen in middle-aged women, and often associated with medical conditions such as diabetes mellitus, rheumatoid arthritis, kidney failure, and pregnancy.

Carpal tunnel syndrome is characterized by numbness and pain over the distribution of the median nerve (thumb, index, middle, and one-half of the ring finger). Generally, these symptoms tend to be worse at night, sometimes bad enough to disturb sleep. Many patients complain of inability to grab small objects due to weakness of the small muscles of the hand. In a simple case, physicians make the diagnosis based on symptoms and physical examination. However, in more subtle cases, doctors may perform a test called electromyography (EMG) to identify the affected nerve.

If symptoms are present for a short duration, nonsurgical treatments are recommended. An immobilizing cast and anti-inflammatory medications such as ibuprofen can help alleviate the pain. In cases where conservative treatments have failed, doctors may offer surgery to release the pressure.

Hip and Leg Pain

Hip

Besides the disorders of the hip joint itself, a common condition that causes pain in this region is bursitis.

- A bursa is a fluid-filled sac that is positioned between the muscles or between muscles and bones to lubricate movement of different surfaces against each other. Direct injury to the area over the bursa or repetitive micro injury by muscle spasm may result in pain and inflammation. Two major bursas around the hip are discussed below.
  - *Ischial Bursitis:* The ischial bursa is located in the buttock area underneath the gluteus muscle. Direct injury to the area, such as falling on the buttock or prolonged horseback riding or bicycle riding, may cause this painful condition. Sharp and "catching" sensation is felt over the buttock region on top of the ischial bony prominence. Sleeping or sitting on the affected side will increase the pain.
  - *Trochanteric Bursitis:* This bursa is located in the outer hip area between the greater trochanter (outer aspect of upper thigh bone) and the muscles overlying it. Direct fall over this area or repetitive micro injury such as prolonged running on a hard and uneven surface may cause this painful condition. Pain is well localized to the upper outer thigh area and is reproduced by direct pressure; therefore, individuals may not be able to sleep on the affected side. Also, weakness of the affected leg is often reported. Therefore, this condition resembles sciatica, which originates from spinal nerve irritation in the back.

In both conditions, conservative (nonsurgical) treatment begins with relieving weight and pressure over the area and anti-inflammatory medications. In
more severe cases, steroid injections directly into the bursa may alleviate
the pain.

o *Meralgia Paresthetica:* While this painful condition resembles trochanteric bursitis in the way that patients feel pain over the upper outer thigh, the cause and
treatment are very different. Meralgia paresthetica is caused by entrapment of
a small nerve called the lateral femoral cutaneous nerve as it courses over a ligament in the groin. Symptoms often begin with burning sensation over the
outer thigh area with skin sensitivity. Pain worsens when sitting, squatting, or
wearing tight belts because these activities increase the compression of the
nerve.

Diagnosis is made primarily on the basis of physical examination. However,
EMG (electromyography) might be indicated for more complex cases to confirm the diagnosis. Treatment begins with avoiding pressure over the groin
area. Wearing loose clothes and having the leg extended (straight) at the hip
may reduce the pain. Anti-inflammatory and anticonvulsant medications can
be recommended. When these treatments fail, steroid injection around the
inflamed nerve at the level of groin may significantly decrease the pain.

Knee

• *Ligament Tears:* Ligaments are tough, fibrous tissue that connect bones. Func-
tionally, four ligaments hold the knee in stable position, and each one is named
based on its location. The anterior cruciate ligament (ACL) is located in the
front of the knee, the posterior cruciate ligament in the back of the knee, the
medial collateral ligament (MCL) in the inner side, and the lateral collateral ligament (LCL) on the outer side of the knee. The most common injuries to the
knee are to the ACL and MCL. They will both be discussed below.

o ACL: ACL tear is the most devastating injury of the four ligaments. It passes
over the front of the knee as it connects the femur (thigh bone) and the tibia
(shin bone). This injury is often caused by excessive rotation of the knee while
the foot adheres to the ground tightly. A distinct pop can be heard at the time of
initial injury.

Treatment begins with compression of the knee, ice pack, and elevation of
the leg. Because knee instability is great with ACL tear, a patient who is
returning to competitive sports requires surgical repair of the ACL ligament.
For individuals with more sedentary lifestyles (minimal physical activity),
aggressive physical therapy might be enough.

o MCL: This ligament connects the femur and tibia over the inner aspect of the
knee. Injury is often caused by sudden inner force on the knee while the foot
is tightly attached to the ground. For example, for a right knee, a right to left
force on the knee while having the lower leg and foot are immobile can cause
sprain and even rupture of this ligament.

Pain is localized over the inner knee area with tenderness in the same
region. In a more severe case, swelling is apparent. X-ray is often taken to
exclude any bone fractures, but MRI is required to fully assess the ligament.
Initial treatment consists of using ice pack and elevation of the leg to reduce

swelling. A knee immobilizer is sometimes required for one to two weeks to provide stability for the knee. Resolution of pain and regaining of the knee stability takes about four weeks. Surgery is rarely required.

• *Meniscal Tears:* The knee has two menisci (cartilages) that are positioned inside the knee joint, one on the inner side (medial) and one on the outer side (lateral) between the femur (the thigh bone) and the tibia (the leg bone). Their function is to absorb shock, disperse the weight of the body, and decrease friction as one moves the knee. A sudden twisting movement of the knee while standing firm on the ground can cause a tear in one or both cartilages. This is a common cause of knee pain. Pain occurs gradually (a day or two after the injury) and is accompanied by swelling. Sometimes, clicking of the knee is heard, and locking of the knee may occur as well.

Initial treatment can be conservative with the use of anti-inflammatory medications, ice pack and relaxation of the knee. For small tears, resolution of pain can be expected in three to six weeks. However, more complex tears may cause recurrent episodes of swelling and pain, and it might require surgery. Also, athletes who engage in competitive sports might opt for early surgical removal of torn tissue as well. Surgery is usually performed arthroscopically (using a small video scope), and injured meniscal tissue is shaved off.

• *Housemaid's Knee (Prepatellar Bursitis):* This is a common source of knee pain and swelling. This was named after the fact that it is common in individuals whose work requires kneeling for a long time. Therefore, wrestlers, carpet installers, gardeners, and housemaids are prone to develop this painful condition. Swelling and irritation originate in the bursa (a cushion sac filled with fluid) between the skin and the kneecap. Treatment consists of avoiding the activities that might worsen this condition, tight knee brace, ice pack, and anti-inflammatory medications to decrease swelling. In severe cases, steroid injection into the bursa may decrease the pain.

• *Patellofemoral Pain Syndrome:* This is also called "patellofemoral arthralgia." It implies that pain is in the joint between the patella (kneecap) and the femur (thigh bone). It is the most common cause of knee pain in younger population. Although it is generally caused by acute injury to the knee, pain can occur gradually and can worsen over time. This syndrome is often caused by excessive running, falling on the knee, or working on the floor kneeling without wearing knee pads.

With repetitive bending of the leg at the knee, thigh muscles can cause patella to move upward, downward, and sideways. Usually, the patella is kept in the normal position by equal opposing force, but pain is caused by abnormal movement of the knee cap due to excessive force to one direction or loss of the opposing force.

Pain is present under the kneecap, and it increases with knee movements or applying pressure over the area. The mainstay of treatment is anti-inflammatory medications such as ibuprofen or naproxen. If the syndrome occurred due to excessive running, it is wise to substitute the exercises for swimming. A knee brace for support and muscle balancing may be helpful as well. In severe cases where the above treatments have failed, trials of steroid injection, acupuncture, or arthroscopic knee surgery might be necessary.

Phantom Limb Pain Syndrome

Phantom limb pain is any painful sensation arising from a missing limb or body part. Ambroise Paré, a French surgeon, first documented phantom limb pain in the 1500s. Since then, many advances have been made in the understanding of this rare medical condition. However, many patients still suffer from its disabling consequences. Phantom pain has been described in cases of missing (amputated) limbs, digits, eyes, nose, teeth, breasts, anus, and genital organs.

Phantom pain must be differentiated from phantom sensation. Phantom sensation is any sensation other than the pain that the patient feels in the distribution of a missing body part. Almost all amputees experience phantom sensation, which generally does not lead to severe problems. These non-painful sensations are interpreted as movements, perceptions of touch, pressure, temperature, itching, and vibration. Also, if internal organs such as the rectum or bladder are missing, patients may report the urge to defecate or to urinate—normal processes that would occur if those organs were still present in the body.

In contrast, phantom pain is described as burning, shocking, shooting, or sharp pain. Also, many patients may feel that their missing arm is twisted or pulled in a wrong direction. They perceive the pain as if an actual arm were positioned in that direction. The importance of differentiation between phantom pain and phantom sensation lies in that painful and non-painful sensations may coincide in the same body part.

Although it is believed that phantom pain is underreported, arm or leg amputees do experience phantom pain the most. Pain usually occurs immediately, though it can occur up to 30 years later. One in 10 women who have their breasts removed experience phantom pain. More than half of children have reported phantom pain, although none of it was described as severe in nature.

Phantom pain usually comes and goes. Emotional stress or injury to another part of the body may trigger phantom pain. Other factors that can provoke phantom pain are weather changes, touching of the stump, and anxiety. Generally, the level of pain and number of attacks will decrease over time.

The human nervous system can be broken down into three groups: the brain, the spinal cord, and the peripheral nerves (any nerve fibers and endings that extend to and from the spinal cord). Traditionally, it was believed that phantom limb pain was due to overactivity of the peripheral nerve endings at the site of amputation. "Neuroma formation," which basically refers to overgrowth of nerve endings, was blamed for pain initiation. However, it is now known that phantom pain is more complex, and it involves all three parts of the nervous system. Development of new connections from peripheral nerves to the brain may start and maintain phantom pain.

It is not surprising that loss of body parts may cause a strong grief reaction, and this psychological distress often manifests as depression. The greater the loss of function due to amputation, the greater the level of interference of daily

activities, and the greater the level of anxiety. Combined with the common soci-
etal belief that phantom pain is just in their heads, psychological stress to
patients who suffer from phantom pain can be extreme. Therefore, it is important for patients to have a strong support group that can provide physical and
mental assistance.

Treatments include pharmacologic (using medications) and non-
pharmacologic options. While various medications have been given to these
patients, none has been found to be universally effective. Different classes of
medications include but are not limited to opiates, anticonvulsants, and antidepressants. The most widely used opiate is morphine. Other medications in this
class are hydrocodone (Vicodin), oxycodone (Oxycontin), hydromorphone
(Dilaudid), fentanyl, and methadone. The mechanism of action of these medications is the same. They stimulate receptors called opioid receptors. These receptors work by reducing the transmission of pain signal. Because all patients
respond differently, various doses and combinations must be tailored to each
patient. All opiates have the potential to cause significant side effects, which
include nausea, sedation, drowsiness, distraction, lack of concentration, and
constipation. These side effects can affect daily functions, and this limits the
amount of medication that can be taken. It is important that patients are closely
watched and followed by physicians who have good knowledge of the effects of
these medications. Anticonvulsants are types of medications that are typically
used to treat patients with seizure. However, for a long time, these medications
were also used to treat pain associated with nerve damage, such as phantom
limb pain. The most widely prescribed anticonvulsant for pain is gabapentin,
and this medicine is shown to be effective for phantom pain.

For non-pharmacologic treatments, transcutaneous electrical nerve stimulation (TENS) units have been used with moderate success. This device is placed
on the affected area of the skin, and then electrical stimulation is generated to
create vibratory sensation. The main advantage of this unit is the absence of
serious side effects and complications. Recently, visual stimulation by means
of a mirror box has been tried with limited success. While no one treatment
modality is fully effective, in order to control the pain for most patients, various
combinations of pharmacologic and non-pharmacologic modalities must be
employed at the same time. Despite the best efforts, many individuals continue
to have significant pain. Further research is currently taking place to better
understand this complex condition, and it is expected to improve the treatment
in the future.

17

GYNECOLOGICAL, PELVIC, AND UROLOGICAL PAIN

Rinoo V. Shah, MD, MBA, and Alan D. Kaye, MD, PhD

INTRODUCTION

Pelvic pain typically refers to pain located in the organs responsible for sex, urination, and defecation. Although the location overlaps with the low back, pelvic pain is not considered to originate from the spine. These patients do not typically see spine or musculoskeletal specialists. They often see gynecologists, urologists, or general surgeons.

Chronic pelvic pain, unlike acute pain, may develop over several months and persist indefinitely. In acute pelvic pain, a specific cause can be identified, such as infection, bleeding, twisting of an organ, or rupture. Chronic pelvic pain may not have a specific cause and carries many synonyms: endometriosis, painful bladder (cystitis), painful vagina (vulvodynia), painful sex (dyspareunia), pelvic congestion, internal scars (pelvic scars), muscle pain (myofascial pain), and nerve injury (neuropathy). Even though there are many names, the underlying causes of these pain syndromes remain a mystery. Unfortunately, these labels bring to memory the story of the five blind men evaluating an elephant; none of them could identify the elephant. Similarly, these labels do not provide greater insight into the cause and treatment of pelvic pain. This can be very frustrating for the patient with pelvic pain.

The risk for developing chronic pelvic pain is 5 out of 100 women. If a woman has a chronic inflammation, such as pelvic inflammatory disease (PID), then the risk rises to 20 out of 100. Many of these patients may undergo surgical treatment before seeing a pain specialist. Men can develop pelvic pain, but this is less frequent when compared to women.

The specific types of pelvic pain surgery include a minimally invasive camera to look into a pelvic cavity (laparoscopy), cauterizing and destroying scar tissue, removal of the uterus, or a selective destruction of vessels leading to the uterus. During laparoscopy, adhesions, endometriosis, fibroids, or no specific pathology may be identified. These findings may be found in patients without pain. Nonetheless, many of these treatments fail, and pain often recurs despite complete removal of the uterus.

A pain specialist may use a different approach in classifying pain: inside (visceral), outside (somatic), musculoskeletal, urinary, or spinal. A pain specialist usually sees patients after they are referred by their gynecologists, urologists, or surgeons.

SYMPTOMS

The doctor may take a medical history to figure out the problem. Chronic pelvic pain is evaluated, first and foremost, by telling a story—the patient's story. The doctor may also use guided questions: "Where is your pain?" "What does it feel like—sharp, stabbing, shooting, twisting, burning?" "On a scale from 0 to 10, with 0 representing no pain and 10 representing the worst pain possible, what is your pain?" "Does the pain go anywhere, such as down to your buttock or leg?" "Is the pain worse with sitting, bending, or walking?" or, "Do you have any numbness in your groin, leaking of urine, or soiling of your underwear?" There may be questions about the pattern of pain, how it started, constant versus periodic pain, the duration of each episode, alleviating factors, and worsening factors. The doctor may inquire about sexual activity, bowel and bladder habits, weight changes, prior surgeries, hormonal changes, prior medications, and pregnancy.

Some types of symptoms may help a doctor decide on the type of pain. Visceral pain is a pain in the softer internal organs. The pain is often hard to describe, difficult to locate, and may be associated with cramping and burning pain. Unlike pain from a cut, which is easy to locate with eyes closed, visceral pain affects a general but deep area in the body. Patients may experience cramping due to stretching of some of the hollow organs. Patients may also have spasms in the muscles around the pelvis. Deep visceral pain can cause a reflex that makes the muscles go into spasm.

DIAGNOSIS

The diagnosis starts with the history. There are some specific conditions that the doctor may wish to consider. Endometriosis is a condition wherein uterine tissue is located outside the uterus. This tissue is active and responds to menstrual cycles and hormonal changes. Patients are of childbearing age and the pain cycles throughout the month. Chronic infection and inflammation of the uterus can lead to pain and infertility. A recent intrauterine procedure, fetal demise, or delivery of a child may be predisposing factors. Multiple sexual partners, use of an intrauterine device (used to prevent pregnancy), and sex with a person infected with a sexually transmitted disease are additional risk factors. Pain is located in the front of the body and in the lower part of the pelvis (suprapubic). The cramping pain may be associated with a low-grade fever, bleeding, urinary urgency, and discharge. Patients may have pain during sex, urination, bowel movements, and gynecological or urological evaluations. Menstrual cycle pain is very prevalent in most women of childbearing age. Sometimes a specific cause, such as a fibroid or intrauterine device, can be pinpointed. Fibroids typically present in patients in their 30s and 40s.

Pelvic congestion is a specific cause of pain attributed to "varicose veins" of the uterus and ovaries. Not unlike varicose veins in the legs, the symptoms of pain worsen with standing. Pelvic adhesions (internal abdominal contents stuck onto each other), especially in patients with prior gynecological surgery, may cause pain. These diagnoses are controversial. Since the physical exam and patient's history cannot distinguish these conditions, additional tests are often needed.

Cancer pain can be due to the direct effects of the tumor on local pelvic structures. This type of pain is unrelenting and devastating. Patients often cannot find relief from this type of pain. This pain may be cramping or burning, and may radiate to other parts of the pelvis.

Men can suffer pain from chronic inflammation or infections of the prostate. A number of terms are used: prostadynia and prostatitis. The urology community has developed a classification system to help diagnose the type of prostatitis. There is a subset of patients who develop chronic pain, but do not have any signs of infection. This is known as chronic nonbacterial prostatitis or prostadynia. Symptoms include pain between the rectum and testicles, pain below the waist, and pain in the penis. The pain can extend to the groin or low back. Patients may complain of urinary symptoms: having to run to the bathroom; frequent trips to the bathroom; and urination characterized by stops and starts. These symptoms have to last more than three months in order to be considered chronic. The exam is typically remarkable for pain during a prostate exam and "touch-me-not pain" (allodynia) along the external genitalia. The prostate may be normal in size or enlarged. The consistency may be uniform and soft.

There are certain musculoskeletal chronic pelvic pain syndromes. Piriformis syndrome refers to a spasm involving a muscle in the buttock—pain may spread down the thigh. Levator ani syndrome refers to pain around the anus, due to a muscle sling that is in spasm. Coccygodynia refers to chronic tailbone pain, with or without a broken tailbone. There are some soft tissue chronic pelvic pain syndromes, typically found in women. These have a strong association with sexual, spousal, or physical abuse. They can cause significant pain during sexual, bowel, and bladder activities. Vulvodynia, pain of the vagina, is one such entity.

Interstitial cystitis is a chronic pelvic pain syndrome that has been heavily studied. This problem has the duality of causing chronic pain and urinary problems. The pain occurs in the pelvis. Patients often have deep and burning pain. They may wake up at night to go to the bathroom and have to make frequent visits to the bathroom. Patients may suffer from poor sleep, abdominal cramps, numbness in the toes and buttocks, nausea, heart pounding, body aches, sweating, and various other body symptoms.

The doctor may be thinking about these conditions when asking specific questions. Doctors are trained to create a differential diagnosis. This is essentially a thought experiment enabling the physician to think about many likely possibilities that could be causing pain. The physician will then attempt to validate and refute these based on your examination. When a few possibilities are left, the doctor will order more tests to figure out which is likely. The physician, based on training, specialty, and experience, will sort through these possibilities in his or her own unique style. This differential diagnosis approach is unique to a medical school or osteopathic school education—it forces doctors to constantly challenge his or her opinions and conclusions. This approach can frustrate patients, since it can be very methodical, cautious, and sometimes slow. This scientifically based approach attempts to reduce speculation and places checks and balances on a doctor.

The doctor may conduct a physical exam; a patient may ask for a chaperone. The physician will ask the patient to point to the area of pain. A range-of-motion assessment of the hip and buttock bones (sacroiliac joint) may be conducted. The doctor may palpate certain areas to pinpoint the area of pain. Is there tenderness over the sacroiliac joint (sacroiliac pain), pubic bone (symphysis pubis osteitis), or tailbone (coccygodynia)? Is there tenderness over some of the muscles in the pelvic floor or buttock (piriformis syndrome, levator ani syndrome)? Is there an altered sensation over the groin region, suggesting a nerve entrapment (ilioinguinal neuralgia)? Are there scars, and are these tender (neuroma)? Is there tenderness over sitting part of the buttock (bursitis)? Does tapping the skin evoke an electrical sensation to the area underneath and between the legs (pudendal neuralgia)? A rectal exam may reveal a painful prostate (prostadynia), be able to assess continence, and detect a tumor. A pelvic exam is usually performed by a gynecologist or family physician. The exam typically consists of several parts: visual inspection, a bimanual exam, and use of a speculum. The bimanual exam involves placing two fingers into the vagina and using the other hand to press down on the outer part of the lower abdomen. This bimanual exam is used to feel for abnormalities, to evaluate the shape and mobility of the uterus, and to evaluate pain.

The doctor may perform blood work and a urine sample analysis. For prostadynia and interstitial cystitis, urine cultures and urine cell analysis may be ordered. This is to look for abnormal cells and bacteria. Imaging studies such as an ultrasound or a CT scan may be needed. An ultrasound uses high-frequency sound waves and captures an image based on the echoes. This test does not use radiation and is used during pregnancy. The ultrasound may detect fluid collections, tumors, and abscesses. The ultrasound is performed by placing a lubricating jelly on the abdomen and using a noninvasive probe. This test can look for specific causes of pelvic pain such as fibroids, cysts, and cancer. A special probe may be inserted inside the vagina for a more detailed analysis of the lining and muscles of the uterus. Specific painful conditions include scarring, polyps, tumors, fibroids, and cancer. In men, the ultrasound can evaluate the prostate. In both men and women, the ultrasound can evaluate the kidney and bladder. A urologist may study the flow of urine in patients with interstitial cystitis and prostadynia with a urodynamic study.

A CT scan is a special test that can "look" inside the body and is noninvasive. CT scans can be done fairly quickly. CT scanning uses X-rays and computers to make detailed pictures inside the body. This study is fundamentally an anatomic study: "Is the architecture of the body normal or abnormal?" Many doctors can look at the CT scan and an official radiology report to explain the findings to the patient. The patient can point to the pain, and the doctor can scroll to that exact location. This detailed analysis can look for an infection (appendicitis, kidney infection), cancer, kidney and bladder stones, fluid collections, postsurgical changes, fibroids, blood clots, hernias, and muscle bleeds. The test is fairly versatile and can be performed in a hospital or outpatient facility.

Gynecologists may be able to perform a "look-and-see procedure," such as a laparoscopy. Under general anesthesia, a small incision is made under the belly button. A small videoscope (like a flexible telescope) is inserted. The doctor is able to see the internal organs, such as the uterus and ovaries. Endometriosis, pelvic infections, ovarian cysts, adhesions, and scar tissue can be identified. The laparoscope can also evaluate the gastrointestinal organs, such as the gallbladder and appendix. Unique to this diagnostic tool is the ability to treat the problem, while looking. Adhesions, cysts, and endometriotic tissue can be removed. Fibroids can be removed at times, as well. One caveat is that adhesions may not cause pain and there is a risk of overreaching; a tendency for the doctor and patient to blame adhesions for chronic pelvic pain. Hysteroscopy involves placing a flexible telescope inside the uterus and looking for polyps, fibroids, or other intrauterine abnormalities. These invasive approaches have an advantage in obtaining tissue for further analysis. The disadvantages are the risks with any surgical procedure, including pain, bleeding, infection, and damage to internal organs.

Urologists use a similar look-and-see-type procedure: cystoscopy. Usually, cystoscopy is not used for prostadynia unless the urologist suspects another cause of pain. Cystoscopy is often used to evaluate interstitial cystitis.

TREATMENT

There are a variety of treatments for chronic pelvic pain. The fundamental challenge for the doctor will depend on the diagnosis. Gynecologists can employ a variety of drug or surgical strategies to control pain if there is a specific cause.

Laparoscopy can be used to cauterize scar tissue for pelvic adhesion pain. A pelvic infection may be treated with antibiotics. Endometriosis may be treated by manipulating the hormones involved. Certain drugs can be utilized, including some birth control pills to reduce the influence of a hormone-estrogen. Surgery to remove the endometrial tissue with heating-type devices or lasers may be used. Some patients may opt for a hysterectomy or nerve ablation (pre-sacral neurectomy). Fibroids may be treated with selective removal of the fibroid, removal of the uterus, or sometimes, by blocking the blood supply to shrink the fibroid. Cancer requires a multipronged approach that may involve surgery and cancer drug therapy (chemotherapy). Gynecologists have access to less invasive surgical approaches and should be contacted for specific conditions. Interstitial cystitis may be treated by "washing out the bladder" with a special solution. DMSO is a solvent that may have anti-inflammatory and pain-relieving abilities. Other agents to wash out the bladder include steroids, a blood thinner (heparin), and bicarbonate. Interstitial cystitis may be treated by filling up the bladder under mild and sustained pressure. A number of surgical approaches exist for interstitial cystitis and prostadynia.

Often, chronic pelvic pain has no specific cause, and surgery may compound the problem. The challenge is that these patients must continue to seek regular gynecological care—the pain, however, requires a different approach. A team of providers may be involved. A psychologist may provide counseling. A special type of therapy, cognitive behavioral therapy, is often used. This focuses on modifying a patient's behavior, reducing pain fears and frustrations, enhancing coping skills, and reframing one's attitudes and beliefs about pain. Chronic pelvic pain patients may learn to fixate on the negative aspects of their pain. Conditioning and coaching can be used to shape "well" behaviors, so that patients can increase their endurance and activity level. Family members may be encouraged to motivate a patient and to avoid expressing concern every time the patient hurts. Relaxation can be used to manage stress and overreaction to pain, as can deep breathing, looking at peaceful vistas or pictures, and tensing/relaxing specific muscle groups. The psychologist may look into family life and prior youth. Problems in general life may affect response to pain treatment.

A special noninvasive technique, known as biofeedback, may help reduce pain. It is discussed in detail in Chapter 8.

Hypnosis aims to put a patient into a hypnotic state. The patient is awake and focused, but unaware of the surroundings and is open to suggestion. The hypnotist attempts to maintain this state. This may provide a degree of self-relaxation. Many chronic pelvic pain patients may benefit from psychological interventions, especially if they have depression and anxiety.

Physical therapy may be used to recondition the muscles in the pelvic floor. Different pain relieving techniques such as heat or a transcutaneous electrical nerve stimulator (TENS) unit may be used. There are physical therapists specializing in pelvic pain. Some believe that the techniques used in back pain can be applied to pelvic pain. They may attempt to locate the pelvic floor muscles and their insertion points. There may be specific areas that are very painful, known as trigger points. The medical community continues to debate the existence and relevance of these trigger points. Therapists may use directed pressure or massage to alleviate the muscle pain. Patients may be educated to voluntarily contract, hold, and release these muscles. This is known as an isometric contraction, because the muscle is contracting and no joints are moving. Physical therapists may use a cooling agent to spray the muscle and stretch it. There are other techniques that involve mobilizing the muscles, deep tissues, and skin: skin rolling, myofascial release, and massage. Due to the location of pelvic pain, clearly this may be beyond the comfort zone of the patient and therapist. Patients should not be ashamed to voice their concerns if this type of physical therapy seems inappropriate. Nonetheless, the physical therapists have increased the awareness that pelvic pain may originate from the muscles and not just the deep internal organs.

Holistic approaches are numerous. They include acupuncture, nutritional counseling, stress management, yoga, meditation, chiropractic adjustment, vitamin therapy, and magnets. Many patients seek these treatments, partly due to their frustration with the poor outcomes of conventional medical care. Some specialists contend that this is just a placebo, but this may not be reassuring to a patient who has undergone multiple, perhaps unnecessary surgeries. Clearly, many patients are willing to seek these holistic providers. A physician should be sympathetic and help patients research these therapies. Patients should understand the safety, cost, and research associated with therapy. Patients should understand their expectations with holistic care.

Medications for chronic pelvic pain control are not unique to just pelvic pain. A gynecologist may advise specific hormonal therapies to manage specific gynecological symptoms. An oncologist may advise specific anticancer therapies. A pain specialist, however, will use an array of different drug classes to help manage pain. For better or worse, pain physicians generally hold a view that drugs from different classes will help target different pathways in pain. An anti-inflammatory drug, such as ibuprofen or etodolac, may be used with inflammation. An antiseizure drug may be used to treat nerve pain. Many of these drugs are used in an "off-label" fashion by physicians to help with pain. Gabapentin, carbamazepine, and lamotrigine are used as antiseizure medications. These can be used to treat severe nerve pain in the pelvis. Muscle relaxants such as cyclobenzaprine, methocarbamol, and baclofen may be used to promote muscle relaxation, either directly or indirectly. Older antidepressants such as amitryptiline and nortriptyline (not to be confused with gabapentin) may be used. Newer agents, such as duloxetine, are used to treat depression and neuropathic pain. Some sedative agents, such as clonazepam, are used to treat nerve disorders. In some cases with very severe pain and disability, certain narcotic agents can be used. This is a controversial area, since there is a risk of drug dependency, addiction, and in some cases, drug diversion for profit.

A number of medications, not actually considered pain medications, are used by gynecologists and urologists. These underscore the complexity of chronic pelvic pain. In cases of pelvic pain due to bladder inflammation, immune system–weakening drugs, blood pressure–lowering drugs, antibiotics, steroids, hormones, vitamins, antihistamines such as diphenhydramine (Benadryl), and even stomach acid–lowering drugs can be used. These require close follow-up with a dedicated specialist.

An interventional pain management specialist may use different procedures to figure out the cause of the pain. Many of these pain specialists utilize an "algorithm." The procedure is used to find the pain generator. Once the pain generator is identified, further treatment is tailored to this pain generator. There are different levels of invasiveness, but all procedures carry risk. The doctor may ask the patient to sign a specialized form informing of the risks, benefits, and alternatives. This form and its development are integral to the practice of medicine and have a long history. The informed consent levels the playing field and empowers the patient. Many of these procedures can be conducted without sedation. However, some patients are very nervous about needles and may request sedation. Sedation can provide comfort during the procedure, but must be conducted in a proper setting. The doctor may use specialized equipment to monitor breathing, heart rate, blood pressure, and alertness. Many doctors will not honor a request to be "out cold" or "completely out." These are relatively short procedures, and verbal feedback from the patient is important for success.

Here are some procedures used by pain specialists for chronic pelvic pain:

1. *Trigger Point Injection*: This involves placing a small needle into a muscle that hurts or is in spasm. The doctor may use a numbing agent, such as lidocaine. The outcome is hard to predict and often short-lived. This can break the pain cycle and is a reasonable alternative to managing a flare-up of pain. There are some deep pelvic floor muscles that can be injected with muscle recordings (EMG) and patient participation (voluntary contraction). The levator ani muscle is a sling that can move the rectum up and down. This muscle may cause severe pelvic pain. The piriformis muscle is in the buttock and can cause pain that can radiate to the thigh. One promising area to target these muscle pains is to use botulinum toxin type A. This is an area of active research.

2. *Nerve Block*: This involves placing a needle next to a nerve that may be responsible for your pain. The doctor may inject a combination of a numbing medication, such as lidocaine, and an anti-inflammatory agent, such as a steroid. There are some nerves that will be targeted depending on the location of the pain. If the pain extends into the groin, the ilioinguinal nerve may be pinpointed. This is a nerve that is injected near the front and outer part of the hip (anterior superior iliac spine); this is near where the lap belt tightens. The iliohypogastric nerve heads toward the belly button. The cluneal nerves are near the buttock. They are in three groups (upper, middle, and lower). The genitofemoral nerve is near the middle part of your groin, just above your private parts. The pudendal nerve is deep, because we sit on it every day—this nerve is important in

providing sensation to the area near the vagina, base of the scrotum, rectum, and bladder opening. A block of this nerve can be performed under x-ray guidance (fluoroscopy), with high-frequency echoes (ultrasound), by feel and palpation, or nerve stimulation. The coccygeal nerve can be blocked near the tailbone. There are some spinal nerves, better known as sacral nerves, which come out of the sacrum (a keystone bone in between your buttocks). Usually, the #3 nerve (S3) can be blocked for pelvic pain, and the #4 nerve (S4) can be blocked for rectal pain. X-ray guidance is necessary to block these nerves. The pain physician may be able to administer a block of some deeper nerves that are involved in deep pain. Another nerve system in our body that acts as an alarm system is the sympathetic nervous system. The sympathetic nerves are located just outside the spine bones, on the left and right. They make a chain and are important in "fight-or-flight" situations or high-alert situations. They can cause pain. They can be blocked at different locations in this chain. The superior hypogastric plexus is part of this chain of sympathetic nerves. This is an important target in the presence of pelvic cancer. Under x-ray guidance, a needle is placed right in front of the transition from the lowest back bone to the sacrum. This may help with deep pelvic pain. Another target is the ganglion impar. The name is intimidating, but refers to the end of the sympathetic chain—the last stop. This is just in front of the tailbone and behind the rectum. The needle is placed through the tailbone joint. This ganglion impar injection can help with rectal or coccyx pain.

3. *Implanted Devices*: A specialized pain pacemaker wire can be advanced through a needle to help with pain. The "lead" is placed under x-ray guidance through the sacrum. This is placed alongside the #3 or #4 sacral nerve. This can be a powerful tool to help with pain. The procedure is conducted, firstly, as a test drive. Unlike surgical procedures, this gives the patient an opportunity to evaluate the effectiveness of the procedure. If the test works, then the leads are implanted with a small incision and hooked up to a small battery—all under the skin. The battery can be recharged. Furthermore, this procedure doesn't interfere with future surgeries. This is important since many of these patients may face laparascopies or cystoscopies.

4. *Internal Drug Delivery Systems*: The literature on this advanced intervention is more robust for cancer pain than for non-cancer pain. A pump is connected to a very soft and durable tube. The tube is inserted into the spinal canal, and the pump is implanted in the abdomen, just under the skin. The pump is not implanted into the body cavity or near internal organs. A potent painkiller, such as morphine, is trickled into the spinal canal. This mixes with the spinal fluid. The spinal cord has special docks (receptors) for the morphine. This can lead to tremendous pain relief, at a fraction of the dose needed by mouth. There may be fewer side effects. As with any surgery, there are risks. Bleeding, infection, pump malfunction, catheter breakage, erosion through the skin, fluid collection around the pump, persistent spinal leak, confusion, sedation, breathing problems, drug programming errors, and drug refill errors have been reported. Patients with these devices, also known colloquially as "intrathecal morphine pumps," must have their pumps refilled with a specialized office procedure. They cannot simply refill the medication at a pharmacy. These patients must closely follow up with their pain physician.

5. *Destructive Procedures*: These procedures use chemicals or heat energy to destroy nerve tissue. They are a desperate attempt to treat someone with devastating cancer pain. A chemical agent can be inserted into the lower part of the spinal canal to kill the sacral nerves, but this will cause permanent incontinence. A chemical can be placed to destroy some of the nerves discussed above. A neurosurgeon can cut the spinal cord near the base of the skull to afford pain relief. These techniques are exceedingly rare and will never be performed on an individual without invasive cancer.

PROGNOSIS

The sobering aspect of chronic pelvic pain is that many patients will continue to have chronic pain. Chronic pelvic pain is difficult to estimate given the population sampled. Many patients may feel uncomfortable discussing this problem and may not seek medical attention. Once the chronic pain develops, the probability of complete remission is remote. Chronic pelvic pain is best thought of in terms of a chronic disease, like diabetes or high blood pressure. These diseases are rarely curable, but can be managed. Effective management requires a multipronged approach: counseling, physical therapy, holistic treatment, medications, nerve blocks, advanced pain procedures, and surgery. The most important aspect in chronic pain involves transforming the patient, so that they can cope with this disease burden.

Early in the course of the disease, the patient may have expectations of a cure. Late in the course, patients may come to terms that this is a chronic disease. Those patients that can keep a positive attitude, understand the role of different pain therapies, and continue to cope will do the best. Navigating the treatment environment for chronic pelvic pain can be very challenging. Patients may feel victimized or, sometimes, stigmatized. This only compounds recovery. Patients that can stay focused, develop adaptive behaviors, cope well, and understand their treatments will do well. Those patients that can engage support groups and engage family, friends, and community will improve. Those that decompensate, catastrophize, panic, and become fearful will do worse. When suffering from pelvic pain, it is important to remain optimistic and hopeful.

18

CHEST PAIN

Zach Nye, DO

INTRODUCTION

Chest pain accounts for 6 million emergency room visits each year, making it the second-most common reason for people to go to the emergency room.

Chest pain may be caused by a variety of health-related issues. There are several structures in the chest that may cause pain, and it is important to determine the cause of chest pain because the treatment varies significantly depending on the structure or disease process involved.

There are two general types of structures in the chest, and they may cause two different types of pain. "Visceral" structures are organs, such as the heart and lungs. Pain in these organs may cause visceral pain, which tends to be dull, harder to localize, and not usually reproduced by touching the outside of the chest. "Somatic," or musculoskeletal structures, are things like the bones, muscles, skin, and ribs that make up the structural components of the chest. Musculoskeletal pain tends to be sharp, more specific, and may be reproduced by touching the outside of the chest.

The main organs in the chest are the heart and lungs, but other organs may also cause pain in the chest, such as the stomach, liver, gallbladder, and esophagus. The musculoskeletal structures in the chest that may cause pain include the ribs, diaphragm, sternum, and skin.

Diseases that may produce pain from the heart include coronary artery disease (narrowing of the arteries in the heart), pericarditis (inflammation of the lining surrounding the heart), aortic dissection (a tearing of the layers of the aorta), or disorders of the valves in the heart, for example aortic stenosis (narrowing of one of the valves in the heart).

Diseases that may produce chest pain from the lungs include pneumonia, pleuritis (inflammation of the lining of the lung), bronchitis (inflammation of the airways going to the lungs), lung cancer, or other systemic diseases such as rheumatoid arthritis, or systemic lupus erythematosis that are autoimmune diseases.

Some diseases may produce chest pain by affecting the lungs as well as the musculoskeletal structures of the chest. For example, asthma or chronic obstructive lung disease may produce chest pain by causing inflammation of the airways in the lungs as well as causing the need to use muscles in the chest and neck to help with breathing. Both factors may result in chest pain.

Factors that may produce pain from the esophagus and stomach include heartburn, acid reflux, and gastritis. Tumors of the esophagus may also cause pain in the chest.

Factors that may cause chest pain from musculoskeletal structures include trauma, infections, tumors, and inflammation of the ribs and sternum. Some systemic diseases that may cause musculoskeletal chest pain include rheumatoid arthritis, fibromyalgia, or costochondritis.

Chest pain may result following surgery. Persistent chest pain following open heart surgery can occur. Another postsurgical pain syndrome is called post-thoracotomy pain syndrome. Thoracotomy is a general term used for any surgery that involves opening the chest wall. This is typically performed for surgery on the lungs or esophagus. During a thoracotomy, an incision is made in the chest wall, and the ribs are typically spread apart in order to gain access to the organs underneath the rib cage. Immediately following surgery, most patients have some degree of postoperative pain. However, in up to 50 percent of patients two years after thoracotomy, the pain continues after the chest has healed.

A specific infection known to cause pain in the skin that frequently occurs in the chest is called shingles. Shingles is caused by the varicella zoster virus. This is the virus that causes chickenpox. Once the initial illness associated with chickenpox resolves, the virus lays dormant in a part of the nerve called the dorsal root ganglion. The virus can become reactivated and causes a rash and blisters in a segmental distribution of the skin called a "dermatome." While the most common area to experience shingles is in the chest or flank, occasionally shingles can affect the nerves that supply the eye and may even cause blindness. The initial rash is often very sensitive and painful. The blisters typically crust over in 7–10 days; however, the pain can persist for several months or even years following the initial rash. This condition is known as postherpetic neuralgia (PHN), which may occur in 15–20 percent of patients who develop shingles.

The probability of developing PHN increases with age. In adults younger than 60 years of age, the probability of developing PHN is less than 2 percent. People older than 60 account for 50 percent of the cases of PHN. Risks for PHN include age, greater initial pain, and greater rash severity.

SYMPTOMS

It is sometimes difficult to distinguish where chest pain is coming from. Chest pain caused by the heart, esophagus, or musculoskeletal structures of the chest may feel similar, or be described as the same type of pain, by different patients. Frequently though, pain from organs in the chest is described differently than from the musculoskeletal structures of the chest.

Symptoms of Chest Pain Related to the Heart

People with coronary artery disease may have chest pain described as squeezing, crushing, or pressure. The pain is often in the chest and may radiate to the arm, jaw, or back. Other symptoms may include shortness of breath, sweating, nausea, or weakness. Pain associated with aortic dissection is often described as severe tearing pain that develops suddenly. The pain often will radiate to the back and sometimes the neck or jaw. Pain from pericarditis usually starts suddenly and tends to be sharp, worsen when taking a deep breath, and may improve by leaning forward. However, the pain may also be dull and achy. Symptoms of valvular diseases such as aortic stenosis include chest pain, shortness of breath, and fainting.

Symptoms of Pain Related to the Esophagus

People with esophageal pain from acid reflux often describe the pain as burning behind the sternum. The pain may radiate to the back or neck and jaw. Pain from masses or tumors may be associated with difficulty swallowing or regurgitation.

Symptoms of Chest Pain Related to the Lung

Symptoms of pneumonia include fevers, chills, shortness of breath, and coughing up sputum. Symptoms of lung cancer include cough, coughing up blood, and shortness of breath. Depending on the type of lung cancer, other symptoms such as pain in the shoulder or pain in the bones in other parts of the body as a result from spread of the tumor may occur. Symptoms of pleuritis may include a sharp pain that is worse with inspiration. At times, the pain from the lung pleura may be felt at the skin.

Symptoms of Chest Pain Related to the Musculoskeletal Structures of the Chest

Pain of the musculoskeletal structures (muscles, bones) of the chest is typically sharp, well localized, and may be modified by things like positions or movements. Symptoms of rib injuries include sharp pain that is made worse with breathing or deep breaths. Typically this is associated with some type of trauma or surgery. Musculoskeletal chest pain due to other diseases such as autoimmune diseases may present with diffuse pain as well as fevers and swelling of the joints in the ribs and sternum.

Symptoms of shingles include a painful rash. The majority of patients have pain in the area of the rash before the rash develops. The pain is often described as burning, stabbing, or throbbing. Some patients also have itching. Frequently, patients have pain with light touch such that the rubbing of their clothing is very uncomfortable.

The rash of shingles typically starts with several raised, red bumps, which then develop into a continuous rash with blisters that may become quite large. These blisters typically crust over in 7–10 days. The rash usually involves a single segment of skin on one side of the body. A minority of people may have other symptoms, such as headache, fever, or fatigue. In postherpetic neuralgia, the rash heals; however, the same pain persists months to years after the rash resolves.

DIAGNOSIS

The diagnosis of chest pain typically involves a combination of history (symptoms of chest pain), risk factors (age, family history, smoking, etc.) physical exam, and diagnostic testing. Any one of these components alone is often not enough to make the diagnosis.

Musculoskeletal chest pain is typically not life threatening; however, diseases of the heart and lungs may be. Therefore, tests are often done first to determine whether the organs of the chest are involved, and if not, then other diagnoses are sought.

Diagnosis of Chest Pain Coming from the Heart

The diagnosis of coronary artery disease may be made by several different tests in addition to the history and physical. An EKG or echocardiogram (which is an ultrasound of the heart) may be used to determine whether the heart is getting an adequate blood supply. A cardiac stress test may be ordered by a cardiologist to help rule in coronary artery disease. This test is not 100% accurate, which means that it can be normal even when life-threatening heart disease is present. Coronary angiography is the "gold standard" procedure where a small flexible catheter is inserted into a large artery in the groin and passed up the aorta to the heart. Dye is then injected, which allows the detection of narrowing of the arteries of the heart. This is considered the best test used to diagnose coronary artery disease.

The diagnosis of aortic dissection is again based on history and physical exam but is confirmed with imaging such as angiography, computed tomography (CT) scan, or echocardiography.

Aortic stenosis is also diagnosed by history and physical exam. A history of symptoms as listed previously with exam findings such as a heart murmur may lead to imaging of the heart (such as an echocardiogram) to visualize the movement and function of the valve.

Pericarditis is diagnosed based on history, physical exam, laboratory tests, and tests such as EKG.

Diagnosis of Chest Pain Coming from the Lung

In addition to a history and physical exam suggestive of pneumonia, the sputum may be collected and cultured for bacteria. A chest x-ray may also be helpful to determine the presence and extent of the pneumonia.

Lung cancer diagnosis is made with a history, physical exam, and imaging. A history of chest pain with unintentional weight loss and risk factors for lung cancer such as smoking or exposure to cancer-causing materials such as asbestos may warrant imaging studies such as a chest x-ray or a CT scan. If a nodule is noted in the lungs, this may be biopsied (a small sample taken) to determine if it is cancer.

Diagnosis of pleuritic chest pain is typically made by history. Occasionally, pleural fluid can be examined to help determine the cause of pleuritic chest pain.

Diagnosis of Chest Pain Coming from the Esophagus

The diagnosis of pain caused by esophageal disorders is often made by a combination of history, physical exam, and studies such as endoscopy where a flexible camera is placed into the esophagus and stomach, and signs of reflux disease and esophagitis are noted. Biopsies may also be taken to determine the cause of the symptoms.

Diagnosis of Musculoskeletal Chest Pain

The diagnosis of musculoskeletal chest pain is often made by history and physical exam. A history of sharp, focal pain that is reproduced by pressing a particular area in the ribs or sternum is suggestive of musculoskeletal chest pain. However, there are times where the exact diagnosis of chest pain can be difficult, and as such, the diagnosis of musculoskeletal chest pain is sometimes made after disorders from other organs are ruled out.

A history of trauma to the chest increases the suspicion of damage or fractures of the ribs or sternum. In this case, an x-ray and/or CT scan may help determine the extent of damage and if any fractures exist. Likewise, suspicion of tumors in the musculoskeletal structures of the chest may warrant imaging to aid in the diagnosis. Laboratory tests may be helpful to determine if the pain is caused by other factors such as infection or an autoimmune disorder.

Diagnosis of Shingles

The diagnosis of shingles is often made by history and physical examination alone. In cases where the rash that develops is not characteristic of the disease, laboratory tests may be needed to confirm the diagnosis. The diagnosis of post-herpetic neuralgia is made by continued pain after the rash of shingles resolves.

TREATMENT

The treatment of chest pain varies depending on the cause of the pain. Often the treatment of chest pain from the organs of the chest involves treating the disease process of these organs. Once the disease is treated, the pain is often improved. There are times, however, when the disease is either untreatable or the treatment does not decrease the pain. In these cases, the pain may be treated separately from treatment of the disease.

For example, cancer has the potential to affect many structures in the chest. Patients may have chest pain as a result of cancer of the lung or bones. As a result of the cancer, patients may have pain. In some cases, treating the tumor to shrink or eliminate it may alleviate the pain. In other cases, chemotherapy, radiation, or surgery may be needed, which have the potential to create new or different pain issues. In these cases, the treatment of pain then becomes focused on the pain caused by the treatment, as opposed to treating the disease process itself.

The treatment of specific disease processes will be discussed first, followed by treatment for pain that may persist as a result of treating these issues.

Treatment of Diseases of the Heart

As far as treatment for specific disease processes in the heart, there are several considerations. Many conditions start with mild symptoms, and as such, the treatment may be more focused on conservative therapies. As the disease progresses and the symptoms worsen, treatment may become more aggressive and include interventions such as surgery.

The treatment of coronary artery disease involves either medications, placing a balloon or stent in the narrowed arteries, or surgery to take vessels from elsewhere in the body and place them in the heart to bypass the narrowed vessels (coronary artery bypass grafting). Medications help improve the blood supply to the heart and/or decrease the work of the heart to decrease the amount of oxygen that the heart demands. Stents may be placed in the narrowed arteries in the heart percutaneously, meaning the stent is introduced in the artery in the groin via a small wire, moved up to the heart via the aorta, and placed across the narrowed part of the artery. This is done in conjunction with angiography so both the stent and the narrowed arteries can be seen using x-ray and dye. Angioplasty is a type of intervention that involves placing a small balloon that is attached to a wire in the narrowed artery. The balloon is then inflated, and the narrowing in the artery expands. Coronary artery bypass grafting is a surgery where the chest is opened and other vessels (such as veins in the legs) are taken and used to provide blood to the heart instead of the narrowed coronary arteries. This is often done when there are multiple arteries narrowed.

The treatment of aortic dissection involves either placing a stent across the aorta percutaneously, or surgery to open the chest and replace the diseased aorta with a synthetic tube.

Treatment of aortic stenosis involves medications or, in severe cases, surgery to replace the valve.

Treatment of pericarditis depends on the cause. Pericarditis due to viral infections often improves on its own and doesn't require specific treatment. Pericarditis due to other systemic inflammatory diseases may respond to medications that decrease inflammation, such as nonsteroidal anti-inflammatory medications or steroids.

Treatment of Diseases of the Lung

Treatment of pneumonia typically involves antibiotics. Once the infection is controlled, the painful symptoms usually subside. Treatment of pleuritis involves treating the cause, whether it is due to infection or inflammation. Infection may be treated with medications and drainage, whereas inflammation may be treated with anti-inflammatory medications.

Treatment of gastroesophageal reflux disease involves behavior modification such as avoiding foods that worsen reflux symptoms, elevating the head of the bed, etc. Medications may be used that decrease stomach acid secretion. In severe cases, surgery may be recommended.

Treatment of musculoskeletal pain depends on the cause. For example, if trauma has caused rib fractures, treatment of the rib fractures may involve watchful waiting while they heal, or may involve surgery depending on the location and severity of the fractures.

Treatment of musculoskeletal pain, including pain from chostochondritis (inflammation of the cartilage that connects ribs to the breastbone), fibromyalgia, or following surgery, may include heat, ice, topical agents such as capsaicin cream, anti-inflammatory gel or patches, or lidocaine cream or patches in addition to medications.

Treatment of shingles may include antiviral medications as well as medications to help control the pain. Additionally, nerve blocks may be used to help the pain associated with shingles.

Postherpetic neuralgia may be treated with medications, topical creams or patches, or procedures that destroy the nerves that process the pain in the area where the shingles rash occurred.

Regardless of the initial cause of chest pain, it will often improve when the disease process associated with the pain is treated. However, if the pain continues despite treatment of the cause, treatment options include interventional procedures, medications, physical therapy, psychology, and other modalities such as manipulations, acupuncture, massage, heat, or ice.

Medications used to treat chest pain depend on the type of pain. Nonsteroidal anti-inflammatory drugs (NSAIDs) and acetaminophen (Tylenol) may be used for mild pain. Opioid medications may be helpful for acute pain such as that following trauma or surgery, or pain due to cancer. If neuropathic pain (pain caused by nerve irritation or injury) is present, as in shingles or postherpetic neuralgia, antiseizure medications such as gabapentin or pregabalin may be effective. Antidepressant medications may also be helpful for neuropathic pain as well as for musculoskeletal diseases like fibromyalgia.

Physical therapy is often important not only for decreasing pain in general, but also to help increase function. This may be especially helpful for chest pain. For example, if the chest pain is due to coronary artery disease, physical therapy may be helpful in increasing conditioning, thus eventually helping oxygen supply and demand on the heart.

Interventions for chest pain may include things such as nerve blocks; for example, nerves that run under the ribs are often affected by things like trauma or surgery. Other interventions include spinal cord stimulation, which is a procedure where electrodes are placed in the back and cause a tingling sensation where the patient feels pain. The patient then feels the tingling instead of the pain. This may be done for both musculoskeletal pain as well as pain from organs such as the heart, in situations where chest pain is significantly limiting yet there are no other treatment options.

Persistent pain may affect several aspects of patients' lives. Therefore, strategies for coping with the pain may be beneficial. Pain psychology may help provide such strategies and help modify the negative thinking that may accompany pain.

Prognosis

As with most aspects of chest pain, the prognosis depends on the disease causing the chest pain. With respect to the prognosis of pain (as opposed to the disease itself), the pain caused from many of the diseases affecting the organs in the chest improve with treatment of the disease. There are some situations in which a chronic pain condition may develop following the initial issue, however. Examples are chronic pain that develops after surgery, or postherpetic neuralgia following shingles.

Additional Resources

American Gastroenterological Association: http://www.gastro.org
American Heart Association: http://www.americanheart.org
American Lung Association: http://www.lungusa.org
American Pain Society: http://www.ampainsoc.org
Medline Plus: http://www.nlm.nih.gov/medlineplus
WebMD: http://www.webmd.com

19

FIBROMYALGIA, ARTHRITIS, AND JOINT PAIN

Nathan Perrizo, DO, and David E. Fish, MD, MPH

FIBROMYALGIA

Introduction

Fibromyalgia is a chronic pain condition that affects 3–6 percent of Americans and is becoming increasingly recognized due to the effects on daily functioning. It is characterized by functional activity deficits due to widespread pain in upper and lower extremity muscles, tendons, and ligaments, but also includes other symptoms such as fatigue, depression, stiffness, and sleep disturbances, which have led to the term Fibromyalgia Syndrome. Although women tend to be affected nine times more than men, it is seen in men, women, and children of all ages and races. Without proper management, fibromyalgia can have a debilitating effect on one's life physically, mentally and socially.

Although the scientific understanding of how and why fibromyalgia develops is still being worked out, research is closer to understanding the mechanism of its causes and also the best treatment methods for fibromyalgia.

Symptoms

The most prominent feature of fibromyalgia is the significant widespread pain that affects both sides of the body, above and below the waist. Sleep disturbance and functional deficits can occur in addition to pain, but these symptoms may not occur in every individual. Other symptoms include fatigue; decreased concentration, attention, and memory; heightened sensitivity to touch, sound, or light; depression or anxiety; irritable bowel syndrome; and joint pains.

The pain of fibromyalgia can vary in its intensity throughout the day and can also change from day to day. Often, those with fibromyalgia will complain of pain that is worse in the morning and may also say that some days are good and some days are bad. The pain is often described as deep muscular aching, throbbing, twitching, stabbing, shooting, stiffness, or tingling. The pain is typically aggravated by poor sleep, fatigue, inactivity, psychological anxiety or stress, and cold or humid weather.

Fatigue in fibromyalgia is more significant than that which accompanies everyday tiredness from a busy day or a poor night's sleep. It is characterized by exhaustion and poor stamina that can interfere with work, personal relationships, and social activities.

Many individuals with fibromyalgia do not get restful sleep and may have an associated sleep disorder. Researchers have shown that the most important and restorative stage 4, or deep sleep phase, is affected most.

The list of other associated symptoms seen in fibromyalgia is quite extensive and includes:

- Irritable bowel syndrome
- Migraines
- Anxiety, depression, and/or posttraumatic stress disorder
- Neurologic symptoms, such as dizziness, ringing in the ears
- Restless leg syndrome
- Joint pains such as those seen in lupus or rheumatoid arthritis
- Endometriosis
- Cognitive impairments in memory, concentration, and attention

Diagnosis

The American College of Rheumatology has set forth specific diagnostic criteria for fibromyalgia, which includes widespread body pain for at least three months. A physical exam must also demonstrate that there is tenderness or pain with fingertip pressure at 11 out of 18 predetermined points throughout the body, which are located on the head, neck, chest, back, arms, and legs. The point is considered positive if pain is provoked with 4 kg of pressure, which is approximately the amount that will blanch the physician's fingernail. A device, called an algometer, can be used by the physician to measure the amount of pressure for a more accurate determination if necessary.

There are no laboratory tests available to diagnose fibromyalgia; therefore, the physician must rely on the patient's history, account of his/her symptoms, and the detailed examination to make a diagnosis. It is also important for the physician to ensure that there is not another disease or medical condition that can explain the various symptoms. In this case, lab testing, x-rays, or other diagnostic tests may be very important. Due to the complexity of the syndrome and its similarities with other medical conditions, the diagnosis can sometimes be delayed for months if not years. However, there is a growing awareness in the medical professional community.

Treatment Options

The most important factor for a patient to achieve meaningful relief is a better understanding of the syndrome and the recognition of the need for lifestyle adaptation. The majority of patients are resistant to initial treatment recommendations regarding lifestyle change because it implies effort, discomfort, and adjustment. Once undertaken, these changes can lead to meaningful improvement in symptoms, functional abilities, and quality of life.

An important aspect of treatment includes a knowledgeable physician who understands all facets of fibromyalgia and can sympathize and connect with the patient and their individual needs. This will allow for meaningful communication through trust and respect and will translate to more effective treatment. The physician may be a primary care physician such as a family practitioner or internist, or may include a specialist such as physiatrist, rheumatologist, or neurologist. A comprehensive approach can be critical in the care of more complicated scenarios and would include a psychiatrist, psychologist, physical and occupational therapists, or nutritionist and may also utilize complementary treatments (acupuncture and chiropractic or osteopathic manipulation).

Pain

An important factor in minimizing pain is regular exercise and stretching, which improves muscle tone and conditioning and therefore reduces pain and stiffness. There are many medications that may be prescribed by your physician. The first FDA-approved medication was pregabalin (Lyrica), the second was duloxetine (Cymbalta), and the third was milnacipran (Savella). There are other medications that are still in the FDA development phase and may be available in the future. Other medications that are not FDA approved for the treatment of fibromyalgia pain but can be very helpful in the management of the various other symptoms include antidepressants (commonly used in the treatment of other pain disorders at lower doses or for the treatment of depression at higher doses), non-opiate pain medications such as Tramadol, and Lidocaine injections for localized pain. Over-the-counter pain medication such as ibuprofen and acetaminophen can also be helpful. With a lack of scientific support for its use in fibromyalgia pain, opioid medications are not recommended. Opioid medications also carry a high risk of addiction, abuse, dependence, and significant side effects.

Sleep Management

A good sleep regimen is critical for improving sleep. This entails going to bed and getting up at the same time each day, ensuring a peaceful place to sleep that is free of loud noise, bright light, and other distractions. Patients must also avoid caffeine, sugar, and alcohol before bed, and eating within two to three hours of bedtime. Engaging in some type of light exercise during the day and implementing relaxation exercises while trying to fall asleep have been shown to be very helpful. On occasion, sleep medications are prescribed, some of which can be especially helpful for restless legs or periodic limb movement disorder.

Psychological Support and Coping

Learning how to live with fibromyalgia is the biggest challenge for most patients, as the treatment is considered a management strategy instead of a cure. Individuals have often been misunderstood and mislabeled by family, friends, and medical professionals. Their relationships, work, school, and functional abilities may have been significantly impacted. Obtaining a diagnosis is only the first step toward improvement. Emotional and psychological support can be achieved via multiple approaches. There are many community and Internet support groups, which can reassure individuals that they are not alone. Hearing about other people's shared symptoms and treatment outcomes can provide the reassurance that one may need. Educating and communicating with family and friends about fibromyalgia can also be of significant benefit. Some patients will require professional counseling with a mental health professional with specific emphasis on coping strategies, relationship building, and stress reduction, among others, and this may take place in a group or individual format.

Other Treatments

Complementary therapies can be very beneficial, and some have been proven in clinical trials. These may include:

- Physical therapy
- Myofascial release, therapeutic massage, acupressure
- Osteopathic or chiropractic manipulation
- Superficial warm or cold packs
- Aquatic therapy
- Acupuncture
- Tai chi
- Yoga
- Relaxation exercises, breathing techniques, aromatherapy, cognitive therapy, biofeedback
- Herbal remedies and nutritional supplements

Prognosis

Although there is no cure for fibromyalgia, it is not a progressive or a fatal condition. There has been a huge increase in the medical community and public awareness of fibromyalgia as well as research in determining the cause and best treatment approaches. This research has led to three new medications receiving FDA approval since 2007 for the treatment of fibromyalgia. While fibromyalgia still remains a significant challenge for sufferers and clinicians, patients have been able to better control their symptoms with newer treatment strategies.

ARTHRITIS AND JOINT PAIN

Introduction

Arthritis includes a group of many diagnoses, all of which lead to destruction or damage to the joints of the body and thereby cause pain. There are many different types and causes of arthritis and joint pain; however, the most common type is osteoarthritis. Other common forms of arthritis include rheumatoid arthritis, systemic lupus erythematosus (SLE), crystal deposition diseases such as gout and pseudogout, and septic arthritis, among many others. The mechanisms of each are different. Osteoarthritis results from wear and tear of the joint's protective cartilaginous surface. Rheumatoid arthritis and other rheumatologic diseases result from the body's own antibodies, which attack some aspect of the normal joint architecture. Crystal deposition diseases cause joint pain when crystals form in the joint fluid and thereby cause inflammation to the lining of the joint known as a synovial membrane. Septic arthritis results from an infection within the joint, which leads to a significant amount of inflammation.

This section covers the more common primary arthritic conditions; however, arthritis may arise in other diseases such as ankylosing spondylitis, inflammatory bowel disease, sarcoidosis, psoriasis, hemachromatosis, hepatitis, vasculitis, and Lyme disease, to name a few. The primary arthritic conditions can appear similar, but each has different characteristics in symptoms, exam findings, radiographic images, and even lab analysis, which can be helpful for the physician to differentiate among the types of arthritis.

Osteoarthritis

Osteoarthritis (OA) can occur in both large and small joints of the body and results from wear and tear of the cartilage surface of the bones within the joint. It is not considered an inflammatory condition, and over time the bones will eventually become in direct contact with one another. As osteoarthritis progresses, it can have a significant impact on an individual's ability to do any type of physical activity. OA typically occurs in elderly individuals, and the risk of acquiring osteoarthritis increases with age. OA can occur in almost any joint in the body. The most commonly affected joints are the spine, thumb, finger, hip, knee, and big toe joints. Risk factors for developing OA include obesity, female sex, age, genetic predisposition, repetitive use of joints, and a sedentary lifestyle.

Rheumatoid Arthritis

Rheumatoid arthritis (RA) is the second-most common form of chronic arthritis and is considered an inflammatory condition that affects approximately 1 percent of the adult population. RA affects all ethnic groups, with females 2.5 times more likely than males to develop the disease. RA is classified as an autoimmune disease, which means the body's own antibodies are misguided to attack various tissues in the body. One of the tissues involved in RA is the cartilage surface, which is considered a lining of a joint. This attack leads to destruction of the cartilage, erosion of the bony surface, weakening of certain ligaments, and eventually deformity of the joint. Inflammation develops within the joint and aggravates the pain in RA. The most commonly affected joints in RA are fingers, wrists, knees, and elbows; however, other joints are less commonly affected.

SLE (Lupus)

Systemic lupus erythematosus (SLE) is a multi-organ system autoimmune disease that can cause symptoms in most of the major organ systems of the body. The most commonly and dramatically affected parts of the body are the skin, kidneys, brain and nerves, blood vessels, and the joints. SLE affects women nine times more commonly than men, and average age of onset is 15–45 years.

Gout and Pseudogout

Gout is a form of arthritis that results from the accumulation of uric acid crystals in the joints. Similarly, pseudogout results from the accumulation of calcium pyrophosphate crystals. Gout tends to affect men two times more commonly than women, and pseudogout tends to affect women more commonly and those with prior trauma to a joint. Gout typically affects the big toe (called Podagra) but is also seen in other joints less commonly. Pseudogout is more common in large joints, with the knee being the most commonly involved joint. Gout may have periods of time during which crystals are still in the joint; however, they do not cause any pain. Furthermore, crystals may also deposit in the connective tissues under the skin, causing nodules termed tophi.

Septic Arthritis

Septic arthritis is caused by an infection, usually bacterial, which finds its way into the joint by either traveling through the bloodstream, by direct infection from outside the body, or by spread from adjacent bone structures. This is a medical emergency, and delaying treatment can lead to destruction of the joint and increased risk of death. There are about 2–10 cases of septic arthritis out of 100,000 people in the general population every year. There is a slightly higher risk in children.

Symptoms

Osteoarthritis

Initially, the pain is mild; however, it will increase as the degree of cartilage loss increases. The pain typically is worse with activity and is relieved with rest. Eventually, as the process advances, the pain may occur at rest or even at night while lying in bed. Joint pain also tends to be worse upon awakening in the morning or after periods of inactivity during the day and is characterized as stiffness. The joints will demonstrate swelling just as it will with most forms of arthritis; however in OA, the swollen joint does not typically have increased warmth. A grinding sensation or sound may also be present, which is called crepitus.

Rheumatoid Arthritis

The most common initial symptom is morning stiffness with fatigue. The joints are painful with swelling and usually involve the smaller joints, equally on left and right sides:

- Wrists
- Finger joints
- Toe joints

Larger joints generally become painful or swollen after small joints. Initially, only a few joints may be involved, but then it may progress to involvement of multiple joints within a few weeks to months.

SLE (Lupus-Related)

The joints in a patient with SLE tend to be painful and swollen and can wax and wane over years. In addition to joint pains, those with SLE may have a facial rash, other rashes, fevers, weight loss, fatigue, pain in the chest, sensitivity to light, seizures, or headaches.

Gout and Pseudogout

During the acute gout "attack," the affected joint is red, swollen, and hot to the touch. In addition, it is exquisitely tender to touch and is very painful to move. With pseudogout, patients typically experience pain, stiffness, swelling, and a limited motion at the involved joint. There is a varying degree of redness and warmth. Pseudogout tends to be less painful and take longer to reach peak intensity than gout.

Septic Arthritis

The most commonly involved joints are the hip and the knee, but any joint can be affected. The joint becomes extremely swollen and red within hours to days. There is an increase in the warmth of the skin over the joint, and the joint will become painful to move. Many people with septic arthritis will also have a fever.

Diagnosis

Osteoarthritis
OA is diagnosed by x-rays, which show joint space loss and bony changes.

Rheumatoid Arthritis
The diagnosis of RA is based primarily on clinical features and must include four of the following:

- Morning stiffness in a joint that lasts at least 30 minutes
- Arthritis in three or more joints for at least 6 weeks
- Arthritis of the hand joints for at least 6 weeks
- Symmetric arthritis for at least 6 weeks
- Rheumatoid nodules (subcutaneous over bony prominences)
- Positive blood test for rheumatoid factor
- X-ray changes

SLE (Lupus-Related)
Lab tests are most commonly used in addition to the clinical history and physical exam.

Gout and Pseudogout
Withdrawing a small sample of joint fluid for evaluation under a special microscope will definitively make the diagnosis of gout or pseudogout, depending on which type of crystals are seen. Blood tests can monitor progress in gout but is not very helpful in making the diagnosis.

Septic Arthritis
The diagnosis of septic arthritis is suggested by a change in some of the normal blood counts such as an increased white blood cell (WBC) count and an increased in the markers of inflammation, which are the erythrocyte sedimentation rate (ESR) and the C-reactive protein (CRP). Your doctor should order all the necessary tests during your visit. Blood cultures can be helpful in identifying the organism when positive. Any time a joint is suspected of being infected, the joint fluid must be withdrawn or aspirated for analysis. This analysis will not only show an increased WBC count, but the actual organism can be identified from a culture.

Treatment Options

For all types of arthritis, treatment may include physical therapy, bracing, and a prescribed or self-directed exercise regimen. Specific treatment will be tailored based on the type of arthritis you have.

Osteoarthritis

Weight loss and regular physical activity coupled with conditioning and stretching are keys to improving symptoms and preventing progression. Acetaminophen and nonsteroidal anti-inflammatory medications (NSAIDs) are the most commonly prescribed medications for treatment. Other treatment options include the use of a brace, and when the pain becomes severe, constant, or debilitating, joint replacement surgery is an option. Joint replacement has become much more common in recent years with growing success.

Rheumatoid Arthritis and SLE (Lupus-Related)

As in all types of autoimmune arthritis, certain medications may be required and are usually prescribed by a rheumatologist. These medications include chemotherapies and immune-modulating medications, which can inhibit the body's immune system and thereby decrease the destruction and inflammation within the affected joints. While these medications can work very well in treating the symptoms and preventing progression of the disease, consideration is always given to the risk of these medications, as side effects are higher than over-the-counter medications.

Gout and Pseudogout

Gout and pseudogout are typically treated with medications that reduce inflammation such as colchicine, NSAIDs, and corticosteroids. In certain cases, other medications are used to treat gout such as allopurinol, which decreases uric acid production in the body. One of the goals in preventing gout attacks is to lower blood uric acid levels. Patients with gout are also advised to decrease beer consumption.

Septic Arthritis

Effective treatment with antibiotics must begin as soon as possible to prevent joint destruction. These are often given in the intravenous forms. The joint is usually aspirated with a needle to decrease the amount of fluid, and when the pain and swelling starts to improve, the joint will need to be mobilized through its range of motion to prevent contractures.

Prognosis

Osteoarthritis

Osteoarthitis is a progressive disease that can lead to significant limitations in functional ability and can have negative impacts on a person's healthy lifestyle and quality of life. While most people think that OA will continue to worsen, there are some cases where the disease and symptoms have periods of stability. Maintaining the joint's range of motion, strengthening and conditioning the adjacent muscles, and regular stretching can limit the progression of osteoarthritis.

Rheumatoid Arthritis

Patients unfortunately experience poor long-term outcomes, as 70 percent of RA patients have damage to the joints that can be seen on x-ray within two years. RA is clearly a disease that shortens survival and produces significant disability. Over 33 percent of RA patients who were working at the time of onset of their disease will leave the workforce within 5 years. Overall, RA shortens the lifespan of patients by 5–10 years.

SLE (Lupus-Related)

The prognosis for SLE is better now than ever before and varies widely based on the severity of the disease. The 20-year survival rate for SLE is near 70 percent, and improved when treatment is initiated early. Although some people with lupus have a severe form with recurrent attacks and are frequently hospitalized, most people with lupus rarely require hospitalization. Generally, SLE that develops in a younger person carries a more serious prognosis than SLE diagnosed in an older person.

Gout and Pseudogout

Some people will rarely have gout attacks, while others may suffer from repeated attacks. The degree to which gout impacts one's life is highly correlated with adherence to a proper treatment regimen. While there is no cure for gout, the attacks can be significantly minimized with proper diet and taking the appropriate medications. Often, the inflamed joints heal without any residual problems, but in many people, permanent joint damage can occur, with some joints becoming severely destroyed.

Septic Arthritis

Despite better antibiotics, the death rate from septic arthritis can approach 15 percent, but many of those who die also have other serious medical problems. The majority of patients who are treated effectively and early will not have any residual functional abnormalities within the affected joint.

ADDITIONAL RESOURCES

http://arthritis.webmd.com/
http://www.arthritis.org
http://www.fibromyalgia.com/
http://www.fmaware.org/

http://www.fmnetnews.com/
http://www.gout.com/
http://www.lupus.org
http://www.niams.nih.gov
http://www.nlm.nih.gov/medlineplus/fibromyalgia.html
http://www.rheumatology.org

20

Ischemic Pain in Diabetes and Other Metabolic Disorders

Michael Harned, MD, and Paul Sloan, MD

Introduction

In this chapter, pain is discussed as it relates to two types of disease: *metabolic* and *ischemic*. While there are many different metabolic disorders, usually only a handful will cause pain. Diabetes is by far the most common metabolic disorder resulting in pain. Diabetic pain results from damage to the nerves themselves; uncontrolled diabetes causes this damage. On the other hand, ischemic pain results when muscles try to perform their usual duties while not getting enough blood; this lack of normal blood flow results from blockages in the arteries.

Diabetes and Pain

Currently there are almost 18 million Americans diagnosed with diabetes, almost 6 million diabetics who are as yet undiagnosed, and 57 million people with *metabolic syndrome*, that is, who are at risk for the development of diabetes. *Diabetes* is a group of diseases defined by increased blood glucose as a result of defects in the body's ability either to make or use insulin; it can cause damage to many different organ systems. For example, the risk of heart attack and stroke is between two and four times higher in diabetics. Diabetes is also the number one cause of kidney failure, which results in the need for lifelong dialysis. Damage to the nerves and blood vessels can result in blindness, amputations, and the development of painful *neuropathies* (problems with the nerves). Approximately 60–70 percent of people with diabetes will have some form of nerve damage, usually affecting the feet and lower legs (the *peripheral* parts of the body). Therefore, the term commonly used is "diabetic peripheral neuropathy," or DPN. It is estimated that seven percent of newly diagnosed diabetes patients will already have symptoms of neuropathy. While not life threatening, the development of diabetic neuropathy can be so painful and disabling that it significantly reduces the patient's quality of life.

Peripheral Vascular Disease (PVD)

Peripheral vascular disease (PVD) is most often caused by *atherosclerotic* (cholesterol plaque) buildup along the inside of arteries. This buildup leads to a narrowing of the *lumen* (the space within the artery), with the resulting constriction of blood flow to the muscles and tissue supplied by that artery. As the muscles continue to work with a poor blood supply, they suffer *ischemia* (lack of blood circulation) resulting in pain. While PVD can theoretically occur in any artery outside of the heart, it is the arteries in the legs that are the most frequently affected. Major risk factors for the development of PVD include being over 40 years old, cigarette smoking, high cholesterol, hypertension, and diabetes. Approximately three percent of men and two percent of women over the age of 60 report symptoms consistent with PVD. Unfortunately, though the symptoms of PVD are relatively benign, most PVD patients also have concomitant *coronary artery disease* (disease of the arteries of the heart), which places a significant risk of morbidity and mortality on the patient.

Symptoms

Diabetic Peripheral Neuropathy (DPN)

The development of *diabetic peripheral neuropathy* (DPN) is thought to result from chronically high blood sugar levels. This complication occurs in type 1 diabetics after many years of disease progression, whereas in type 2 diabetics, the symptoms of neuropathies can present after a few short years of poor glucose control. As stated above, symptoms of neuropathy are often already present upon diagnosis of type 2 diabetes. In either case, neuropathy can occur along a wide spectrum of symptoms. Patients may have changes in *sensory* nerves (the way things feel), *motor* nerves (loss of muscle strength), or in the *autonomic nervous system* (processes that occur without conscious effort, such as digestion or sweating).

Sensory symptoms are the most common presenting complaint in patients with undiagnosed diabetes. These symptoms can be categorized as either *positive* (new sensations) or *negative* (a loss of feeling). Positive sensory symptoms often include burning, electrical shocking, or pins-and-needles sensations. Patients may also experience *dysesthesia* (unpleasant sensations, such as that of bugs crawling on the skin) or *hyperalgesia* (normally painful sensations may become much more painful). Negative symptoms include numbness or the feeling of deadness. Patients will often report feeling as though they are wearing a sock or glove on the affected extremity. These negative symptoms put diabetics at risk of incurring minor injuries, which, because of high blood glucose levels, are more likely to become infected.

Motor (muscle) neuropathies can result in loss of coordination. In the upper extremities, this results in difficulty with tasks such as unscrewing a jar top or using keys. In the lower extremities, patients often report frequent tripping and toe-stubbing. Patients will also have a loss of balance due to the inability to feel their feet.

Autonomic symptoms can affect multiple different systems in the body, ranging from simple nausea to severe, life-threatening complications. Patients can develop unusually dry or unusually sweaty skin, depending on which nerves are damaged. Patients may also experience problems with digestion such as diarrhea, constipation, or nausea and vomiting with eating.

Peripheral Vascular Disease

Rarely an acute event, the symptoms of PVD tend to be more gradual and chronic in onset. The most common symptom of PVD is called *claudication.* Claudication has its root in the Latin word "to limp." Each time you begin to walk, the muscles of your legs require more oxygen to keep up with the increased metabolic demand of walking. The delivery of oxygen occurs in the form of increased blood flow. PVD reduces blood flow through the arteries to parts of the body, especially the legs. As blood flow is constricted during times of need, the muscles suffer from a lack of oxygen and develop *ischemia.* This ischemia results in pain in the muscles of the legs, usually in the calves. Patients will often note that they are able to walk predictable distances before symptoms come on. The pain is usually relieved with rest, and then they can continue further. Patients will often be symptom-free during times of rest, such as in bed. When the disease is severe, patients may experience pain even during periods of lying flat; they may need to hang their feet off the side of the bed in order to improve blood flow to the extremities.

Diagnosis

Diabetic Peripheral Neuropathy

The diagnosis of painful diabetic peripheral neuropathy can be difficult, as symptoms can vary from patient to patient. A thorough history and physical are required, along with a detailed neurologic evaluation, in order to rule out many of the other causes of peripheral neuropathy. Blood tests will be required to diagnose diabetes and may be required to rule out other causes of neuropathy such as toxins, bacterial or viral infections, or vitamin deficiencies.

Following blood tests, imaging may be used to further elucidate the cause of the neuropathy. *Computed tomography* (CT) and *magnetic resonance imaging* (MRI) are both painless tests that provide information about the structures of the body. MRI is especially useful in detecting abnormal changes in the nerves of the brain or body. Another diagnostic tool that may reveal the cause of neuropathy is called *electromyography* (EMG) and *nerve conduction velocity* (NCV). These tests are usually used in combination. The EMG test uses a fine needle inserted into the muscles, whereas the NCV places electrodes on the skin. The EMG portion measures the amount of electric activity present when muscles are at rest and when they contract. This helps the doctor differentiate between a muscle and a nerve disorder as the cause of the neuropathy. The NCV portion can determine where along the nerve the damage has occurred, which can help the provider determine the cause of the neuropathy.

Peripheral Vascular Disease

The diagnosis of pain secondary to peripheral vascular disease (PVD) starts with a thorough history and physical. Patients with high blood pressure, diabetes, high cholesterol, a history of smoking, and older age are at more of a risk. Pain in the legs, especially pain brought on by activity, could be the result of other health problems, such as narrowing of the *spinal canal* (the space around the spinal cord), or complications from diabetes. Therefore, the doctor may need to perform several tests to determine the exact cause of leg pain. For example, an MRI of the spine may be needed to determine whether narrowing of the spinal canal has occurred. Patients may need blood tests to rule out diabetes. Finally, nerve conduction tests (*see above*) may help determine the cause of lower extremity pain.

On physical examination, the doctor will pay special attention to the pulses in the legs and feet. Weakened pulses in the extremities are often a good indication that somewhere in the vascular system, there is a narrowing that prevents adequate blood flow to the muscles. Next, the doctor will compare the blood pressure in the arm to the blood pressure in the ankle. This is an objective test of any differences in circulation due to this narrowing. Finally, more sophisticated tests can be performed, usually in a hospital laboratory, where ultrasound is used to see the arteries or x-rays are taken after the injection of dye to map the arterial blockages.

TREATMENT OPTIONS

Diabetic Peripheral Neuropathy

There are currently no specific treatment options that can repair damaged nerves. Therefore, the treatment goals are centered on modification of the symptoms for optimal improvement in quality of life. Tight *glycemic* (blood glucose) control is necessary not only for the overall health of the individual, but also to prevent further damage to the nervous system. Pharmacologic therapy is used to modify symptoms and improve pain control. Often, different kinds of drugs will be used in combination to achieve these goals.

There are many different classes of medicines that may help treat DPN. The typical first-line analgesics for acute pain, such as acetaminophen and nonsteroidal drugs (e.g., naproxen), are not usually effective for DPN. The *antiseizure class of medicines*, of which gabapentin is the most common, has proven beneficial in modifying the painful symptoms. Given that the painful symptoms result from nerve damage, many of the medicines work to modify the way in which nerves "talk" to one another. Gabapentin and pregabalin, a more potent and effective form of gabapentin, as well as other medicines in this class, help control pain by stabilizing and reducing the nerve firing that transmits pain signals. It should be noted that pregabalin is one of only two medications to have received FDA (Food and Drug Administration) approval for the treatment of DPN. While these medicines will rarely relieve all of the pain associated with diabetic neuropathy, they are extremely helpful. Common side effects include dizziness and sedation.

Antidepressants are also used for DPN. While *Tricyclic antidepressants* (TCA) are typically used to treat clinical depression, they have also been demonstrated in multiple studies to be beneficial in relieving nerve pain. Tricyclic antidepressants work by blocking much of the body's normal loss of many different molecules including serotonin, norepinephrine, and sodium. While each individual drug has slightly different effects, the entire class has demonstrated pain relief in painful nerve conditions. A newer class of medications, SNRIs (*serotonin and norepinephrine reuptake inhibitors*), recently gained FDA approval for the treatment of painful diabetic neuropathy. Duloxetine, the first of the SNRIs, has been proven to give effective analgesia as well as alleviate the psychological stresses associated with long-term chronic pain. Duloxetine is the second medication that currently has FDA approval for the treatment of DPN.

Opioid (*narcotic*) medications are strong analgesics that have morphine-like effects. Morphine is a commonly used opioid, as are oxycodone, hydromorphone, oxymorphone, and methadone. In recent years, evidence has shown that opioids are somewhat effective in the management of nerve pain; however, unusually high doses are often needed. The opioids are a *second line* of treatment, meaning they should not be used unless antiseizure and antidepressant medications have only partially controlled the pain, or have failed altogether. Side effects such as constipation, nausea, and sedation may develop with use of opioid analgesics. These side effects may diminish over time, or may be treated with other medications. The patient may be switched to another opioid drug until finding the one with the fewest side effects for that person. Careful dose titration by the treating physician is necessary to avoid serious side effects such as respiratory depression.

Peripheral Vascular Disease

The treatment goals for patients with claudication are to relieve exertion-induced symptoms and improve quality of life. Patients should begin very conservatively by modifying their *lifestyle choices*. Patients should immediately stop smoking. With the help of a physician, high blood pressure and cholesterol should be reduced. If a patient has diabetes, then blood sugar levels should be managed tightly.

After modifying the risk factors, beginning a walking program is the best therapy for symptom improvement in the long term. Patients are encouraged to walk up to the point of pain and then rest until the pain goes away. This is to be done in increasing increments of time until the patient can walk four times per week, for 30–60 minutes each time. Often, patients will begin to notice symptom improvement within two months. Additionally, there are drugs available that change the shape of red blood cells so they can more easily pass through narrowed areas in the vascular system. Pain from PVD can also be treated with surgery to improve blood flow to the muscles and tissues of the limb. Vascular surgical procedures reroute the blood flow around areas of blockage and provide more blood flow to the legs and feet. This increased blood flow usually provides relief from the chronic pain. In rare cases in which surgery does not provide pain relief, or in cases where the patient is not a candidate for surgery, the antidepressant medications and opioid drugs may be tried (see above).

When more conservative measures fail in the management of DPN or PVD, there are more invasive treatments, termed *neuromodulation therapy*, which can help control painful symptoms. Neuromodulation refers to medical technology that allows direct alteration of the nervous system to help control pain. The choice of therapy depends on which type of pain is being treated. As a general rule, spinal cord stimulators are more beneficial for neuropathic pain, while intrathecal pumps are effective for mixed pain syndromes, which include both neuropathic and mechanical pain.

Spinal cord stimulation (SCS) uses pulsed electrical energy applied near the spinal cord to control pain. The most common type of stimulation uses small electrodes placed in the epidural space, which is below the bones of the spine, adjacent to and outside of the spinal cord. A small generator then sends electrical energy to the leads. The effect for the patient is a replacement of the body's own painful nerve firings with a pleasant vibratory sensation in the affected area. This type of treatment has proven extremely beneficial for neuropathic pain secondary to painful diabetic complications, and for ischemic pain due to peripheral or coronary artery disease.

The second interventional technique, *intrathecal drug delivery*, involves placing extremely small amounts of medication, usually opioids alone or in combination with local anesthetics and other medications, directly into the spinal fluid. This drug delivery route bypasses the oral or intravenous route, thus reducing side effects and improving efficacy. The system is comprised of a small catheter (plastic tube) placed between the bones of the spine, and a small pump placed below the skin. This device is refilled by placing a small needle through the skin about once every three months, but is otherwise maintenance-free.

PROGNOSIS

Diabetic Peripheral Neuropathy

When patients present with the painful complications of diabetes, this is often a late warning sign of the damage diabetes has already caused in the body. Currently, there is no way to restore nerve function lost to chronically high blood glucose levels. However, when patients make significant changes in their lifestyle choices, this disease progression slows significantly.

When pain management is approached methodically, most patients will achieve at least a moderate amount of pain control. Often, each medication added to the patient's regimen provides yet another increment of relief from pain. This trial process of selecting different medications and interventions can be time consuming and frustrating for the patient. Bear in mind that it is not unusual for the doctor to prescribe several different medications within each medication class or category before the patient reports on the one that best balances side effects with pain relief.

More invasive therapies such as SCS and intrathecal drug delivery are capable of providing some degree of pain relief in patients who have exhausted other options. These therapies, while not without potential side effects, have great potential to improve quality of life in diabetic patients.

Peripheral Vascular Disease

The prognosis for pain secondary to peripheral vascular disease depends greatly on the severity of the disease upon diagnosis. By the time most patients experience pain with ambulation, there is already a significant amount of atherosclerotic disease in the extremity. Patients need to make significant and sweeping changes in their lifestyle choices if there is to be any hope of slowing the disease process. Surgical correction is sometimes a treatment option for PVD, after which the patient may be pain-free. Even with a completely successful operation, however, the disease is very likely to recur without changes in diet, exercise, and smoking cessation.

For patients who are not candidates for this surgery, the treatment path is much less clear. For the motivated patient, a rigorous walking program will lead to symptom improvement as exercise prompts the body to find alternate routes to send blood to the affected extremity. In addition, pain medications may reduce painful symptoms to a small degree. However, medications rarely provide complete relief from pain.

Finally, interventional therapies such as SCS and intrathecal drug delivery have proven beneficial when more conservative measures have failed. SCS has been especially effective for PVD, not only controlling painful symptoms, but also actually improving blood flow through ischemic areas.

ADDITIONAL RESOURCES

Patients and families can find helpful additional information from the following websites:
http://www.canadianpaincoalition.ca.
http://www.diabetesmonitor.com
http://www.livestrong.com
http://www.painrelieffoundation.org.uk

21

REFLEX SYMPATHETIC DYSTROPHY (RSD) PAIN

Matthew Hansen, MD, and Jianguo Cheng, MD, PhD

INTRODUCTION

Brittany, a 16-year-old high school junior, had suffered from left leg pain for four months after twisting her ankle. Her left leg became extremely sensitive, and she felt pain in that leg at even the slightest touch that was persistent, excruciating, and burning. The area had frequent color changes and swelling as well. After visiting her family doctor and an orthopedic surgeon, she was referred to a pain specialist and was given a diagnosis of reflex sympathetic dystrophy. She wanted to know more about this disease and sought a cure for her condition before starting college.

Reflex Sympathetic Dystrophy (RSD) is one of a multitude of names given to a very complex and debilitating syndrome. During his tenure in charge of nervous diseases at the Hospital at Turner's Lane, Philadelphia, the great American physician and novelist Dr. Silas Weir Mitchell published the first description of Reflex Sympathetic Dystrophy in his 1864 essay, "Gunshot Wounds and Other Injuries of Nerves." In it, Mitchell observed the peculiar behavior and inexplicable physical findings of seven soldiers who sustained upper-extremity gunshot wounds during the Civil War. Taken from the Greek words for burning and pain, this condition became known as causalgia.

During World War II, Dr. John Bonica, an American anesthesiologist, noted similar symptoms among the wounded infantry, and this condition was renamed Reflex Sympathetic Dystrophy based on the theory that a dysfunction of the nervous system was the root of the problem. The term Complex Regional Pain Syndrome (CRPS) was created in 1993 to be a more comprehensive description of the syndrome with RSD and causalgia pertaining to specific subtypes, Type 1 and Type 2, respectively. Alternative names include algodystrophy, Sudeck's atrophy, transient osteoporosis, and acute atrophy of the bone.

In this country alone, Complex Regional Pain Syndrome afflicts somewhere between 200,000 and 1.2 million people. Predominantly occurring in females between the ages of 30 and 50, CRPS can occur at any age or gender. The first known pediatric diagnosis of CRPS occurred in 1971, with the youngest case found in the left arm of a 2.5-year-old Turkish female in 2003. On the other end of the spectrum, RSD has been diagnosed in octogenarians, though the median age at diagnosis is 42. The incidence of CRPS is not entirely known. A recent study suggests that the rate of CRPS is 26.2 per 100,000 persons/year, with females affected three times more frequently than males. Regardless of gender or age at diagnosis, patients suffering from this condition are impacted, not just from the physical symptoms, but from the emotional and psychological stresses placed on themselves and their loved ones.

SYMPTOMS

As the pain increases the general sympathy becomes more marked. The temper changes and grows irritable; the face becomes anxious and has a look of weariness and suffering. The sleep is restless, and the constitution condition, reacting on the wounded limb, exasperates the hyperaesthetic state, so that the rattling of a newspaper, a breath of air, another's step across the ward, the vibrations caused by a military band, or the shock of the feet in walking, give rise to increase of pain. At last the patient grows hysterical, if we may use the only term which covers the facts.

—Silas Weir Mitchell

In his landmark paper on causalgia, Dr. Mitchell eloquently described the symptoms of his newly discovered syndrome. One of the more intriguing behaviors he noted was the observation of patients carrying wet sponges in their hands or pouring water into their boots before handling objects or walking in attempts to counteract the burning pain they were experiencing. This unpleasant, abnormal sensation is a defining characteristic of RSD.

After the inciting event, symptoms tend to develop within hours to weeks in close proximity to the initial injury site. In the past, it was believed that CRPS progressed through three stages. The length of time at each stage was variable, with progression occurring over days to years, if at all. Adding further confusion was the fact that the symptoms did not necessarily occur in sequential order through the stages. Upon further evaluation, it is now believed that the differences in symptoms seen in CRPS may be variants of the condition and not time-dependent stages. In any case, the pain associated with CRPS may be constant and can certainly be affected by emotional or physical stress. Symptoms of CRPS typically occur in the limbs, though it is possible for any body area to be affected.

Stage I (acute) is characterized by an intense burning, aching pain at or near the initial injury site. Patients themselves may describe the pain as having their limbs on fire. Common complaints include muscle spasms, joint stiffness, and restricted mobility secondary to limb edema (swelling). Patients may also note an acceleration of hair and nail growth as well as changes in both the color and temperature of affected limbs due to blood vessel constrictions.

Stage II (dystrophic) is described as having an increase in the intensity and frequency of the pain when compared to Stage I. The limbs may be cool to the touch and hairless, the tissue firm, the joints stiff. The skin may sweat excessively. The nails become cracked and brittle. It is not uncommon for affected muscles to atrophy. Radiography shows signs of bone density loss or osteoporosis.

Stage III (atrophic) is defined by irreversible tissue damage to the skin and bone. Pain may spread from the initial site of injury and may include other extremities. The skin thins and takes on a shiny appearance. Muscle atrophy is severe, and tendon contractures limit joint mobility. Radiographs show severe osteoporosis (thinning of bone tissue) and demineralization of the bones.

DIAGNOSIS

Diagnosing Complex Regional Pain Syndrome can be somewhat challenging. There is no definitive test for CRPS, meaning the diagnosis must be based on the patient's symptoms and physical exam. While a history of trauma is common, it is not essential. This has led to the creation of subtypes of CRPS, namely Type 1 (RSD) and Type 2 (causalgia). In Type 1 (RSD), which accounts for 90 percent of CRPS cases, symptoms may develop after non-traumatic events or injuries without specific nerve injury, such as sprains, fractures, and surgery. In Type 2 (causalgia), the diagnosis is defined by an established nerve injury.

While a definitive diagnosis may be difficult to obtain, there are characteristics in the patient's history and physical that may help. Typically, patients with CRPS have some form of severe unexplainable pain, a sensitivity to touch, and signs of abnormal sweating and blood flow. On physical exam, the physician may find swelling of the extremities, decreased range of motion in the joints, and temperature changes of the skin as well as the abnormalities of the skin and nails described above. Keeping these traits in mind, the International Association for the Study of Pain (IASP) developed criteria for the diagnosis of CRPS.

In diagnosing CRPS Type 1 (RSD), patients must have the following characteristics:

1. The presence of an initiating injuring event or a cause of immobilization
2. Continuing pain, allodynia (perception of pain from a nonpainful stimulus), or hyperalgesia (an exaggerated sense of pain) disproportionate to the inciting event
3. Evidence at some time of edema (swelling), changes in skin blood flow, or abnormal sweating activity in the area of pain
4. The diagnosis is excluded by the existence of any condition that would otherwise account for the degree of pain and dysfunction

According to the IASP, CRPS Type 2 (causalgia) must have the following characteristics:

1. The presence of continuing pain, allodynia (see above), or hyperalgesia (see above) after a nerve injury, not necessarily limited to the distribution of the injured nerve
2. Evidence at some time of edema, changes in skin blood flow, or abnormal sweating activity in the region of pain
3. The diagnosis is excluded by the existence of any condition that would otherwise account for the degree of pain and dysfunction

While no test can definitively diagnose CRPS, there are some tests that may provide supportive evidence to the IASP criteria. Thermography, a technique that measures heat emitted from a body to determine blood flow, often will appear abnormal in the area affected by CRPS. The QSART test measures sweat response and will be abnormal in most CRPS patients. Measuring differences in resting skin temperature or resting sweat output may be helpful. Once again, radiographs may show signs of osteoporosis and demineralization. This may also be seen with bone scans or bone densitometry. MRI and CT scans are not routinely used in the diagnosis of CRPS. Diagnostic interventions that block the hypersensitive and hyperactive portion of the nervous system causing the syndrome may provide both relief and guide future treatment.

Treatment Options

After identifying CRPS, Dr. Mitchell developed a wide variety of methods to treat his newly discovered disease. Utilizing the cutting-edge techniques of the age, patients were treated with applications of leeches, electricity, and massage. After hypothesizing that pain resulted from an alteration in patient blood flow, Dr. Mitchell utilized ammonia and cantharis to induce blistering of the patient's skin. Interestingly, this treatment resulted in a reported 90 percent success rate in patients. Inspired by these results, Dr. Mitchell instituted aggressive blistering in all his afflicted patients.

Fortunately, medicine has advanced since the 19th century, and blistering is no longer the treatment of choice in the management of CRPS. It goes without saying that the best treatment of a condition is prevention. Though seen in patients following stroke or heart attacks, data suggests that early mobilization may reduce the risk of developing CRPS. While not understood, there is some evidence that taking vitamin C following wrist fracture may also reduce this risk. Cigarette smoking is a known risk factor for CRPS and should be avoided regardless of whether signs of CRPS are present or not.

Similar to prevention, a foundation for the initial treatment of CRPS involves mobilization and strengthening of the affected body part. It is worth remembering that the pain caused by this condition is an abnormality of the nerves themselves and does not mean tissue damage is actually occurring. Therefore, it is important to maintain flexibility and strength of the extremities to prevent the development of joint stiffness and contractures. Naturally, this is easier said than done. Pain often limits a patient's ability to participate in physical therapy. Nonetheless, maintaining function of the affected limb is imperative and bears repeating. Physical therapy is important when combating a condition like CRPS.

Another interesting component of CRPS is the ability of your emotions and daily stresses to increase the sensation of pain. For this very reason, stress management techniques may be useful in managing the symptoms of CRPS. In more complex cases, evaluation by a clinical psychologist and treatment with cognitive behavioral therapy may be warranted. In cognitive therapy, the focus of treatment involves reshaping how you perceive your symptoms in regard to yourself and your environment. In behavioral therapy, patients are taught to control behaviors that may be influencing their symptoms. Cognitive behavioral therapy combines these principles and teaches the patient how their thoughts and behaviors may influence their symptoms and how best to control them.

Pharmacologic (e.g., medications) management is a mainstay of treatment. Some current regimens include a combination of antiseizure medications, as well as antidepressants, nonsteroidal anti-inflammatory drugs, and muscle relaxants. While it may seem unusual, antiseizure agents and antidepressants have been shown to be rather effective in treating pain originating from the nerves. In particular, antiseizure medications are helpful in controlling the burning, sharp, electrical-type pain seen with CRPS. Less successful therapies include calcium channel blockers, steroids, and opioids (narcotics). Applications of numbing creams to the skin have also had some success. Additionally, the infusion of medications such as local anesthetics and magnesium may provide temporarily relief.

Other nontraditional treatments include acupuncture and mirror box therapy. Mirror box therapy, which was first seen in treating phantom limb pain in patients with amputated extremities, involves placing a mirror in between the affected and unaffected limbs. When a patient moves the unaffected limb, it appears in the mirror as if the affected limb is moving painlessly. Patients note that after this therapy, the pain is decreased when actually moving the affected limb.

If symptoms are not controlled with medications and physical therapy, more invasive therapies may be required. Painful areas of muscle spasm may be treated with injections of these points with local anesthetic and steroid. Known as trigger point injections, this method may be able to break the muscle spasm and is considered to be a relatively safe procedure.

Another treatment option involves the delivery of medication though an epidural catheter. Commonly used to treat labor pain in pregnant women, epidural catheters allow for the delivery of medications close to the affected nerves. While the catheter could be buried beneath the skin, the risk of infection makes this only a short-term solution lasting several weeks.

One of the major hypotheses regarding the mechanism of action behind CRPS involves the derangement of an aspect of the central nervous system. The sympathetic nervous system helps regulate everyday bodily functions below the level of consciousness. When stressed, the sympathetic nervous system activates a "fight-or-flight" response. Under such stimulation, the heart rate accelerates, blood vessels constrict, and blood pressure increases. In CRPS, the sympathetic nervous system is inadvertently activated in the affected limb, causing both pain and the changes seen in temperature and color when compared to the unaffected limb.

Keeping in mind that increased sympathetic activity in the affected limb may be the source of pain, blocking this stimulation may prove both beneficial in diagnosing and treating CRPS. Oral pharmacologic agents that block sympathetic input have not proven to be particularly useful. However, by injecting medication directly at the sympathetic nerve clusters, pain transmission can be stopped, allowing for both diagnosis and treatment. Patients with skin and temperature changes are candidates for such procedures. Depending on the affected limb, injections could be performed either in the neck or the lower back to treat upper and lower extremity pain, respectively. If pain relief occurs, the physician would be able to diagnose the sympathetic nervous system as the cause of the pain and provide guidance in treating the symptoms. These injections can be performed multiple times a year and may provide relief lasting weeks to months.

In 1965, psychologist Ronald Melzack and neuroscientist Patrick David Wall published a theory that provided a novel way to look at the transmission of pain. While working at the Massachusetts Institute of Technology, Wall and Melzack hypothesized that both nerves that transmit pain and nerves that transmit touch meet at a point in the spinal cord. They proposed that if more of the nerves that transmit touch were stimulated, they would in effect block the transmission of pain. This came to be known as "gate control theory of pain."

The gate control theory helped usher in the era of electrotherapy for pain management. While it took modern medicine centuries to discover this theory, Scribonius Largus, the court physician to the Roman emperor Claudius, was treating pain with electrical torpedo fish. With this in mind, patients may benefit from transcutaneous electrical nerve stimulation (TENS) units. A TENS unit is a portable device that supplies a current from a battery to externally placed electrodes on the skin of the affected area. Developed by the Medtronic Company in 1974, these units are able to vary the intensity, width, and frequency in such a way as to diminish the sensation of pain.

Taking this principle a step further, a spinal cord stimulator is an implantable device that can provide more permanent relief. In fact, the first TENS unit was developed to test the chronic pain patient's tolerance to electrical stimulation prior to implantation. Developed by Norman Shealy, a neurosurgeon in Cleveland, Ohio, the first implantation of a spinal cord stimulator occurred in 1967. Prior to implantation, patients undergo both a psychological evaluation and an external generator trial to determine whether there will be a 50 percent or greater reduction in pain, a reduction in pain medication, or an increase in daily activity. After a successful trial, the procedure is performed under conscious sedation in an operating suite. Utilizing x-ray guidance, electrodes are placed close to the spinal cord and connected to a pulse generator and battery. Patients are able to increase and decrease stimulation as needed, providing long-term, effective, and adjustable pain control.

Another implantable device that may provide benefit is an intrathecal drug delivery pump. Similar to the epidural, these implantable pumps allow for the delivery of medication, such as local anesthetics, opioids, or muscle relaxants, directly to the nerve roots and spinal cord. A medication derived from the toxin of the cone snail has shown promising results in the treatment of CRPS. Overall, intrathecal drug delivery allows for much smaller amounts of medication to be used, thereby limiting side effects and adverse reactions.

Surgical sympathectomy is a treatment of last resort. In this therapy, either surgical technique or chemicals are used to destroy the sympathetic nerves in patients who have had a good response to sympathetic nerve blocks. The evidence regarding the effectiveness of this treatment has been inconclusive, with some patients reporting improvement and others noting a worsening of symptoms. In fact, there may be adverse reactions like increased pain and sweating.

While all options are clinically useful, the treatment of CRPS requires "multimodal" therapy. Multimodal means a combined approach of stress-reducing techniques, physical therapy, oral medications, interventional injections or device implants will provide relief of pain, increase in flexibility, and a return of function of the affected limb.

PROGNOSIS

The prognosis is generally favorable for patients with CRPS. In fact, there are instances of spontaneous remission, particularly in young patients. For the most part, treatment effectiveness generally improves with early diagnosis and management of symptoms within the first three months. However, if CRPS is allowed to spread, then muscle, nerve, and bone changes can be irreversible and can lead to unremitting pain despite treatment. Nonetheless, when provided with appropriate and timely multimodal therapy, effective treatment may be able to provide remission in 25–90 percent of cases, according to researchers.

In the case of our vignette, after thorough evaluation, Brittany underwent comprehensive multimodal treatment leading to remission of her symptoms. She is currently enjoying a productive and rewarding experience in college.

ADDITIONAL RESOURCES

American Chronic Pain Association (ACPA): http://www.theacpa.org
American Pain Foundation: http://www.painfoundation.org
American RSDHope Organization: http://www.rsdhope.org
International Research Foundation for RSD/CRPS: http://rsdhealthcare.org/
Mayday Fund (For Pain Research): http://www.painandhealth.org
National Foundation for the Treatment of Pain: http://www.paincare.org
National Institute of Neurological Disorders and Stroke: http://www.ninds.nih.gov
The Reflex Sympathetic Dystrophy Syndrome Association: http://www.rsds.org

22

Shingles and Postherpetic Neuralgia

Lowell Reynolds, MD, and Jonathan Geach, MD

Introduction

Postherpetic neuralgia is a chronic pain syndrome that occurs following a herpes zoster outbreak. This outbreak is frequently referred to as shingles. The herpes zoster virus is the same virus that causes chickenpox. When someone develops chickenpox early in life, it lays dormant in the spinal cord long after the chickenpox lesions have healed. Frequently, it will stay dormant in our spinal cords for the remainder of our lives. However, at some point the virus may awaken and travel from the spinal cord to a nerve and then to the area of our skin supplied by that nerve. Usually this means the patient will have a strip of skin with a significant rash consisting of lots of red vesicles.

The rash is usually located on the chest wall, but can involve an arm, leg, or even the face. This rash is generally very painful. Typically, patients will not want to wear clothing that brushes against the rash or even allow bed sheets to touch the rash. It can be painful to bathe the affected skin area, and it can make it very difficult for them to sleep. Frequently, patients will appear very tired and disheveled, as a result of their painful condition interfering with sleep and hygiene.

After the rash heals, usually the pain will subside. Unfortunately, in some people the pain persists in the region of the rash. If this pain continues for more than three months after the rash has disappeared, then this chronic pain condition is referred to as postherpetic neuralgia.

Symptoms

The symptoms of postherpetic neuralgia are typical of any chronic painful nerve condition. Patients generally describe chronic nerve pain as burning, sharp, and lancinating in nature. Frequently, this pain will be quite severe. As with the acute shingles outbreak, just a brush of clothing or bed sheets to the area of involved skin may be unbearable. Many people will not want to have water from the shower running over this portion of their skin as well.

Usually, as with the initial shingles outbreak, the symptoms of postherpetic neuralgia are limited to the surface of the skin. Unfortunately, the herpes zoster virus may also cause muscle weakness. For instance, although rare, a herpes zoster outbreak in the leg may not only cause a rash and severe skin pain, but may also cause muscle weakness in the leg. Rarely, this weakness can persist into and throughout the postherpetic period. Likewise, people who have this type of rash in the face may also have a facial droop, which results from involvement of a nerve that goes to the muscles of the face.

As with any chronic pain condition, patients may suffer from depression due to their chronic pain. Serious insomnia due to the pain is also very common. Of course, issues like insomnia and depression make it that much harder to cope with a chronic pain condition.

Diagnosis

When a patient goes to a doctor's office to discuss their painful condition, generally the doctor will ask the patient to rate the pain on a 0-to-10 scale, 0 being no pain and 10 being the worst possible pain imaginable. The doctor may ask about pain descriptors, such as the quality of the pain, the frequency of their pain, the duration of the pain, what makes the pain better and worse, whether or not the pain moves around, and, in the case of postherpetic neuralgia, whether the rash was associated with the painful area prior to or preceding the chronic pain condition. Usually due to the fact that shingles generally involves only one nerve, the patient's pain will be located on only one side of their body and usually in a very well demarcated area. However, it can involve more than one nerve; it can involve, for instance, two adjacent nerves, or it can be on both sides of the body, but usually involves a single nerve on one side of the body. Generally, this clinical information is the most important part of diagnosing postherpetic neuralgia. The doctor may also look for objective findings such as scarring over the painful area caused by the rash. Next, the doctor may gently stoke the skin to see if light touch elicits a painful response. He or she may also want to check and see if there is any muscle weakness associated with this painful area.

Generally no specific tests such as x-ray, MRI, or laboratory studies need to be done to make this diagnosis, as it is generally thought to be a clinical diagnosis. Usually the herpes zoster outbreak arises due to no particular reason. However, a patient's doctor may want to explore potential causes for the herpes zoster outbreak.

Some of these associated causes may include a stressful situation such as changing of a career, moving, death of a loved one, etc. However, it may not only be caused by a stressful psychologic situation, but may be due to a physiologic stressful situation such as a chronic disease state. The doctor may be interested in ruling out infection, cancer, or some other disease state that may be physiologically stressing the patient's body.

Treatment Options

Treatment options for postherpetic neuralgia are now quite extensive. Of course, as mentioned above, the first line of treatment is to shorten the duration and severity of the herpes zoster rash. If this is done by aggressively treating with antiviral agents and/or nerve block injections, the patient may be less likely to develop the chronic pain condition known as postherpetic neuralgia.

Many patients can take medications to shorten the length and severity of the outbreak. As the name implies, herpes zoster is closely related to herpes simplex virus, which causes cold sores around the mouth and sores in the genital region. Therefore, it is not surprising that a herpes zoster outbreak can be effectively treated in a similar fashion. Antiviral medications such as acyclovir, valcyclovir, and other agents are frequently used.

Also, various nerve block injections have been shown to shorten the duration of the shingles rash. As a result, these patients seem less likely to develop the chronic pain syndrome, postherpetic neuralgia. Unfortunately, many patients do not seek medical attention until after it becomes a chronic nerve condition. Even so, there are still quite a few treatment options available to them to manage their chronic pain.

Some medications used for the treatment of postherpetic neuralgia include lidocaine patches, pregabalin (Lyrica), gabapentin (Neurontin), and duloxetine (Cymbalta). These medications are all FDA-approved for the treatment of postherpetic neuralgia. These are all fairly new medications, and your doctor may choose an older medication that is similar to these FDA-approved medications and prescribe it for "off-label" use. These medications can be grouped into several broad categories such as local anesthetics, antiseizure medications, and antidepressants.

Sometimes patients will respond well to nerve block injections. This may be thought of as an attempt to reset the nerve or retrain the nerve. Generally this type of nerve pain will respond quite well to local anesthetics that are injected around the nerve, which blocks the pain sensation. For instance, if somebody has postherpetic neuralgia in the face area, their doctor may refer them for a trigeminal nerve block, sphenopalatine block, or a stellate ganglion block. There are also small nerves that can be anesthetized in the face, which may provide significant pain relief. The local anesthetic that is used for blocking the nerve transmission generally lasts for only a couple of hours. However, the pain reduction may greatly exceed the two hours of local anesthetic duration.

A stellate ganglion block may also work well for nerve pain in the arm. The stellate ganglion is a bundle of nerves in the front of the neck that supplies sensation to the face and arm. By injecting this bundle of nerves with local anesthetic, the doctor can provide significant pain relief to the patient. This injection is done by having the patient lie on the back, while the injection is administered in the front part of the neck, just to the side of where the thyroid gland is located.

For somebody who has nerve pain in the chest or legs, a spinal injection known as an epidural or an injection just outside the spine which is known as a paravertebral block, may be beneficial in reducing the pain. The doctor may also decide to numb the nerves that run underneath each rib. This is known as an intercostal nerve block. All of these injections can have significant complications and side effects. These injections are only to be performed by doctors who have received specialized training. With repeated injections, the hope is that the pain reduction will outlast the local anesthetic duration and provide the patient with some significant long-term benefit.

Nerve stimulation techniques have been frequently used for the treatment of postherpetic neuralgia. This may involve the use of a transcutaneous electrical nerve stimulator (TENS unit). A TENS unit is basically EKG-type pads that are stuck onto the skin. These pads then are connected to wires, which connect to a battery pack. When turning the stimulator unit on, the patient will generally feel a tingling or pulsating feeling. This type of stimulation can trick the mind into feeling the stimulation, rather than the underlying postherpetic pain. There are a variety of these types of units on the market, each with some subtle differences. Some are distinguished by different waveforms, and some, instead of having pads that affix to the skin, may actually have a garment such as a glove or a sock that may be worn, or a sleeve that may be placed on the body to stimulate a larger area. If this type of external stimulation is not effective, an implantable spinal cord stimulator may be considered.

As discussed elsewhere in the book, spinal cord stimulation involves a surgical procedure where wires are placed inside the spinal column, on top of the spinal cord, in what is known as the epidural space. These wires are then connected to a pacemaker-type battery, which is also placed under the skin. The patient then has a remote control that can turn the battery on and off or turn the stimulation strength up or down. The patient will hopefully feel the stimulation pattern covering their painful area. If the stimulation is not felt where the patient's pain is located, adjustments can be made to change the stimulation area.

As with the external stimulator, it is hoped that the brain will find the stimulation more pleasing than the underlying painful condition. This may be likened to someone who smashes their finger with a hammer. The person's finger will, of course, be quite painful and throbbing. If, however, the person rubs their finger, the brain will frequently pick up the rubbing sensation rather than the throbbing painful finger. Unfortunately, when the person stops rubbing the finger, the brain again recognizes the throbbing pain in the hand.

Unfortunately, not everybody benefits from medications, injections, or stimulation. However, most people can benefit from a so-called cognitive behavioral approach to chronic pain. This may be thought of as a mind-over-matter approach to chronic pain. This is something that neuropsychologists routinely provide to patients to reduce their pain and suffering.

Various techniques that can be used for the cognitive behavioral approach include, but are not limited to, biofeedback, visual imagery, relaxation, and almost a self-hypnosis approach to chronic pain. Biofeedback can take many forms. In a classic setting, a patient may be hooked up to a blood pressure machine and an electrocardiogram (EKG) machine, and a temperature probe may be placed on their skin. The patient then learns how to use their mind to lower their blood pressure, heart rate, and skin temperature. Then this is taken one step further, and the patient is taught how to lower their pain level. Obviously, this is not like flipping a light switch, but takes a lot of practice. For this reason, it is generally reserved for those patients who are highly motivated and willing to practice biofeedback techniques on a daily basis.

Of course, prevention is the best medicine. With this in mind, we must not forget that there is a vaccine that adults may receive to reduce the risk of developing shingles (herpes zoster) outbreak. Unfortunately, most people do not realize this and never get the vaccine.

PROGNOSIS

Prognosis for postherpetic neuralgia can be quite good, especially when it is diagnosed early and treated fairly aggressively. Like any chronic medical condition, it is difficult to eliminate a chronic pain condition. However, if the patient's expectations and goals are appropriate, success can be achieved. For instance, a diabetic patient frequently understands that insulin may be required to achieve the goal of blood sugar control. Someone with high blood pressure expects to use medication, exercise, and diet to achieve better blood pressure control. Likewise, a patient with chronic pain may require chronic medications and other interventions to achieve the goal of pain control. Elimination of chronic pain, like the elimination of diabetes and hypertension, may not be a reasonable goal.

With the understanding that pain management success is usually greatest when a multidisciplinary approach is used, your doctor should consider this approach early on in your pain condition. This means that you should probably start not only with medications, but also consider nerve blocks, electrical stimulation, and biofeedback-type techniques. Frequently attacking the problem from more than one angle increases the likelihood of success.

ADDITIONAL RESOURCES

There are many articles, chapters, and even books written on postherpetic neuralgia. Unfortunately, most of these are written in quite technical terms and are geared toward people working in the medical field. These can sometimes be very difficult for patients to understand. Fortunately, with the advent of the Internet, there is quite a bit of information available to patients. Likewise, there are also many postherpetic neuralgia support groups, both in cyberspace and in local communities. Sometimes realizing that one is not alone in their suffering, but that there are others out there dealing with the same thing, can be beneficial in helping deal with this type of chronic pain condition. If one lives in a small community, sometimes just a general chronic pain support group can be beneficial. People in this type of a pain support group may include people who suffer from headaches, back pain, or other types of chronic pain conditions.

23

FOOT PAIN

Vanny Le, MD, and Tamer Elbaz, MD

The foot is comprised of 26 bones, 33 joints, and hundreds of muscles, ligaments, and nerves. It is not unexpected that with time, aging, and normal wear and tear, foot pain may develop for various reasons. Athletes, understandably, are more prone to pathological conditions due to trauma, physical overload, and repeated exertion. Acute injuries causing open fractures or obvious deformities should immediately be evaluated by medical personnel. Acute injuries should be distinguished from persistent foot pain and will not be discussed in this section.

Chronic foot pain may be secondary to nerve damage, arthritis, trauma, or disease processes that affect the entire body, such as diabetes or multiple sclerosis. However, the main cause of foot pain is biomechanical due to an intrinsic deformity (e.g., heel spur), external overload such as obesity, or an imbalance between the forces acting on the foot.

AGE-RELATED CHANGES CAUSING PAIN

The type of foot pain is often determined by growth and stresses faced at different stages of life. Children under the age of seven years rarely require postural correction due to the high degree of foot flexibility and the ability to adapt. Stress is rarely due to excess weight and pressure, but rather from strain at points of tendon insertions into immature bone formation sites. Osteochondrosis, a disease process of growing bones, is characterized by degeneration or death of the bone tissue followed by regeneration (regrowth) and calcification (deposition of calcium). It occurs most often in children between 8 and 12 years of age.

As children age into the teens and through to the mid-thirties, common causes of foot pain are due to sports-related activities. At this point in life, injury can be secondary to the discrepancy between growth and increased load placed on the maturing bones. Stress fractures are common in this age group and may need to be evaluated by a sports physician, orthopedic surgeon, or podiatrist to determine if the fracture requires surgical correction or stabilization.

Osteoarthritis, also known as degenerative arthritis or degenerative joint disease, is a condition of chronic inflammation and breakdown of the cartilage between the joint surfaces, causing pain, swelling, and stiffness. It tends to present in people in their thirties but can be seen in younger individuals who are active in sports that require intense running and jumping loads. Overall, the most common cause of foot pain is a condition called plantar fasciitis. Plantar fasciitis is an irritation and swelling of the thick tissue on the bottom of the foot. It is seen in 10–15 percent of all persistent foot pain cases and usually presents in this age group.

In people in their 40s and older, foot pain is usually a result of years of continued postural stress on the tendons, ligaments, and bones causing overload and anatomical deformities. Foot pronation is when the foot turns inward and flattens out the arch. Mild pronation occurs naturally when taking a step and the heel touches the ground to stabilize the foot and distribute the forces of impact. However, overpronation can lead to excessive stress and stretching on the inner ligaments and bones of the foot leading to adult-acquired flatfoot and arthritis of the ankle. Flatfeet can cause the foot to lengthen, which creates an imbalance between the muscles that flex and extend the foot and toes. This may eventually produce tension on the weaker muscles in the toes and cause claw toes or hammertoes. However, underlying systemic diseases such as diabetes, neuromuscular disorders (multiple sclerosis, cerebral palsy, Charcot-Marie-Tooth disease), and inflammatory conditions (rheumatoid arthritis, psoriasis) must also be considered as risk factors for toe deformities.

Other abnormalities seen in older people include bunions (first toe) and bunionettes (fifth toe) from wearing shoes that are too tight. As people age, there is deterioration of the fat pads underneath the ball of the foot and the heel that cushion the impact when taking a step. Osteoarthritis affecting the midfoot and ankle joints develops after years of wear and tear but may develop earlier in overweight people and athletes. Finally, inflammation of the tendon on the inside of the ankle (tibialis posterior tenosynovitis) produces significant pain and possible collapse of the ankle. This condition generally occurs in people in their 50s and 60s.

SPECIFIC CONDITIONS

Table 23.1 shows common causes of foot pain divided into areas of the foot. The major conditions causing foot pain will be covered in this section.

Table 23.1
Common Causes of Foot Pain

Heel Pain	Arch Pain	Ball of Foot Pain
• Plantar fasciitis	• Plantar fasciitis	• Neuroma
• Heel spurs	• Flat foot	• Metatarsalgia
• Sever's disease		• Plantar warts
• Bursitis		• Freiberg's disease
• Haglund's deformity		• Sesamoiditis
Toe Pain	**Big Toe Pain**	**Ankle Pain**
• Ingrown toenail	• Bunions	• Sprained ankle
• Claw toes	• Bunion surgery	• Tarsal tunnel
• Hammer toes	• Gout	syndrome
	• Hallux rigidus	• Achilles tendinitis
		• Achilles tendon rupture
Whole Foot Pain	**Nerve Pain**	**Skin Pain**
• Burning foot	• Neuroma	• Cracked heel
• Poor circulation	• Burning foot	• Foot corns and calluses
	• Tarsal tunnel syndrome	• Ingrown toenail
	• Peripheral neuropathy	• Chilblains
	• Charcot's foot	

Heel Pain

Plantar Fasciitis/Heel Spurs

Plantar fasciitis is the most common cause of heel pain complaints. It is also known as heel spur syndrome or plantar fasciosis. The plantar fascia is a thick, fibrous band underneath the foot that attaches at the inner heel, spans under the arch and spreads out to the ball of the foot. Weight-bearing overload produces a downward force on the foot that can cause stress to the heel bone and stretch the plantar fascia. Overpronation, where the foot turns too far inward and the arch flattens out, will also overextend the fascia. The continued tension on the plantar fascia generates pain from inflammation and tearing of the fibers away from the heel bone. Over time, the body tries to reattach the band by depositing new calcium at the heel, which may produce a heel spur or bony protrusion. The body may eventually reabsorb the calcium deposits, but if it doesn't, the heel spur itself can be a source of heel pain. Only about 5 percent of heel spurs cause pain, and therefore, not all heel spurs need to be removed. The presence of a heel spur seen on x-ray usually means that the condition has been present for longer than six months.

- Risk factors for plantar fasciitis
  - High arch
  - Tight calf muscles that make it difficult to bend ankle upwards
  - Obesity
  - Repetitive high impact sports such as running

- Symptoms
  - Isolated heel pain
  - Pain with weight-bearing, especially when taking the first step and after periods of rest
  - Pain when walking barefoot or with thin shoes
  - Pain when pressing on the bottom of the foot near the heel
  - Pain when turning the ankle up towards the head
  - Pain when stretching the foot and pulling the toes up
- Treatment
  - First line—Conservative (no procedures) treatment should be tried for six weeks prior to moving on to second-line treatment
    - Rest
    - Ice
    - Regular Achilles tendon/calf muscle and plantar fascia stretching exercises
    - Over-the-counter orthotic insoles for arch and heel support
    - Changing to appropriately padded shoes with modest heel; avoid flat shoes and walking barefoot
    - Anti-inflammatory medications (aspirin, ibuprofen, etc.)
    - Corticosteroid injections in the bottom of the foot to decrease inflammation
    - Home physical therapy
  - Second line—Patients should follow second-line therapies for at least six months before considering more invasive treatment. Eighty-five to 90 percent of people have resolution of symptoms in two to three months using first- and second-line therapy and 90–95 percent have complete resolution within one year.
    - Continue first-line treatments
    - Orthotic devices
    - Night splints to stretch and keep the foot extended during sleep
    - Repeat corticosteroid injections
    - Botulinum toxin injections
    - Physical therapy
    - Short-term cast immobilization or walking boot
    - Weight loss
  - Third line
    - Surgical correction—plantar fascia release or calf muscle release
    - Possible nerve release if nerve entrapment is also implicated in pain syndrome
    - Extracorporeal shock wave therapy (ESWT)—noninvasive shockwaves to the bottom of the foot may stimulate healing

Sever's Disease

Sever's disease or calcaneal apophysitis is a condition seen in children and adolescents ages 8–12. Usually, it occurs more in children who are active in sports, but can occur in less active children. Chronic injury or compression of the growth plates in the heel from overuse and repetitive activity can cause both inflammation and pain. Sever's disease typically resolves on its own with rest in three to six weeks.

- Risk factors for Sever's disease
  - Obesity
  - Athletic children, especially in soccer, basketball, track, and running
  - Tight calf muscles
  - Pronated feet (turned inwards)
- Symptoms
  - Heel pain worse with activity, especially running and jumping
  - Pain over the back of the heel where the Achilles tendon attaches to the heel bone
  - Tightness of the Achilles tendon
  - Weakness when flexing the ankle upwards
  - Pain on the inside and outside of the foot at the heel
- Treatment
  - Rest
  - Ice
  - Short-term immobilization or restricted weight-bearing
  - Over-the-counter analgesics
  - Heel cups, pads, or lifts for pain relief
  - Home or professional physical therapy to stretch and strengthen calf muscles

Heel Bursitis

Bursitis is inflammation of a bursa (fluid-filled sac) that provides a cushion between bone and tendons or bones and muscles. Heel bursitis can occur in the bursa that protects and lubricates movement of the Achilles tendon over the heel bone. Bursitis may occur from constant rubbing and pressure on the heel from ill-fitting shoes. It is more common in young women in their 20s and 30s who wear heels. In addition, it can also occur in people with Haglund's deformity, which is a bony protuberance on the back of the heel caused by repeated friction. Haglund's deformity is also known as "pump bump" because it is often seen in women who wear high-heeled shoes (i.e., pumps) or anybody who wears shoes with rigid backs. The protuberance may or may not cause pain. However, it is frequently associated with heel bursitis because it is a common site of irritation where the bone rubs against the shoe.

- Risk factors for heel bursitis
  - Females, aged 20s–30s
  - Obesity
- Symptoms
  - Pain aggravated by shoe wear
  - Pain relieved when barefoot or with backless shoes
- Treatment
  - Open-back shoes
  - Nonsteroidal anti-inflammatory drugs (NSAIDs)

- o Injection into the bursa
- o Orthotics to pad the heel or heel lifts
- o Physical therapy
- o Weight loss
- o Surgical resection of inflamed bursa and/or removal of Haglund's deformity if conservative treatments are ineffective

Arch Pain

Adult Acquired Flatfoot

There are multiple causes of adult acquired flatfoot. The most common etiology is a mechanical dysfunction and loss of the structural support of the foot arch. The posterior tibial tendon is a tendon that runs just behind the inner ankle bone and underneath the foot. It is one of the major support structures for the foot arch. When it contracts, it causes the foot to flex downward and turn inward, and the arch to heighten. This allows for the mid- and rear-foot to become rigid and to stabilize the foot when walking. If there is dysfunction of the posterior tibial tendon, the ligaments and the joints in the foot weaken, and flatfoot develops.

Other important causes must be ruled out, such as fractures and dislocations. Rheumatoid arthritis, osteoarthritis, or other degenerative changes in the ankles and foot joints can lead to flatfoot. Systemic diseases like diabetes and leprosy that cause nerve damage are also conditions that may cause adult acquired flatfoot. Evaluation by a physician is recommended to ensure that untreated underlying diseases are not missed.

- • Risk factors for adult acquired flatfoot
  - o Congenital flatfeet
  - o Obesity
  - o Hypertension
  - o Middle-aged women
  - o Steroid injections around the tendon
  - o Inflammatory diseases (e.g., rheumatoid arthritis, psoriasis, ankylosing spondylitis)
  - o Previous surgery or trauma
- • Symptoms
  - o Pain and/or swelling behind the inner ankle bone and along the arch
  - o Change in the shape of the foot or worsening flatfeet
  - o Instability when walking or inability to walk long distances
  - o Weakness and difficulty standing on toes
  - o Foot turns out or "too many toes" sign
- • Treatment
  - o Rest
  - o Nonsteroidal anti-inflammatory medications by mouth
  - o Short-term immobilization in a cast or walking boot
  - o Orthotics to support heel and arch

- ○ Physical therapy
- ○ Surgery

Ankle Pain

Achilles Tendon Disorders

The Achilles tendon is the strongest tendon in the body. It attaches the calf muscles to the heel bone and is located behind the ankle and must withstand considerable forces. Disorders of the Achilles tendon, or tendinopathies (which means "disorders of the tendons"), are known as Achilles tendinitis or Achilles tendinosis. Tendinitis implies that inflammation occurs, while tendinosis refers to a pathological condition where the tendon sustains micro-tears and other structural changes. Most tendon disorders do not involve inflammation.

There are three types of Achilles tendinopathies based on location in the tendon and are considered either insertional or noninsertional disorders. Noninsertional tendinopathies are two to three times more common than insertional tendinopathies. The younger and more active people usually sustain noninsertional tendinosis injuries that are located higher up in the ankle and further away from where the tendon attaches to the heel bone. These injuries occur from sports, chronic noninflammatory degeneration from repetitive damage, and overuse. On the contrary, poor training techniques, improper warmup, overpronation of the foot, and inappropriate footwear all contribute to Achilles tendinitis, which occurs in the same location. The second type of Achilles tendinopathy, located in the upper heel/ankle, is associated with Haglund's deformity or pump bump. This was previously discussed in the heel pain section. Lastly, the third type of tendinopathy is age-related and occurs at the tendon insertion site above the heel bone. This insertional tendinopathy occurs in the elderly population from degeneration and calcification of the tendon and the heel bone.

Partial or complete rupture of the Achilles tendon is characteristically seen in athletes or the "weekend warrior" (participating in sports only on weekends). The latter are people in their 30s–50s and who are normally sedentary (physically inactive or minimally active) but who also participate in sports. The sudden acceleration of certain movements such as basketball or racket sports injures an already damaged tendon with micro-tears and calcification. There is also an association with Achilles tendon ruptures and certain types of antibiotics usage. This group of antibiotics is collectively called fluoroquinolones (e.g., ciprofloxacin).

- • Risk factors for Achilles tendon disorders
  - ○ Noninsertional
    - ■ Sudden increases in the amount or intensity of exercise
    - ■ Tight calf muscles
    - ■ Bone spurs or Haglund's deformity
    - ■ Ill-fitting shoes
    - ■ Overpronated foot (excessive pronation)

- Symptoms
  - Pain and stiffness along Achilles tendon in the morning
  - Pain along the tendon that increases with activity
  - Pain the day after exercising
  - Thickening or enlargement of the tendon
  - Swelling of the tendon
  - Decreased ability to move the foot, especially flexing the ankle upwards
- Treatment
  - Rest
  - Ice
  - Nonsteroidal anti-inflammatory medications for pain relief
  - Immobilization with a fracture boot for severe cases
  - Exercise and stretching of calf muscles
  - Physical therapy
  - Proper-fitting shoes
  - Orthotics for heel support or heel lifts
  - Surgery can be considered if pain does not subside after six months

Tarsal Tunnel Syndrome

Tarsal tunnel syndrome in the ankle is similar to carpal tunnel syndrome of the wrist. Characterized by pain on the inner ankle, it is caused by compression of the posterior tibial nerve in a thick, fibrous sheath called the flexor retinaculum. Tarsal tunnel syndrome can be confused with plantar fasciitis or heel spurs. However, the pain of tarsal tunnel syndrome is more diffuse than plantar fasciitis. It can be caused by various reasons, including trauma from severe ankle sprains or crush injuries. In addition, any mass that takes up extra space within the tarsal tunnel can compress the nerve. For example, cysts, tumors, blood vessels, or ganglions can all be the source of tarsal tunnel syndrome.

- Risk factors for tarsal tunnel syndrome
  - Rheumatoid arthritis
  - Poor circulation causing foot swelling
  - Fractures
  - Hypothyroidism (decreased activity of the thyroid gland)
- Symptoms
  - Pain, burning, or tingling behind the inner ankle bone, over the base of the heel, or on the sole of the foot
  - Pain can occur at rest as disease progresses
  - Tapping or touching behind the inner ankle bone or at the heel can produce tingling further down the foot
- Treatment
  - Strapping the foot or wearing an orthotic to keep the foot turned slightly inward relieves pressure on the nerve
  - Steroid injection to reduce inflammation
  - Surgical excision of the mass causing the pain
  - Surgical release of flexor retinaculum

Ball of Foot Pain

Metatarsalgia/Morton's Neuroma

Metatarsalgia refers to pain in the ball of the foot. It is often called a disease in itself, which is a misnomer. Metatarsalgia is actually the symptom of overuse injuries that cause stress on the metatarsals or the bones located in the ball of the foot at the base of the toes. There are multiple etiologies for metatarsalgia, including Freiberg's disease, sesamoiditis, and toe deformities, but the most common cause of metatarsalgia is Morton's neuroma. The term neuroma suggests that there is an abnormal growth of nerve tissue. However, Morton's neuroma is in fact due to compression and irritation of the nerves that innervate the area between the toes and is also called interdigital neuritis. A palpable mass can sometimes be felt due to a thickening of the fibrous sheath surrounding the nerve. It usually occurs at the ball of the foot between the second and third toes (80–85 percent) and between the third and fourth toes (15–20 percent).

- Risk factors for metatarsalgia
  - Middle-aged women 4:1 or 78 percent
  - Wearing poor-fitting and constricting shoes
  - Chronic and excessive toe flexion such as in prolonged running, walking, squatting, or ballet
- Symptoms
  - Pain and/or burning and tingling in the web spaces (areas at the base of the toes)
  - Pain worse with walking, especially in high heels or shoes with a narrow toe-box
  - Pain is intermittent and can last for minutes to hours
  - Numbness in the toes surrounding the neuroma
  - Compression of the forefoot with simultaneous pressure between the web space will reproduce the pain; sometimes a click will be heard (Muldur sign)
  - Massage of the area relieves the symptoms
- Treatment
  - Change to low-heel shoes with a wide toe-box
  - Shoe padding at the ball of the foot
  - Stretching
  - Ice
  - Deep tissue massage
  - Cryotherapy
  - Ultrasound therapy
  - Medications for tingling/numbness
  - Surgical removal

24

Cancer Pain and Palliative Care

Arash Asher, MD

Introduction

Cancer pain can be complex as it can be due to the cancer itself, the cancer treatment, or possibly unrelated causes. Whatever its cause, pain can affect many aspects of a person's life, including physical functioning, ability to think clearly, emotional outlook, and ability to socialize. About 30–50 percent of cancer patients experience pain. The prevalence is much higher with advanced disease (over 80%). Given that pain is frequently associated with cancer, *all* cancer patients should be routinely screened for pain.

Palliative care specialists are doctors who specialize in a type of care whose goal is to prevent and alleviate suffering. They help people with serious illnesses, such as cancer, relieve pain and other symptoms and make informed decisions about treatment. Working as part of a team, they help patients and their loved ones with the emotional, physical, and spiritual needs to address the whole person and not just the disease.

Palliative care is sometimes erroneously confused with end-of-life care and shortening life. In fact, a recent study shows it not only improves the quality of life, but it actually extends it. This may be because of its holistic approach to care, its focus on keeping people as active as possible, and treating symptoms such as pain, nausea, shortness of breath, and the anxieties and worries that are common among cancer patients. People whose pain is treated often sleep better, eat better, connect more with friends and family, and therefore may also live longer as this recent important study suggested. Palliative care is for people of any age, at any stage of illness—whether the illness is curable, chronic, or life-threatening. Palliative medicine specialists work in collaboration with other doctors, who may be providing treatments to cure or reverse the illness. Regardless of the prognosis, the goal is to improve the quality of life as best as possible for the patient and family.

It is extremely important that you communicate openly with your physician so that your symptoms, including pain, can be well managed. The importance of controlling pain is not only to alleviate unnecessary suffering, but also to promote healing. What follows is an overview on cancer pain management. Hopefully, it will allow for a more informed and thoughtful discussion with your health care provider regarding your needs or the needs of a loved one.

SYMPTOMS

Pain is not objective and cannot be measured easily as is blood pressure or body temperature. Since there are no blood tests for measuring pain, clinicians often use some type of scale to help understand the intensity of pain. For example, the visual analogue scale is often used. With this scale, zero is no pain and 10 is the worst imaginable pain. In this way, your pain can be tracked over time using the same scale so that your clinician can know whether your treatment is working or not. Especially in the cancer setting, pain is often not an isolated problem. For example, pain can affect sleep, appetite, and energy. Alternatively, depression and anxiety can worsen pain. For this reason, it's important to not only discuss not only your pain, but other commonly associated symptoms for optimal treatment.

Once the intensity of pain and other symptoms has been established, the pain will need to be better described to help determine the best treatment. Where is the pain located? Does it radiate or spread anywhere? What makes the pain worse? What makes the pain better? Is it constant? Or is the pain triggered with certain activities, such as walking, coughing, or moving an arm? Constant pain that is steady regardless of activity or movement may be treated very differently from pain that is minimal or absent at rest, but worst with certain movements or positions (often called "incidental pain").

For physicians, it is also often helpful to differentiate between two broad categories of pain: "*nociceptive*" pain versus "*neuropathic*" pain. Nociceptive pain is pain caused by injury to tissue. For example, a cancer growing into lung tissue or bone may cause injury and therefore pain. Nociceptive pain may be described as "aching," "stabbing," "throbbing," or "crampy." In contrast, neuropathic pain is pain caused by injury to the nervous system. Neuropathic pain is often described as "burning," "electrical," or "shock-like." It may be worse at night. Approximately 40 percent of cancer-related pain involves neuropathic pain, which can be a result of the cancer or its treatment. Many patients have a combination of both "neuropathic" and "nociceptive" pain. Packaging all this information will help your physician better determine the cause of the pain and determine the best treatments.

DIAGNOSIS

Oral Mucositis

Our digestive tracts, including our mouths, are lined with a protective layer called mucous membranes. Mucositis is the painful inflammation and ulceration of these protective membranes. It can be a result of many different chemotherapy regimens and typically becomes evident after the first week of chemotherapy. The severity can range from mild mouth soreness to severe pain with an inability to eat or drink. Remember, chemotherapy can affect normal, non-cancer cells as well! The agents most commonly associated with mucositis include doxorubicin, fluorouracil, bleomycin, cytarabine, and methotrexate, although other chemotherapy drugs may also cause this problem. Virtually all patients who receive radiation therapy to the head and neck region also develop mucositis. In addition, since these mucous membranes line the entire digestive tract, mucositis can develop throughout the entire tract. This can result in (1) difficult or painful swallowing (when the membranes in the esophagus or food pipe are affected); (2) abdominal pain (when the membranes in the stomach are affected); and (3) diarrhea (membranes in the colon and small bowel are affected). Fortunately, the pain resolves in most patients within one to two weeks after chemotherapy, and radiation therapy ends as the mucous membranes regenerate.

You and your physician can take a number of steps to minimize the risk and severity of mucositis. Make sure to have a comprehensive oral examination with a dentist that is familiar with cancer care. Taking care of any oral problems such as cavities, teeth that need extracting, and other oral hygiene as recommended by your dentist may reduce your chances for complications (such as infection) related to mucositis. Speak to your physician about medications that can prevent the severity of mucositis, such as palifermin and L-glutamine. These strategies are now being actively studied and may prove to be useful in preventing this self-limited but painful condition.

Bone Pain

Bone metastasis, or the spread of cancer to the bones, is the most common reason for chronic pain among cancer patients. However, it is important to realize that 75 percent of patients with bone metastasis have *no pain* whatsoever. We don't really know why some individuals have bone pain and others do not. Therefore, try not to convince yourself you have pain solely because an x-ray shows a mass in your bones! Lung, breast, and prostate cancer are cancers with the most frequent spread to the bone. The most common site of bone metastasis is the vertebrae (the bones along the spine). If the cancer spreads beyond the vertebrae and into the spinal cord, this can cause potentially irreversible nerve damage. Since back or neck pain almost always occurs *before* any nerve damage, it is very important for any cancer patient to be evaluated with any new back or neck pain to rule out this significant complication.

Magnetic resonance imaging (MRI) is the best way to look at the bones and spinal cord. Other bones may be involved as well. For example, metastases to the bones in the pelvis and hips may occur, which can feel like pain in the hip, groin, or thigh and is worst with walking. Pain in the sacrum (tailbone) may feel like pain in the buttocks or back of the thigh.

Visceral Pain

Visceral pain refers to pain of any of the internal organs, such as the lung or liver. These pain syndromes are most common in those with gastrointestinal cancers (such as pancreas or liver) and gynecologic cancer (such as ovarian or cervical). Pain is experienced when the tumor causes obstruction of any of the tubes of the body, such as when the bowel or ureter (tube that propels urine from the kidney to the bladder) is obstructed. Pain due to obstruction may be "colicky" and "wave-like." Pain can also be experienced if the tumor injures or irritates another pain-sensitive structure. For example, a liver mass may be painless, but if it irritates the capsule (which encases the liver) or the blood vessels of the liver (which do send pain signals), then the mass may be painful.

Soft Tissue Pain

Soft tissues refer to our tendons, ligaments, and muscles. Some cancers, such as sarcomas, can arise from muscle and may result in pain at that local area. Some patients with lung cancer can experience pain along the tissues of the chest wall, which may be worse with coughing or deep inspiration. Muscle pain may also be due to muscular cramps, which may be due to electrolyte abnormalities or nerve injury.

Neuropathic Pain

Cancer and its treatment may cause a number of neuropathic pain syndromes (pain involving the nervous system). Our nervous system includes the nerves of the brain, spinal cord, and all the nerves that leave the spinal cord to connect to our organs, arms, and legs. What follows is a brief overview of some of these syndromes.

Leptomeningeal Disease: Leptomeninges refer to the thin membranes that surround the brain and spinal cord. Any cancer can potentially spread to this region, but the most common tumors are lung and breast cancer, leukemia, and lymphoma. The symptoms may be vague, such as headache, back pain, or neurological symptoms such as weakness, numbness, or difficulty with thinking. An MRI of the brain or spinal cord may show evidence for leptomeningeal disease. The definitive diagnosis is made by a lumbar puncture or "spinal tap."

Cranial Neuralgias: This involves pain related to the nerves from cancers of the head, neck, or sinuses. The pain may feel like a severe, one-sided, stabbing, or electrical pain, depending on which nerve may be affected.

Radiculopathy and Plexopathy: The brain sends motor commands through our spinal cord and through nerves, such as to clinch a fist or move a leg; there are also return signals from the arms and legs that tell our brains whether we may be experiencing heat or cold, pain, or vibratory senses. We have 31 pairs of nerve roots that connect our brains with our arms, legs, and trunks. A nerve plexus is a network of some of these intersecting nerves, which combine sets of nerves that serve the same area of the body into one large grouped nerve. The two largest are the brachial plexus, which serves the chest, shoulders, arm, and hand, and the lumbo-sacral plexus, which serves the thighs, legs, feet, buttocks, and genitals.

Inflammation, irritation, or compression of a nerve root is called a radiculopathy. When the nerve plexus is involved, it is called plexopathy. Either a radiculopathy or plexopathy can be caused by a cancer or sometimes as a complication from radiation therapy (i.e., if radiation therapy caused damage to one or some of the nerves as an innocent bystander). The pain may be burning or electrical-like and will spread in the direction of the involved nerve. For example, if a cervical nerve root is irritated, pain can radiate from the neck to the part of the arm or hand that the particular nerve root serves. In addition to pain, some may experience weakness and/or changes in sensation in the involved part of the nerve.

The diagnosis of radiculopathy or plexopathy is typically made by an MRI of the involved region of the nervous system. Further testing with electromyography and nerve conduction testing, which uses a computer and special equipment to study the functioning of the nerves, may help clarify the diagnosis by pinpointing which nerves may be exactly involved.

Peripheral Neuropathy: Some chemotherapy medications cause pain because they damage the ends of the nerves that reach our feet and hands. The nerves that go to your toes are the farthest away from the spinal cord (which has its nutritional stores) and therefore are most susceptible to the toxicities of chemotherapy. The pain may be described as "burning," "numbing," or "electrical-like." It is called "peripheral" neuropathy because the nerves are in the periphery, or far away from the spinal cord. Typically, the pain from chemotherapy-related peripheral neuropathy improves with time, but some patients have persistent pain. In addition, although the pain improves with most patients, some may have residual numbness and difficulty with balance as a result of the neuropathy.

Postsurgical Pain Syndromes: A number of pain syndromes have been described after various types of cancer surgeries. These include post-mastectomy pain syndrome, post-thoracotomy (lung surgery) pain, phantom limb pain, and post-radical neck dissection. These syndromes seem to be primarily neuropathic, which means they involve irritation of the nerves and usually involve burning, electrical, or tingling pain. Please see Chapter 16 for a more detailed discussion of phantom limb pain, which is very similar in nature to these other syndromes.

Paraneoplastic Syndromes

Paraneoplastic syndromes are not caused directly by the tumor. Sometimes our immune system reacts to the tumor or substances released by the tumor. Rarely, the immune response can inadvertently attack some of our healthy cells as well. This may result in syndromes that cause pain. *Hypertrophic osteoarthropathy* is one example, which may result in joint pains, such as in the hands, ankles, and legs. This is most often associated with lung cancer. Another example is *subacute sensory neuronopathy*, which is a result of inflammation of the nerve roots as it exits the spinal cord. It typically results in "pins and needles" or "electrical shocks" in the arms, legs, or trunk over the course of a few weeks to months.

TREATMENT OPTIONS

For many, a cancer diagnosis comes with an immediate flood of fears and worries. Images of uncontrollable, severe pain and other symptoms such as nausea and vomiting are automatic for some. Many of these fears are not unfounded, since in the past, proven and effective pain management often was not available or understood. Today, pain physicians have a vast armamentarium of medications, interventions, and approaches to cancer pain. Adequate pain relief can be achieved in over 90 percent of cancer patients by following well-accepted international treatment guidelines. Unfortunately, over 40 percent of cancer patients' pain is undertreated today due to inadequate skills or knowledge from the health care provider, barriers from the health care system, and even patients' fears of utilizing effective treatments due to concerns for addiction or even an irrational sense of defeat.

It is fair to say that pain results in unnecessary suffering, reduces the ability to spend quality time with loved ones, makes it difficult to reintegrate into the community, and may result in extended or repeated hospital admissions. Therefore, it is incumbent upon pain management physicians to work closely with their patients to develop a personalized plan to manage pain as effectively and quickly as possible with the goal of maximizing quality of life.

Although this chapter has focused exclusively on the management of cancer pain, it must be emphasized that cancer pain is *best* managed in the context of palliative care, which focuses on a broad array of other symptoms (such as fatigue, appetite, anxiety, sleep, depression, etc.) and also integration of social, emotional, physical, and existential needs as part of the comprehensive, individualized plan. What follows is a discussion on some of the general principles of cancer pain management with some recommendations on select cancer pain syndromes.

The first step in cancer pain management is to determine whether any cancer treatment (such as surgery, chemotherapy, or radiation therapy) may help the pain as long as it is in line with the patient's goals. Even if active cancer treatment is being pursued, oftentimes your symptoms may need to be treated symptomatically while this is undertaken.

Mild to Moderate Pain

If your pain is mild, simple acetaminophen or a nonsteroidal anti-inflammatory agent (NSAID) such as ibuprofen or naproxen may be adequate and inexpensive. You should discuss with your physician if there are any reasons why these medications may be unsafe for you. For example, you will want to avoid NSAIDs if you have kidney disease or a history of stomach ulcers. You will want to avoid or limit acetaminophen if you have liver disease. Even if you have more severe pain that requires stronger medication, using one of these medications may be a very useful adjunct that may lower the amount of other medication that you may require. In fact, some stronger pain medications combine acetaminophen or an NSAID with a mild opioid to increase its efficacy. For example, Vicodin combines hydrocodone (a mild opioid) with acetaminophen. The main limitation is that there are specific limits on how much of acetaminophen or an NSAID that you can take each day safely.

Other medications that are considered for mild to moderate pain include tramadol and codeine. Tramadol should be avoided if you have a history of seizures and used cautiously with many antidepressants. Codeine is a mild opioid that is often combined with acetaminophen and may provide adequate pain relief with mild to moderate pain.

Moderate to Severe Pain

The cornerstone of moderate to severe cancer pain management is *opioids* (narcotics). Typical examples of medications in this category include morphine, oxycodone, fentanyl, hydromorphone, and methadone (see Chapters 6 and 7). Before discussing their use, it is important to clarify concerns regarding abuse or misuse of these medications (see Chapter 9). Addiction refers to the continued inappropriate use of a medication, such as opioid, with significant craving and loss of control with continued use despite the harm it may be causing. All of these medications are *potentially* abusable or addictive. Sometimes addictive personalities run in some families. If you have a history of alcoholism or drug abuse, there is a concern for potential addiction to opioid medications. This does not mean that opioids cannot or should not be used to control cancer pain! It simply means that these medications need to be discussed with your physician and used in a thoughtful manner, taking into consideration your individual background. Everyone taking opioid medications should be cognizant about using these medications to treat physical pain and not emotional, spiritual, or psychological suffering. This requires a level of introspection and careful assessment with your physician. These caveats said, addiction is *very uncommon* in the cancer setting, and opioids should not be withheld since they are extremely useful in cancer pain management. It's also worth pointing out that addiction is entirely different from "tolerance," which means that the medication may be less effective over time and you may require more of the same medication to produce the same effect over time. Your physician can manage this issue by increasing the dosage or "rotating" to a new opioid.

Opioids are generally *effective, reliable*, and *safe* in treating a wide array of cancer pain syndromes if they are used appropriately. They are most commonly and easily taken by mouth. However, if one is unable to take medication by mouth, opioids can be given intravenously (IV), subcutaneously (SQ), rectally, or through the skin with use of a patch. Among the various opioids that are available, there is no convincing evidence that any one opioid is better than any other. Therefore, if cost is an issue, speak to your physician about using a medication that is less expensive as an initial trial, and then only transitioning to a different one if not working effectively. The only caveat to this rule is that some pain experts feel that methadone may be the most effective pain medication, and it may help both nociceptive pain and neuropathic pain. Prescribing this medication safely and appropriately requires special training and knowledge. Therefore, this medication is typically only used by physicians who have experience with its use.

Opioids come in both long-acting and short-acting forms. If your pain is constant (i.e., it's there most of the day and night), you would probably most benefit from an opioid that lasts a long time and only needs to be taken once or twice a day on a fixed, "around-the-clock" schedule. If you experience breakthrough pain despite taking these long-acting medications, then a very short-acting medication should be used to control your pain. If you need to use a short-acting pain medication more than three or four times a day, then your long-acting pain medication is insufficient. In general, there is no maximum dose of opioid that can be safely given each day, in contrast to acetaminophen or NSAIDs. Your physician may increase the dose of the medication until the pain is reasonably controlled or until a side effect develops—whichever comes first.

Opioid Side Effects

Part of the success of opioid medications will depend on managing potential side effects. The most common and persistent side effect is constipation. Many doctors will start their patients on a bowel regimen prophylactically—before the problem begins—to avoid this problem, which can also make nausea and loss of appetite worse. Typically prescribed medications are docusate and senna, but many bowel regimens can be used to effectively manage this problem. Additionally, some patients can develop mental clouding with opioids. Typically this improves in a matter of days or weeks as your body acclimates to the medication. If it does not go away or if it is severe, the dosage of your medication can be reduced (as long as your pain is still controlled), your doctor can try an alternate opioid, or sometimes your doctor can add a stimulant medication, such as methylphenidate, to help with alertness. Decreasing your breathing rate is the most serious and dangerous side effect of opioids. However, this is virtually *never* a problem when accepted guidelines are followed when prescribing these medications. This problem primarily occurs when opioids are used to treat emotional suffering and not physical pain. In addition, significant sedation always precedes this problem, so there is an opportunity to intervene if necessary. Nausea sometimes occurs when first starting an opioid, which also can be managed with a variety of antinausea medications or choosing an alternate opioid. Typically this goes away within a few days or weeks. A number of other potential side effects include itching and, rarely, muscle spasms or a paradoxical increase in pain due to opioids. These need to be discussed with your physician.

Adjuvant Medications

Adjuvant medications are those that were originally intended to treat other conditions, but may be useful managing some types of pain as well.

All Types of Pain: Corticosteroids such as dexamethasone may be useful for various types of pain, including pain due to bowel obstruction, neuropathic pain, or any pain that's felt to have inflammation associated with it. It's also very useful to help with fatigue and stimulate appetite. Its main limitation is that its use is limited typically to one to three weeks to avoid long-term side effects of corticosteroids, such as increased risk of infection.

Neuropathic Pain: Increasingly, more and more medications are being used with some success for neuropathic pain. Certain antidepressants can be very effective for neuropathic pain as they affect serotonin levels and other substances that modulate pain. They can simultaneously help treat any concomitant depression as well. If there is no depressed mood, a variety of antiseizure drugs are available that can be effective. Most commonly, a medication called gabapentin (Neurontin) or pregabalin (Lyrica) is used, since neither has many side effects. There are numerous other medications that may be useful adjuncts for neuropathic pain that should be discussed with your physician. Keep in mind that typically these medications take several days to a few weeks before knowing if it is working for you.

A variety of topical (applied to the skin) medications can be used for pain that is limited to a defined, small area. For example, a lidocaine patch or capsaicin cream can be applied to the skin and it can provide effective pain relief.

Bone Pain: NSAIDs can work quite well for bone pain if they are deemed safe for you to use by your doctor. A class of medication called bisphosphonates may also be useful for helping some cancers with bone pain. More importantly, it seems to also prevent bone fractures for patients whose cancer has spread to the bone. Corticosteroids can be very effectively used for short periods of time for bone pain that is significant. If one has a single or a few specific areas of bone pain, radiation to the area can provide extremely effective pain relief.

For bone pain that is located in multiple sites that has not responded to other measures, some centers can provide a treatment using radioisotopes, which is a nuclear medicine procedure.

Mucositis Pain: Oral rinses with a weak solution of salt and baking soda (one-half teaspoon of salt and one teaspoon of baking soda in a quart of water) every four hours are important in order to keep the area clean. Try to avoid foods that make the pain worse, such as acidic, salty, or dry foods. With mild pain, symptoms can usually be controlled with a combination of topical medications that coat the membranes of the mouth. These are prepared in many hospital pharmacies and include a combination of diphenhydramine (Benadryl), oral antacids, lidocaine, or other agents. Sometimes the pain is so severe that some require opioids to be given intravenously and even nutritional feeding intravenously for a short period of time.

Interventional Approaches (Procedures)

Over 90 percent of cancer pain can be well managed with medications. When it cannot, one can consider any increasing array of available procedures and interventions. These include delivering medications directly into the spinal cord area, a vast array of nerve blocks, and orthopedic and neurosurgical procedures. The details of these procedures are beyond the scope of this chapter, but should be kept in mind for pain that cannot otherwise be well managed using the principles discussed above. See Chapters 26 and 27 for more information.

Alternative and Nonpharmacologic Options

Exercise is emerging as one of the most important tools we know about to decrease cancer-related fatigue, boost your mood, support your immune system, and improve sleep. Exercise also promotes the production of natural endorphins, which can decrease pain overall. In addition, most oncologists look at your physical capacity to determine how much further anticancer treatment you can tolerate. Therefore, continuing to remain as engaged and active as possible in a safe matter is paramount. You need to find the right exercise type and intensity for you, because engaging in exercise that is too strenuous can also be harmful. For example, if your bones are fragile because of large bone metastasis, you may need to avoid high-impact exercise. Your physician can help delineate a program that can best meet your needs.

There are many nonpharmacologic options to treat pain and improve wellness. Ultrasound, acupuncture, psychological therapies, hypnosis, massage, ice or heat packs, nerve stimulation techniques (such as transcutaneous electric nerve stimulation or TENS), guided imagery, and biofeedback are all approaches that may be useful in certain circumstances for some patients. Because of historical precedent, many oncologists prefer some of these modalities, such as massage for example, to not be used over the area of the tumor.

Prognosis

A cancer prognosis depends on many factors, including the type of cancer, the stage, and overall health as well as many other factors. Only your oncologist and medical team can comment on your prognosis. Some cancer patients may be cured, others can expect to live with cancer for a long time as a chronic illness, and unfortunately, some may succumb to this terrible illness. Whatever the prognosis may be regarding the cancer, it appears that the prognosis regarding effective pain and symptom management can be very good. More than ever before, there is a wide interdisciplinary team of trained physicians and allied providers that have developed ever more sophisticated treatments for cancer pain and symptom management. This team may include palliative care specialists, physical medicine and rehabilitation specialists, psychiatrists, anesthesiologists, psychologists, and others who care deeply about the quality of life and dignity of cancer patients. The notion that cancer patients are destined to suffer should now be relegated to the past.

Additional Resources

American Cancer Society: http://www.cancer.org
Lance Armstrong Foundation: http://www.livestrong.org
National Cancer Institute: http://www.cancer.gov
National Comprehensive Cancer Network: http://www.nccn.org
The Wellness Community: http://www.thewellnesscommunity.org

25

PSYCHIATRIC DISORDERS AND PAIN MANAGEMENT

Phillip R. T. Weidner, DO

INTRODUCTION

Research has highlighted the link between psychological well-being and response to pain. Intactness of the mind, a sense of self, and relationships with others influence perception of pain and the ability and willingness to seek out care and reap its benefits. The following chapter explores depression, anxiety, posttraumatic stress disorder, and sleep disturbances in relationship to pain management.

Biobehavioral (psychological) studies of pain have shown that disease processes and pain are influenced by emotional factors. Therefore, the presence of psychological issues requires a multidisciplinary approach to pain management. Treatment of psychological problems may help to alleviate pain and response to emotional stressors.

As with any medical care, it is important to keep each health care practitioner informed of changes, progress, and treatment by other practitioners. It is critical to mention medications prescribed, because psychoactive drugs could potentially have interactions with one another. These interactions could enhance or reduce the effects of other medications you are taking and have dangerous consequences.

Below psychological conditions are listed with an outline of characteristic symptoms and diagnosis. The treatment options for each disorder are not exhaustive and include the most common approaches. The interventions employed by individual mental health care practitioners vary and are not mutually exclusive.

DEPRESSION

Symptoms of depression are often more elevated in chronic pain patients than among those in the general population. Depression and pain are often so intertwined that it is difficult for researchers to figure out whether the pain or depression came first in those who are depressed. In fact, pain and depression are signaled through the same neurological pathway. In essence, the experience of chronic pain may indicate or be strongly correlated with the symptoms of depression.

Symptoms of Depression

As stated above, it can be very difficult to differentiate the symptoms of depression and chronic pain, and the two are not mutually exclusive. The usual symptoms of depression include those listed in Table 25.1, which also includes a form of depression called mania, which is generally reserved for hyperactive behavior beyond the scope of general happiness.

Table 25.1
Symptoms of Depression and Mania

Present in most depressions	– Mood varies from mild sadness to intense feelings of guilt, worthlessness, and hopelessness.
	– Difficulty in thinking, including inability to concentrate, ruminations (obsessive thinking), and lack of decisiveness.
	– Loss of interest, with diminished involvement in work and recreation.
	– Headache; disrupted, lessened, or excessive sleep; loss of energy; change in appetite; decreased sexual drive.
	– Anxiety.
Present in some severe depressions	– Agitation.
	– Delusions of a hypochondriacal (delusions of illness) or persecutory nature.
	– Withdrawal from activities.
	– Physical symptoms of major severity, e.g., anorexia, insomnia, reduced sexual drive, weight loss, and various somatic (bodily) complaints.
	– Suicidal ideation.
Present in mania	– Mood ranging from euphoria to irritability.
	– Sleep disruption.
	– Hyperactivity.
	– Racing thoughts.
	– Grandiosity.

Source: Eisendrath Stuart J, Lichtmacher Jonathan E, "Chapter 25. Psychiatric Disorders." McPhee SJ, Papadakis MA: CURRENT Medical Diagnosis & Treatment 2011.

Diagnosis of Depression

The diagnosis of depression can only be made by licensed medical personnel and often requires a psychological/medical history, psychological or psychiatric assessment, and a physical exam. The presence of other mental disorders and physical illnesses must be considered.

Treatment Options

There are three basic categories of treatment: medical, psychological, and treatment of the physical body. The treatment options are not exclusive and should be thought of as complementary.

Medical Treatment

Antidepressant medications can be generally classified into at least four categories: serotonin-norepinephrine reuptake inhibitors (SNRIs, for example Effexor, Cymbalta), the selective seratonin reuptake inhibitors (SSRIs, for example Zoloft), the tricyclic antidepressants (TCAs, for example Elavil), and the monoamine oxidase inhibitors (MAOs, for example Marplan). Different families of medications have very specific side effects, which should be explained in detail by the prescriber and/or pharmacist. It is very important to take medications as

Table 25.2
The Most Commonly Prescribed Antidepressants in the United States in 2007 and Their Respective Types

Antidepressant Type	Prescriptions (in millions) from 2007
SNRIs	
Venlafaxine (Effexor)	17
Duloxetine (Cymbalta)	Unknown
SSRIs	
Sertraline (Zoloft)	29
Escitalopram (Lexapro)	27
Fluoxetine (Prozac)	22
Citalopram (Celexa)	16
TCAs	
Amitriptyline (Elavil)	13
Nortriptyline (Pamelor)	3
MAO Inhibitors	
Phenelzine (Nardil)	Unknown
Tranylcypromine (Parnate)	Unknown

instructed and be aware of side effects. Antidepressant medications can be pre-scribed by a licensed practitioner and are generally considered the first treatment for depressive symptoms. Table 25.2 includes the most commonly prescribed antidepressants in the United States.

Physical Treatment

There are two major physical treatments of depression that are recognized by the FDA: electroconvulsive therapy (ECT), and transcranial magnetic stimu-lation (TMS).

ECT is a generalized nervous system seizure induced with a short burst of an electric charge. It is generally not used for depression associated with chronic pain but is considered when depressive symptoms are resistant to conventional medical treatment or when pharmacological treatment is unsafe. The data sug-gest that ECT is a valid means of treating depression and has long-standing results with maintenance treatments. The most common side effects of ECT are memory deficits and headache.

TMS refers to magnetic stimulation of parts of the brain by temporarily plac-ing two electric coils on the outside of the head. Although TMS is controversial, there are data to support its efficacy in treating major depression. Its uses in treating chronic pain combined with depression have yet to be defined.

Psychological Treatment

Mental health care professionals often provide counseling for people to over-come depression associated with chronic pain. The use of behavioral therapies depends on the individual and the expertise of the provider. Acute depression may be treated using a form of psychotherapy called interpersonal psycho-therapy (IPT). IPT encourages adaptations to new situations and developing new coping strategies.

Cognitive behavioral therapy (CBT) is a form of psychotherapy in which neg-ative thoughts and emotions are identified and modified by the teaching of new coping strategies. It is recognized that individuals cannot avoid certain aspects of life (such as pain or a disease process) but can control how distressing those events are to them. With this technique, patients are often asked to start a diary of their emotions and to examine self-defeating thoughts and compare those to more rational alternatives. The combination of CBT and pharmacological treat-ment has been shown to be more effective at treating depression than either treatment alone.

ANXIETY

Anxiety is defined as an unpleasant state associated with apprehension, fear, worry, or uneasiness. It includes physical, emotional, and behavioral aspects and heightens irritability to all stimuli. High levels of anxiety are often associated with heightened awareness of pain. The anticipation of pain can be anxiety-provoking for patients and lead to lifestyle changes such as avoiding physical activity and/or beneficial therapy (such as physical therapy and even procedures and/or surgery). In the book *The Pain Chronicles*, author Melanie Thernstrom quotes a survivor of torture: "Torture isn't having your leg bit off by a shark, torture is being slowly lowered into the pool." This view shows the constant, threatening attack of pain and its emotional impact.

Symptoms of Anxiety

Anxiety and its symptoms may be the result of an overactive limbic system. The limbic system regulates the sympathetic nervous system, which generates the "fight-or-flight" reflex. This is a primitive reflex that occurs in stressful situations and causes adrenaline release. Physical effects of the high-adrenaline state include racing heart, increased blood pressure, shortness of breath, stomach pain, insomnia, and increased sweating. Emotionally, an individual may experience a racing mind, irritability, jumpiness, and an inability to stop worrying. Given these troubling symptoms, it is not surprising that people who experience pain and anxiety frequent the emergency room and their primary care provider. These visits can be time consuming and costly and rarely contribute to the progress of treatment.

Diagnosis of Anxiety

Anxiety may be difficult to diagnose because of its varied physical manifestations. The complaint of pain paralleled with the feeling that "something isn't right" under certain circumstances can be the acute state. Often an individual will undergo testing to "rule out" serious medical conditions (for example, heart attack for chest pain), and after a negative appropriate workup, anxiety is considered as the cause.

To diagnose anxiety, practitioners may administer a short questionnaire. If the results suggest heightened anxiety, further evaluation by a specialized professional is needed.

Treatment of Anxiety

The management of people with anxiety can involve psychological, environmental, and pharmacological interventions. Patients with pain as the provocation for their anxiety are especially challenging. For most patients, it is more difficult to avoid pain than a certain place or social situation. Understanding pain and the appropriate and timely treatment of anxiety (including pharmacological treatment) are the cornerstones to avoiding a perpetual cycle of pain and heightened anxiety.

The first line of treatment includes helping the patient to avoid substances that are potentially stimulating, such as caffeine and various medications (including over-the-counter cold medications). Self-soothing mental exercises, such as deep breathing, redirecting attention, and keeping a journal may also help with relaxation. Psychological therapies such as CBT may also be used in the treatment of anxiety.

Pharmacological treatments for anxiety include many of the same medications used for depression—SSRIs, MAO inhibitors, and TCAs, with SSRIs being the first line of treatment. In addition to antidepressants, a drug family called the *benzodiazepines* (examples include Ativan and Valium) are frequently used for anxiety. This family of medications increases the sensitivity of receptors in your brain to a neurotransmitter called GABA (*Gamma Aminobutyric Acid*), which has a calming effect. This family of medications can be highly addictive, are sedating (especially in combination with opioids such as oxycodone), and can cause withdrawal if stopped abruptly.

POSTTRAUMATIC STRESS DISORDER

Posttraumatic stress disorder (PTSD) is a type of anxiety disorder that shares many characteristics with generalized anxiety. It differs in that the person re-experiences specific, traumatic psychological events with varying levels of recollection and emotional stress. The original traumatic event or events often involve violence. The disorder is more common in females and in those that serve in the armed forces. Of all mental disorders, PTSD has been shown in recent studies to have the highest prevalence in those suffering from chronic pain.

Symptoms of PTSD

The physiological and emotional responses depicted above for general anxiety attacks are similar to the symptomatic episodes of PTSD. In PTSD, memory of original events is retriggered and may cause hypervigilance, difficulty with sleep patterns and social interactions, and anger.

Diagnosis of PTSD

There is a high incidence of depression and panic disorders in individuals who suffer from PTSD, and it is often difficult to diagnose these separately. What separates PTSD from other mental disorders is the experience of one or more significant life-threatening events leading to distressful thoughts and emotions for weeks or months. The diagnosis is usually made by a mental health care professional. The current diagnosis criteria are outlined by the *Diagnostic and Statistical Manual of Mental Disorders IV* (*DSM IV*) available to all health-care providers.

Treatment of PTSD

The best treatment for PTSD is still undetermined, but psychotherapy and medications in combination are likely to yield the best results. Research has shown that the more quickly treatment is initiated after the inciting event, the better the prognosis. It is important to implement psychotherapy as early as possible, which usually includes cognitive behavioral therapy.

The FDA has approved sertraline and paroxetine (SSRIs) for the treatment of PTSD, although other medications such as carbamazepine (Tegretol) may be employed to target impulsivity and anger. Benzodiazepines such as Valium, Ativan, Klonopin, and Xanax may also be used to control anxiety attacks, but these drugs require monitoring because of their addictive qualities. Opioid derivatives such as morphine and/or hydromorphone are used to treat physical pain, which is often difficult to discern from emotional pain inflicted at the time of the original event. Recent research involving beta blockers has shown promise.

SLEEP DISORDER AND PAIN

Chronic pain conditions can negatively impact sleeping patterns. Disturbances in sleeping patterns can have many causes, including physical obstruction of the upper airway (such as in obstructive sleep apnea), over-sedation for pain management, insufficient pain control, and the presence of anxiety and depression. Abnormalities in sleeping patterns can interfere with effective treatment of pain. Because the causes of sleep disorders are so diverse, it is important to contact a healthcare provider if problems with sleep persist.

Symptoms

Sleep disorders can be characterized by disturbances in any stage of sleep, including falling asleep, staying asleep, and feeling rested. Patients with neuropathic pain may experience a disorder called *restless leg syndrome* in which pain arises in the legs while lying down, but is alleviated by slight movements that occur throughout the night. These painful movements disturb sleep.

Diagnosis

Similar to other psychological disorders mentioned, diagnosis of sleep disorder is made after consideration of possible physical and mental comorbidities, including depression and anxiety.

Treatment

The first line of treatment is to remove things that might disturb sleep, such as eating late in the day before sleep, stressors, and stimulants like caffeine or cold medicines. Other approaches include establishing a regular bedtime, darkening the room, and minimizing noise in the environment. Keeping a sleep diary may also be helpful. Examples can be found at http://www.sleepdiary .com.

Pharmacological approaches include benzodiazepines such as Valium and Ativan, non-benzodiazepine hypnotics such as zolpidem (Ambien), melatonin receptor agonists such as ramelteon (Rozerem), and sedating antidepressants such as trazodone (Desyrel).

Melatonin is a critical hormone that is released from the pineal gland. A synthetic compound that works in a similar manner is available over the counter, typically in a dose of 3–5 mg, although a better dose is 1.5–2.5 mg (3–5 mg makes many people groggy the next day, but the lower dose range does not, so buy a pill cutter and cut in half). This synthetic melatonin-like medication deserves additional attention for older patients with sleep issues. For many older patients, this therapy works very well. Starting from the age of 35 years old, the pineal gland begins to calcify and release less melatonin as we age.

SUMMARY

Psychological disorders often coexist with chronic pain. Because of the significant overlap between different disorders and pain states, therapy needs to be directed by a skilled provider whom you trust and can confide in. Most important to the success of your treatment is clarity and honesty with your providers and communication within the treatment team. There are many options available, and often the prognosis is good.

ADDITIONAL RESOURCES

"Depression and Pain," Harvard Health Publications, http://www.health.harvard.edu/
    newsweek/Depression_and_pain.htm
Mindfulness Meditation for Pain Relief, by John Kabat Zinn, 1994. http://www.amazon
    .com/Mindfulness-Meditation-Pain-Relief-Reclaiming/dp/1591797403/ref=sr_1
    _1?s=books&ie=UTF8&qid=1311811286&sr=1-1
The Pain Chronicles, by Melanie Thernstrom, 2010. http://www.amazon.com/Pain
    -Chronicles-Mysteries-Prayers-Suffering/dp/0312573073/ref=sr_1_1?s=books
    &ie=UTF8&qid=1311811442&sr=1-1

PART III

ADVANCED PAIN PROCEDURES, SURGERY, AND ANESTHESIA

26

INJECTIONS AND OTHER INTERVENTIONS FOR PAIN MANAGEMENT

Jie Zhu, MD, Frank J. E. Falco, MD, C. Obi Onyewu, MD, and Youssef Josephson, DO

INTRODUCTION

Pain is a growing epidemic in the United States. Just about everyone will experience some sort of pain in their life. It is a reflection of our society and, quite frankly, the aging process. In 2000, the Arthritis Foundation reported that 42 percent of all adults in the United States experienced pain on a daily basis and 89 percent experienced pain on a monthly basis. This means that about 105 million of us Americans, or 35.5 percent of the U.S. population, have experienced some form of pain. In 2001, the Mayo Clinic found that close to half of all Americans visit a physician with a primary complaint of pain each year.

Interventional spine is a technical term used to describe injections or other procedures to treat neck, mid back, or low back pain. This approach is typically used when other simpler, less invasive methods of treatment such as medications, physical therapy, chiropractic care, acupuncture, or other forms of treatment fail to provide pain relief. In this chapter, we will describe the common procedures used to treat spine-related pain that might affect you at some point in your lifetime.

EPIDURAL AND NERVE ROOT INJECTIONS

Epidural steroid injections are not just used for pain control during labor, but are also used to treat neck or low back pain and nerve pain that lead to arm and leg (sciatica) pain. Steroids or cortisone with or without a numbing (like novocaine) solution are injected into the spine to provide pain relief from a number of different types of problems. The injected medications spread to nerves in the spine that provide relief by reducing nerve inflammation or swelling from a disc herniation (slipped disc) or arthritis that is pressing on the nerve. The injection is done with x-rays and x-ray dye that allow your pain doctor to see your spine so that he or she can place the needle in your back safely with precision prior to injection. Usually, a sedative and an IV pain reliever are used to relax you and minimize any discomfort that you might feel during the injection. Pain relief from the injection often occurs shortly after the injection due to the local anesthetic and this relief can last for hours. Long-term pain relief begins approximately two to three days after the injected steroid has reduced inflammation around the nerves.

Post-injection local tenderness at the needle insertion site can occur for a few hours or days after the procedure and pain can be reduced by simply applying an ice pack. You will be asked to rest for the remainder of the day on which you have had the epidural injection. On occasion you may feel a temporary increase in your pain that can last for several days after the injection. One can usually return to normal non-strenuous work or recreational activities the next day.

Selective nerve root injections are another way to inject cortisone and a novocaine-like numbing medicine for the treatment of your neck, back and sciatic pain. This injection procedure is similar to the epidural injections in that they work by placing the cortisone and numbing medication directly around your nerves as they exit the spine. The needle is placed along the nerve as it passes outside of your spine. This is an injection that puts the medication around an exact spot that is causing your pain. These nerve-specific injections are also done with x-rays and x-ray dye just like the epidural injection. Sedation is typically provided to reduce any pain associated with the injection. Considerations regarding what is expected regarding pain relief, rest, and return to regular activities are the same as that for epidural injections.

FACET JOINT INJECTIONS

Facet joint injections are used for the neck and back without sciatica. The facet joints are small joints located in your neck and back that provide support to your neck and back. Facet joints can cause neck or back pain from arthritis or from repetitive bending and rotation. Whiplash injuries such as from a car accident or a fall are a common cause for facet joint pain, particularly in the neck.

Facet joint injections are performed by injecting the joint itself or by numbing the nerves that only supply the facet joint. These nerves are *not* the same as the nerves that go into your arms or legs that cause sciatica, as we discussed earlier in this chapter. The facet joint injections or the injection of the nerves are done with x-rays and x-ray dye along with sedation to provide you with pain relief during the injection. Corticosteroids and a numbing medicine are used in these injections. Post-injection course, precautions, and recovery are similar to epidural and selective nerve root injections.

Radiofrequency ablation is a procedure for the treatment of facet joint pain when facet joint injections provide only temporary or short-term pain relief. This procedure uses specially designed needles and equipment that emit radio waves to create heat through the needle around your facet joint nerves. The needles are placed along your facet joint nerves using x-rays. Electrical stimulation is first performed to ensure that the needle has been correctly placed next to your facet joint nerves before they are melted away by the heat created from the radiofrequency energy.

You will receive sedation for this procedure, which typically takes more time to perform than the other injections we discuss so far. It typically takes an hour to complete this procedure. In addition, you are more likely to have stronger sedation compared to what you would receive with the injections because there is more pain involved in doing this procedure. Post-procedure pain will be greater and last longer compared to the injections. Pain relief from radiofrequency is not as fast compared to the injections. It can take up to six or eight weeks before you will notice any significant relief. On the other hand, the duration of your pain relief from radiofrequency is often a lot longer compared to the facet injections. Your post-procedure course precautions and recovery are also longer than compared to the injections.

SACROILIAC JOINT INJECTIONS

Sacroiliac (SI) joint injections are used for the treatment of low back or pelvic pain from the sacroiliac joint. Sacroiliac joints are located in the back of the pelvis and are formed by the sacrum (the large bone at the bottom of your spine) and the pelvis on both sides of the sacrum. The sacroiliac joint gives support to your pelvis when standing, sitting, and walking. This joint along with the other joints in your legs allow for the ability to walk.

Sacroiliac pain is usually on one side when it occurs after an injury. The pain that you feel arises as a result of an injury that sends a jolt-like force from your foot that travels up your leg to your SI joint. This type of injury is seen when you forcefully put your foot on the brake in a car accident. Other injuries to the SI joint can happen when you step down off of a step or curb and strike the ground at an awkward angle with one leg. A fall landing on one or both of your feet can lead to an injury to one or both sacroiliac joints. There are different diseases that can lead to sacroiliac joint pain in one or both joints. These include osteoarthritis and other types of arthritic disorders. Sacroiliac joint pain is typically localized in your buttock area and can spread into your posterior thigh. In rare cases, it can spread from the buttock down your entire leg into the foot.

The sacroiliac joint is injected in the same manner as the other injections that we discussed in this chapter. The injection is done with the use of x-rays and x-ray dye to make sure that the needle is properly placed into your SI joint.

Sedation is given for comfort during the injection. A numbing medication and corticosteroid is injected into the SI joint. As with the other injections the anesthetic should provide you with immediate pain relief, whereas the corticosteroid will provide you with relief in two to three days. Post-injection course, precautions, and recovery are similar to other injections.

Radiofrequency ablation can also be used to treat SI joint pain in a similar fashion in which it is used to treat facet joint pain. Again, this type of procedure is considered as long as there was an SI joint injection that provided good but temporary pain relief. The radiofrequency will provide longer pain relief than the SI joint injections. There will be the same prolonged recovery course and precautions after the SI joint radiofrequency as with any other radiofrequency procedure for pain.

SYMPATHETIC NERVE INJECTIONS

Sympathetic nerve injections are commonly used for treating what is called neuropathic pain, pain that is burning, shooting, lightning-like, or stabbing that involves either your arms or legs. The sympathetic nerves provide the necessary functions for your heart, kidneys, stomach, intestines, bladder, blood vessels, and skin. These nerves can cause you pain when they lose their ability to work normally. This is often seen when there is a direct injury of a nerve in the arm or leg or when the arm or leg is involved in a crush-like injury with no specific nerve injury per se. These types of injuries as well as medical conditions such as stroke or brain injury can lead to a condition known as reflex sympathetic dystrophy (RSD) that causes the neuropathic pain in the arms or legs.

A cervical (neck) sympathetic injection for treating neuropathic arm pain involves placing a needle through the front of the neck until it makes contact with the cervical bones of the neck. The needle for a lumbar (low back) sympathetic injection is placed through the back and positioned along the bones of the back. Both cervical and lumbar sympathetic injections are performed with x-rays and x-ray dye to ensure correct needle placement. You will receive sedation for comfort during the procedure. A long-acting numbing medication is injected through the needle once the needle tip has been confirmed to be in the correct position. You will feel a warm sensation in the arm or leg depending on whether the injection is performed in the neck or back. Typically there will be immediate pain after injection. Post-procedure recovery is usually short, lasting several hours. The duration of pain relief varies depending on diagnosis, how long you have had the pain, and how severe the pain is. Oftentimes, several injections are necessary in order to obtain long-term relief. Although sympathetic injections are helpful in confirming your diagnosis of neuropathic pain, they rarely provide long-term relief for those with severe pain. Therefore, the injection of a neurolytic agent (a solution that destroys insulation material of the nerve) or the use of radiofrequency ablation is necessary in order to give you long-term relief.

Discography

The cervical and lumbar discs are soft tissue structures located between the bones in your neck and low back that provide support and flexibility. Discography was developed to help diagnose herniated discs at a time in medicine when more sophisticated imaging tests such as MRI (magnetic resonance imaging) and CT (computer tomography) scanners did not exist. Today, discography is more commonly used to determine whether you have a disc that is causing your neck or low back pain.

This procedure is like having a "stress test" for discs in the neck or back. It involves injecting x-ray dye into several discs to see if any of the discs reproduce neck or back pain. Needles are inserted into the neck or back discs using x-rays for correct placement. Sedation is given to keep comfortable during the procedure. The disc or discs that recreate neck or low back pain during the injection of the x-ray contrast are recorded throughout the procedure. A CT scan of the neck or low back is done after the discogram for further evaluation of disc anatomy.

Spinal Cord Stimulation

Spinal cord stimulation (SCS) is a device that is surgically implanted in the body to give relief from chronic intractable pain of the neck and arm, or low back and leg. Typically SCS is considered only for those who have failed all other forms of more conservative treatment such as pain medication, physical therapy, chiropractic care, spinal injection, and radiofrequency. It is also considered if there has been no significant pain relief after neck or back surgery. SCS is also recommended if one suffers from RSD, or unrelenting sciatica.

The procedure is performed by placing a small, flexible wire with embedded electrodes, called a SCS lead, through a needle into the spine of the neck or low back using x-rays for correct positioning of the lead. Sedation is provided for comfort during the procedure. Only part of the lead is placed into the spine. The remaining part of the lead that is not in the spine is attached to the neck or low back with special medical tape and attached to an external battery (the size of a small transistor radio) that is worn on the belt. The spinal cord stimulation lead is left in place for a three- to five-day outpatient trial or test to see if the SCS successfully stops the pain. The lead has embedded electrodes that electrically stimulate the spinal cord, which blocks or stops the pain signals from the neck and arm, or the back and leg from traveling to the brain. A successful trial or test is one where the stimulation reduces pain by at least 50 percent. The SCS trial or test also evaluates whether or not one tolerated the stimulation, reduced need for pain medication, allowed one to physically do more activities, and improved one's sleep. The test lead is removed after a trial period and a surgery to implant a permanent spinal cord stimulation lead and internal battery is scheduled if the trial was successful. The surgery for implanting the lead and battery does not require overnight hospitalization and is done on an outpatient basis. Post-procedure course is typically uneventful, with some soreness and incisional pain for one to two weeks.

PERIPHERAL NERVE STIMULATION

Peripheral nerve stimulation (PNS) is an implantable device similar to SCS that is used to treat chronic intractable facial, neck, or low back pain as well as headaches if one has failed all other forms of treatment including pain medication, physical therapy, chiropractic care, spinal injection, and ablation procedures as well as spine surgery. One is not a candidate for PNS if the primary pain involves the arms or legs. If the pain is predominately in the arms or legs one should be considered for spinal cord stimulation.

The procedure employs the same type of stimulation leads that are used for spinal cord stimulation. The PNS leads are placed through a needle into the areas of the face, head, neck, or low back depending on where your pain is using x-rays for correct lead placement. Patients will receive sedation during the procedure for comfort. Only part of the lead is placed into the body. The remaining part of the lead is attached to the skin surface with sterile medical tape and then attached to an external battery. The peripheral nerve stimulation lead is left in place for a three- to five-day outpatient trial or testing period to determine if it successfully stops your pain. The lead electrically stimulates the peripheral nerves which ultimately blocks the pain signals reaching the brain. A successful trial or test is one in which the stimulation reduces your pain by at least 50 percent, the stimulation is tolerable to you, reduces the use of your pain medication, increases function, and improves sleep. Surgery to implant a permanent peripheral nerve stimulation lead and internal battery is scheduled if the trial was successful and is done on an outpatient basis. Post-procedure course is similar to that of spinal cord stimulation.

INTRATHECAL PAIN PUMPS

The intrathecal pump delivers pain medications through a catheter into the sac of fluid surrounding your spinal cord, and the pain medications are able to directly access the pain receptors found in the spinal cord and brain. Typical medications used in the pump include a local anesthetic and opioids such as morphine. Patients will undergo an outpatient trial or testing period similar to spinal cord and peripheral nerve stimulation to determine whether or not you are an appropriate candidate for intrathecal pump therapy. A catheter is inserted using x-ray guidance into the spine sac for the trial. Sedation is provided for your comfort during the catheter insertion. A portable external pump is used for the trial infusion that you wear on your belt or in a sack with a shoulder strap. The testing period can last as short as three days or as long as two weeks depending on titration of the medicine infusion rate to at least 50 percent pain relief or reaching a maximum daily dose. The trial is considered to be successful if it reduces pain by at least 50 percent, one can tolerate the infusion without side effects from the medications, it reduces pain medication, increases function, and it improves sleep. Surgery to implant a permanent pump and catheter is scheduled if the trial was successful. One can have the implant done on an outpatient basis or if necessary with an overnight stay in the hospital. Post-procedure course is similar to spinal cord and peripheral nerve stimulation implants.

Conclusions

Interventional spine procedures play an important role in the evaluation and treatment of your neck and low back pain if your pain does not respond to more conservative care such as medications, physical therapy, or chiropractic treatments. Some of the procedures are simple, such as epidural, nerve root, facet joint, and sympathetic injections that are used for treating less complex problems, establishing your diagnosis, or identifying the source of your pain. Other procedures are more complex, such as radiofrequency, spinal cord stimulation, and peripheral nerve stimulation and intrathecal pain pumps used for treating more complicated pain or spine problems.

27

ADVANCED TECHNIQUES FOR CHRONIC PAIN OF THE SPINE

Rinoo V. Shah, MD, MBA, Sudhir Diwan, MD, and Alan D. Kaye, MD, PhD

Interventional pain management is a medical specialty. Only licensed and appropriately trained physicians should practice this specialty. The procedures pose risks and require a high degree of specialization. If you receive an interventional pain management procedure, make sure that a physician with proper qualifications is performing it. Ideally, it should be a physician who has interacted with you and has outlined a treatment plan with you. Qualifications to practice this field are discussed in another chapter.

The goal of interventional pain management is to diagnose and treat chronic pain. These specialized physicians use minimally invasive techniques (versus open surgery). A needle, electric wand, flexible tubes, and a scalpel are tools of this profession. Interventional pain physicians are trained to diagnose and treat chronic pain, particularly chronic low back pain. A needle can be placed in a targeted area; nerves can be ablated (an electrical current produced by a radio wave is used to heat up a small area of nerve tissue to decrease pain signals from that specific area); electric pacemakers can help with nerve pain; and a delivery pump can deliver a potent drug to the spinal cord. Minor surgery is used for advanced interventional pain procedures; these include shrinking the spine's shock absorber (discectomy), blocking pain with electricity (spinal cord stimulator); delivering medications to the spinal canal (intrathecal pump); or stabilizing a spine fracture (kyphoplasty). These procedures can be performed compassionately, with medications to reduce the anxiety and reassurances to allay fears about the procedure.

Procedures for low back pain are based on the principle of pinpointing and treating the pain generator (the cause of pain). There are many potential pain generators in the low back. There are a number of procedures that can target these pain generators.

The low back has a bunch of structures that work together to allow you to stand upright, twist, bend, and walk. This is a very complex and well-orchestrated function. There are muscles, which move things at your command. There are bones for support. Bones act as struts and anchors. There are tendons, which allow the muscles to connect to the bones. The muscles can move these bones. There are ligaments, which are soft and resilient tissues. Ligaments play a supportive role. Finally, there are the nerves and spinal cord. These are the circuits that allow us to communicate with the muscles. These circuits act as sensors to tell us about pain, touch, and our body position.

There are typically five lower back bones, known as vertebra. They look like a lopsided ring. The front part (vertebral body) helps with load bearing and support. When this is weakened due to bone loss (osteoporosis), a fracture can occur (compression fracture). The ring part (spinal canal) circles and confines the nerves and spinal fluid. The back part has small hooks and shingles, known as facets. In the front, the vertebra are separated by discs. These discs allow us to twist and act as shock absorbers. This disc can age with time (disc degeneration); older discs don't work as well as younger discs. Younger discs can tear and leak out a soft gelatinous material. This is known as a *herniated disc*. The herniated disc can cause back pain by itself. The herniated disc can also touch a nerve and cause the infamous "sciatica" pain. The older discs can wear out and bulge. The bones can rub together in some cases, and the patient may feel that their back is stiff. The older discs can narrow the spinal canal or the tunnels that let the nerves leave the spine, as they go to the legs. The tunnels are on both sides and are known as foramen (singular) or foramina (plural). This narrowing gets worse when the patient stands. This is known as spinal stenosis (crowding of the nerves). The facets help coordinate movements and prevent you from twisting your back all the way around. They snap with a chiropractic adjustment. They can be affected by arthritis. This can cause pain, particularly when bending backwards.

Inside the spinal canal, there is a spinal sac called the dura. The dura contains the nerves and a fluid, spinal fluid. The dura is punctured when you need a spinal fluid tap or when your doctor sends you for a myelogram (x-ray examination that uses an injected dye to detect abnormalities in the spinal canal). Just behind the dura is a ligament, called the yellow ligament. This ligament can buckle inward during spinal stenosis. In between the dura and the yellow ligament is the *epidural space*. This is an important space in interventional pain management—it is one of the favorite places where doctors place medications. The lowest disc separates the lowest vertebral body from a special shovel-shaped bone. This shovel-shaped bone is known as the sacrum. Right above the sacrum is the disc, and off to the side is the sacroiliac joint. This joint, or "hinge" if you prefer, links the sacrum to the pelvis. This joint loosens during pregnancy to allow delivery of a baby.

With this background, we can discuss the different injections.

GENERAL PRINCIPLES

These procedures should ideally be performed using fluoroscopic (x-ray) guidance. In this day and age, fluoroscope machines are readily available. This device enhances the safety of the procedure and helps ensure the needle is placed correctly. Your doctor will position you. Cushions may be used to make you feel comfortable. An IV (intravenous catheter) may be placed, in case you need fluids or sedation. Often, an IV is placed for safety. The area on the skin to be injected is cleaned with a sterile solution. Monitors are placed to watch your breathing, oxygen supply, heart rate, and blood pressure.

There will be several people in the room, depending on your location. Fewer staff are present for office-based procedures, and more staff are present for hospital-based procedures. Hospitals typically have more regulations than offices. There may be a nurse watching you and giving you sedation. Another nurse or scrub technologist will help prepare the equipment and supplies for the doctor. An x-ray tech will move the fluoroscope machine at the doctor's request. Another staff member may be there to help with transportation and cleaning.

The fluoroscope machine is connected to a pair of screens. This gives the doctor a real-time "television" view of what is going on with your back. Special sequences are sometimes used on the fluoroscope to look at blood vessels (digital subtraction angiography). The doctor will numb the skin after deciding where to enter. A needle will be advanced to the specific target. The doctor may then opt to use a special dye, in order to make the "invisible" visible. Bone is always visible on fluoroscopy. Nerves and blood vessels are not. A special dye is used to make these structures visible and to help with accurate needle placement. Depending on the technique, another numbing medicine and a steroid (anti-inflammatory) are injected along the target. The needle is removed and a Band-Aid is applied. You are then brought to the recovery room. The staff will then check your strength, ask about your pain relief, and have you perform previously painful maneuvers.

Rarely, complications can occur. These include bleeding, infection, nerve damage, spinal leak, medication allergy (unexpected), and medication side effects (possibly expected). Pain injections work sometimes, and they fail sometimes. There is a bit of trial and error. Doctors like to use a fancy name: "spine algorithm." This is a step-by-step approach. Different injections are tried to identify the pain generator (the cause of your pain). If it works, repeat. If it doesn't work, go to the next procedure. Patients can be frustrated by this process, but this can be helpful in pinpointing the pain.

1. *Epidural Steroid*: As mentioned previously, the epidural space is a special location between the dural sac and the yellow ligament. What didn't we tell you? The epidural space is like a ring within the vertebral ring. So, you can reach it from the back (interlaminar), from the side (transforaminal), or from below (caudal with or without a catheter). The epidural space has a front. This is where herniated discs can occur. Since this space reaches all parts of the spine, the epidural steroid injection is used to deliver medications into the spine.

   A. *Interlaminar Epidural Steroid:* This was the first type of epidural injection and is the most commonly performed. You will lie on your back. A special needle will be placed between two of your lower back bones. This will depend on where your doctor thinks your pain is located. Due to variations in anatomy, the medication may stay on one side or another. One criticism is that the medication is nonselective—it doesn't get to the right locations. A catheter can be used, or the needle can be placed at a different angle, in order to get closer to the target. If you imagine your spinal canal to be a house, then an interlaminar is similar to entering through the back door.

   B. *Transforaminal Epidural Steroid:* The needle is placed when the nerve is exiting the spinal canal. Sometimes, the doctor may place more than one needle. The second needle may be placed on the other side, one level above or one level below. This injection is popular because it is target specific. This means the steroids can be placed near where the disc meets the nerve. This is similar to entering through the side windows, on the first or second floor.

   C. *Caudal Epidural Steroid Injection:* The needle is placed near the tailbone. Once it enters the tailbone, the steroid can be delivered. This is not selective. Some doctors are trained to use catheters. In our practice, we use catheters to get to where we want to go. The catheter is selective. You can decide on which side and which level you want to access. This approach is akin to entering from the basement. This technique can be especially helpful in patients with spinal stenosis (crowding of the nerves) or prior spine surgery.

2. *Epidural Lysis of Adhesions:* This is a technique that was developed for patients with persistent pain after back surgery. After any surgery, scar tissue develops. As is, epidural injections are more challenging when patients have had prior back surgery. Even then, the scar tissue may prevent the medication from getting to the right location. The medication will take the path of least resistance. If traffic is held up in the right lane, drivers go into the left. They take the path of least resistance. Epidural lysis of adhesions was developed to "soften" the scar and deal with the root cause of pain. Typically, a catheter is placed through the tailbone and advances to the scar tissue. At that location, specialized medications are delivered, in addition to the steroids. These medications soften the scar tissue and reduce nerve swelling. This is similar to an emergency road vehicle helping the cars stalled in the right lane: take the path of greatest resistance, in order to solve the problem. You may believe it or not, but a medical-grade "meat tenderizer" and a concentrated salt solution is used. Sounds hokey? Some practitioners think so. However, there is a large body of excellent research and clinical trials indicating that this technique is highly effective. We use this technique routinely to help patients.

3. *Facet Joint Injection:* A needle is placed into the joint or to the nerves surrounding this joint. The facet joint is actually a "real" joint. Many practitioners
place a needle into this joint, or they block the nerves responsible to this joint.
Clinical trials demonstrate that this injection can help with back pain. Since
there are many (12) facet joints in the low back, these procedures often
require more than one needle. They play an important role in figuring out
whether the facets are causing pain. The joints have a shingle orientation,
and a fluoroscope is needed to ensure accurate needle placement. The medical literature advises blocking the nerves to the joint, not just once but twice.
This is called a double diagnostic comparative block. This helps to figure out
who has facet pain or placebo. These injections can help pain in the short term
and may have to be repeated.

4. *Sacroiliac Joint Injection:* A needle is placed into the sacroiliac joint in the
lower part of your buttock. The sacroiliac joint is a common cause of back
pain, and an injection may help pinpoint the source of the pain.

5. *Discogram:* A needle is placed in the disc to figure out if the disc is causing the
pain. Before the MRI and CT scan, discograms and myelograms were useful to
surgeons to plan surgery on the disc. MRIs and CT scans are now routinely
used. Unfortunately, an MRI and CT cannot pinpoint the source of pain
except in rare instances. For instance, infections, fractures, cancer, or bleeding
can be pinpointed as the source of pain. These are rare causes of low back
pain. Since everyone has aging discs, it is virtually impossible to state whether
one patient has pain or not. A doctor may look for a hint of whether a disc
causes pain or not, but they cannot know for sure. Discograms are useful in
figuring out the source of pain in the back. They are controversial. There
was a sordid and unfortunate experiment on prisoners in the late 1960s,
which cast a shadow on discograms. Over the past few years, the role of a discogram has been challenged. The technique has been improved. The procedure is performed under live x-rays. Pressure recordings are used. The
language to describe what is seen has been standardized. A CT scan is used
after the discogram. Patients are simply asked to report what they feel during
the discogram and if the pain is exactly like the pain they have at home. The
physician is not supposed to cheat and "help" the patient give a report.
Researchers have tried to optimize the results to reduce what is called a false
positive. Imagine an umpire calling a pitch "OK," when the videotape shows
that the pitch was a strike. This is a false positive. Now imagine if the umpire
loses his eyeglasses, the false positives keep adding up. This type of error
can change the outcome of the game. If you have a false positive discogram,
you could get operated upon unnecessarily. The procedure continues to be
hotly debated. When performed properly, this procedure can be useful. Ask
your doctor, "What is a control level?" "Do you get a control level?" "Do you
record pressures?" "Do you ask me specific questions about the intensity of
the pain, the location of the pain, and if it reproduces my exact pain?" and
"Do you do this under light sedation or no sedation?" This will gauge the
physician's expertise and philosophy of discography. Finally, discography is
not a pre-surgical test. It *cannot* predict the outcome of surgery. Surgery has
its own hit-or-miss track record—whether or not you have a discogram. A discogram may be an empowerment tool. It provides closure and gives you

choices about what road in pain management you want to pursue. For instance, if you have a painful tear in the disc that will not heal, you may be tempted to rush to surgery. The reality is that surgery may not work no matter what you do. On the other hand, now you know you have a non-healing small tear in the disc. You have options. You can seek out a minimally invasive procedure, you can consider alternate medications, and you can help decide what your functional limitations will be.

6. *Discectomy:* There are some minimally invasive disc removal procedures. These can typically be performed with mild sedation. They are often outpatient procedures. They avoid going through the spinal canal—this can reduce the risk of a spinal scar. These devices all place a guide into the center of the disc. Then, a special instrument is placed through the guide. Some instruments are augurs that rotate and suck out disc material. Some use proprietary types of heating technologies. Some use a high-speed jet. Others make use of lasers. Some use a flexible telescope and a rasp (like a bird's beak) to remove disc material. The technologies in this area are rapidly progressing and hold promise in facilitating faster recoveries. The research, unfortunately, is not as robust as with other procedures. One should talk to their pain management physician about which technique may be the right one. As a general rule of thumb, these procedures are indicated for specific types of herniated discs and for specific patient populations (younger patients).

7. *Disc Heating Procedures:* Some discs can cause pain due to a small non-healing tear (annular tear). There is not an imminent risk of a "disc leaking out." The tear does indicate a type of weakness in the outer wall of the disc. In rare instances, tremendous pressures can be transmitted across the tear and cause a herniation. A number of devices have been developed to allow heating of this tear. Painful nerve endings grow into the tear, and heating them can alleviate pain. The exact cause of the pain is unknown. Specialized wands, heating coils, and needles have been designed to heat this tear/fissure. The outcomes have been unpredictable, and many insurance companies have denied payment. Nonetheless, published research is optimistic about this approach to injured discs. One device is known as the intradiscal electrothermal catheter. Another is known as "cooled" radiofrequency or disc biaculoplasty. Despite the intimidating names, the procedures focus on generating enough heat to destroy the pain receptors in the disc tears. Patients cannot be "out" for these procedures. The doctor must be able to talk to you and perform a neurological check during the procedure. Treatment failure can be high (30–60%), even when patients are well selected. Since the only other alternative is a spinal fusion, well-trained pain physicians are willing to offer this technique their patients. No one can guarantee a cure and recovery may be prolonged.

8. *Radiofrequency Ablation:* Radiofrequency is a type of energy wave that generates heat when it exits the needle. This type of heat is nothing like that from an open flame. This type of heat creates a very uniform and discrete "cooking zone." This is used to permanently kill a nerve. The nerve cannot be used for moving a muscle—it must only be involved in sensation. If this is used on a big nerve, it can cause numbness and weakness. Extreme caution must be used when "ablating a nerve." The common locations are small branches of the spine nerves that go to the facet. This is called "facet denervation or

ablation." Radiofrequency ablation has been applied to the sacro iliac joint. If a patient gets temporary relief from a sacro-iliac-joint injection, they may be a candidate for ablation of the joint or the nerves to the joint. Specialized needles, wands, probes, and power generators are used. As a patient, the invasiveness is similar to a block; the procedure takes longer than a block. Some physicians believe that the pain relief comes from the electrical current and not the heat. By adjusting the dials on the generator, a special type of nondestructive radiofrequency can be created. This is known as pulsed radiofrequency. Unlike standard radiofrequency, which can reach a temperature of 176 degrees F (80 deg. C), pulsed radiofrequency reaches a temperature of 108 deg. F (42 deg. C). The literature on pulsed radiofrequency primarily consists of isolated success reports. If this technique gains wider acceptance, large nerves can be treated. Pulsed radiofrequency is not thought to damage nerves.

9. *Kyphoplasty, Vertebroplasty:* These are procedures to treat spine compression fractures and cancer that has spread to the spine bones. A series of cannulas are placed into the vertebral body. A bone sample is removed for analysis. Then cement is mixed and placed through the cannula into the vertebral body. Kyphoplasty uses a balloon to create a pocket for the cement. A cavity may reduce the risk of the cement leaking. There may be some height restoration of the vertebral body. One company has developed a gun to deliver plastic type wafers into the vertebral body. This may increase height and reduce the amount of cement utilized. The purpose of these techniques is to reduce fracture-related pain. Many of these frail patients lose height and their spine curve increases. This can cause significant depression and increase fall risk. There was a great deal of controversy in 2009, since two papers in a prestigious journal stated that vertebroplasty is not effective. Another paper, however, stated that kyphoplasty was effective. There are many anecdotal reports of success with kyphoplasty and vertebroplasty.

   In our experience, this is one off the most successful and gratifying pain management procedures. These patients are very appreciative and continue to return to their pre-fracture function levels. Those who are untreated may have to be placed in a wheelchair. These techniques have been applied to the sacrum for treating stable sacral fractures in frail individuals.

10. *Spinal Cord Stimulator:* This is an electrical pacemaker. These leads have multiple contacts. They are placed through a needle into the epidural space. They are right behind the spinal cord in the mid back, not the lower back. The leads are connected to an output device that delivers a low voltage current. The patient may feel tingling going down the back and legs. This may help the pain. This doesn't get rid of all the pain, so emergency-type pains will be felt. The patient has control over the device. Initially, a test drive is conducted to see if the patient likes the leads/soft wires. The patient can give feedback about whether they like the device or not. If they like the device, it can be implanted under the skin. A battery can be connected and fully implanted under the skin. Patients have tremendous leverage to control this device.

11. *Intrathecal Pump:* Internal drug delivery systems are available. The research literature on this advanced intervention is more robust for cancer pain than

for non-cancer pain. The most common patients to receive these pumps are those with failed back surgery syndrome. These are patients who underwent back surgery, but are no better. These patients may have been on high-dose narcotics prior to the pump. A psychologist should evaluate all potential candidates for a pump. A pump is connected to a very soft and durable tube. The tube is inserted into the spinal canal, and the pump is implanted in the abdomen, just under the skin. The pump is not implanted into the body cavity or near internal organs. A potent painkiller, such as morphine, is trickled into the spinal canal. This mixes with the spinal fluid. The spinal cord has special docks (receptors) for the morphine. This can lead to tremendous pain relief, at a fraction of the dose needed by mouth. There may be fewer side effects. As with any surgery, there are risks. Bleeding, infection, pump malfunction, catheter breakage, erosion through the skin, fluid collection around pump, persistent spinal leak, confusion, sedation, breathing problems, drug programming errors, and drug refill errors have been reported. Patients with these devices, also known colloquially as "intrathecal morphine pumps," must have their pumps refilled with a specialized office procedure. They cannot simply refill the medication at a pharmacy. These patients must closely follow up with their pain physician.

In summary, interventional pain procedures attempt to aggressively tackle the source of your pain state and are helpful when medicines and other therapeutic modalities are unsuccessful. Interventional pain physicians have evolved into unique medical experts that have special skill sets which can make a big difference for someone in moderate to severe pain. Understanding your pain and therapeutic options including interventional pain injections may go a very long way in easing your suffering.

28

ANESTHESIA AND SURGERY: WHAT TO EXPECT

Haibin Wang, MD, PhD, and Jianguo Cheng, MD, PhD

INTRODUCTION

The thought of having surgery under anesthesia can be intimidating to many people. The chances are that at some point in your life you will need to undergo a surgical procedure. In fact, even some interventional pain procedures (pump implantation, nerve blocks) require that you are either sedated or completely asleep. It is true that any medical procedure carries certain risks and should not be taken lightly. However, the risks can be minimized, and anesthesia has become much safer with the evolution of science of medicine, vigilant anesthesiologists, better monitoring equipment, and improved anesthetics and other drugs. Indeed, data published by the American Society of Anesthesiologists suggest that an estimated 40 million anesthetics are performed annually in the United States, and complications from anesthesia have declined dramatically over the past half century. For example, the odds of anesthesia-related death 50 years ago were approximately 1 in 1,500. But today, the odds have dropped to almost one-tenth of that number despite the fact that we are taking care of many older and sicker patients. For an otherwise healthy patient, the odds of death attributable to anesthesia are less than 1 in 200,000 when an anesthesiologist is involved in patient care. In contrast, the chance of dying from a motor vehicle accident in this country is 1 in 6,700, according to the risk analysis report by the Harvard School of Public Health. Anesthesiologists are extremely well-trained specialists (they train for at least four years after medical school) who oversee all aspects of your care to ensure your safety within the operating room during surgery and immediately postoperatively. Other anesthesia professionals that may be involved in your care include certified registered nurse anesthetists (CRNAs) and anesthesia assistants (AAs), as well as residents and students. Throughout this chapter, we will refer to your anesthesia provider as "anesthesiologist." It is important for patients to have a good understanding of, and realistic expectation for their forthcoming surgery and anesthesia.

Since the first public demonstration of anesthesia using ether took place at the Massachusetts General Hospital back in 1846, surgery and anesthesia have been interdependent and evolved together. Pain is a part of almost every single medical procedure, from a simple skin biopsy to a sophisticated open heart operation. Anesthesia is dedicated to the relief of pain and the well-being of the patient before, during, and after surgery. It is used to create an ideal condition for the surgeon to operate, while keeping the patient safe, stable, and comfortable utilizing a combination of anesthetics, pain medications, muscle relaxants, and close monitoring. Anesthesiologists closely monitor the patient's basic vital activities such as breathing, blood pressure, heart rate, and temperature. The goals of anesthesia are to achieve the following: (1) stable vital functions; (2) analgesia (no pain); (3) immobility (no movement); (4) amnesia (no memory or recall of the operation); and (5) unconsciousness (which depends on the type of anesthesia). A successful anesthesia is dependent on many steps that include pre-surgery evaluation and preparation, anesthesia care during surgery, and care during recovery from anesthesia. This chapter addresses this process step by step to help you be prepared.

PRE-SURGERY EVALUATION

Preoperative (pre-surgery) evaluation helps your anesthesiologist to develop plans to fit your needs. It also provides an opportunity for you to have your questions and concerns addressed to reduce your anxiety and fear. The American Society of Anesthesiologists classifies patients into five categories based upon their physical status, from normal healthy to severely ill patients. Higher categories can potentially carry higher risks for surgery and anesthesia. So it is critically important for your anesthesiologist to accurately assess your overall health status and put together an anesthesia strategy most appropriate for you. You may not need to know the details of the classification criteria, but it is important to know the anesthesia plan your anesthesiologist has for you. If you are asked to make an appointment at the pre-operation clinic, you will be seen by an anesthesia provider who may not be the one to administer your anesthesia on the day of surgery, but who is nevertheless experienced to evaluate potential challenges during your anesthesia. He or she will review your medical history, surgical history, and anesthesia history. It is important to answer all the questions truthfully and clearly, to the best of your knowledge. Bring a list of prescribed or over-the-counter medications and dietary supplements or herbal products. Many herbals, for example, can cause bleeding or interact with anesthesia drugs and should be discontinued two to three weeks prior to surgery. A survey performed by one of the editors of this book, Dr. Alan Kaye, MD, PhD, demonstrated that one-third of patients coming for surgery were taking one or more herbal products (over 29,000 of these products are available), but 70 percent of these patients did not disclose this information to their anesthesia providers.

Other important information you will be asked to provide is whether you smoke cigarettes, drink alcohol, or use illicit drugs; whether you are allergic to any medications or latex; and whether you have a personal or a family history of adverse reaction to anesthesia. This information will help the anesthesiologist determine the choice of anesthetics and other medications. For example, Demerol, a type of opioid (narcotic) commonly used during anesthesia, should not be given to patients taking monoamine oxidase inhibitors (such as Selegiline), a class of medications used to treat depression, since it can result in a life-threatening reaction.

The anesthesiologist will also perform a physical exam, focusing on your heart, lungs, mouth, and throat. The doctor will hear if there are any irregular heartbeats or abnormal breathing sounds, and will examine your ranges of mouth opening and neck flexion-extension. Your teeth and the shape of your throat will also be examined in order to estimate how easy or difficult it may be to insert a breathing tube, if needed. An evaluation of spine curvature may also be performed if spinal or epidural anesthesia is planned.

Your current laboratory test results will be reviewed to ensure safe anesthesia. If indicated, further tests may be ordered. For instance, if you have a history of coronary heart disease and have a recent experience of shortness of breath after walking a short distance, you may need an echocardiogram or a stress test to further investigate your heart function. You may also need to see a cardiologist to optimize your heart condition before surgery. At the end of the visit, the anesthesiologist will usually explain to you the options for anesthesia based on the type of surgery and the risks and benefits associated with the anesthesia. He or she will also answer your questions, address your concerns, and obtain your consent to the anesthesia plan. Please make sure you understand what is explained to you before signing the "informed consent."

PRE-OPERATION FOOD AND LIQUID RESTRICTIONS

It is necessary to have an empty stomach before receiving anesthesia to reduce the risk of aspiration. Under anesthesia, protective reflexes are usually suppressed, and aspiration could occur when stomach content regurgitates and spills into your airway. As a general rule, you should withhold eating and drinking after midnight before your surgery. However, the fasting time requirement varies depending on the types of anesthesia and surgery and age and other factors. Under some circumstances, you may drink clear liquids (water, apple juice, black coffee, or tea) up to two hours before your anesthesia. Your anesthesiologist will usually give clear instructions, and adhering to the instruction is essential to your safety.

Pre-Operation Management of Medications

If you take any medicines regularly, you should ask your surgeon and anesthesiologist whether you should continue taking those medicines before the operation. Generally speaking, some blood thinners (but not all) are stopped prior to the operation to minimize the risk of excessive bleeding. Oral hypoglycemic medications for diabetes, such as metformin and glyburide, generally should be skipped on the day of surgery. Medications for high blood pressure or rate disturbances, such as metoprolol, should be continued on the day of surgery. However, these general principles may not apply to every patient. For example, it may not be wise to stop a blood thinner in a patient with a high risk of stroke without initiating an alternative blood thinner. Communication and coordination between anesthesioligists, surgeons, and other specialists is critically important to ensure safe and effective patient care.

Painkillers are particularly relevant in patients with chronic pain. Abrupt discontinuation of pain medicines may cause exacerbated pain and even precipitate withdrawal reactions if opioid medications have been used for a long time. Surgical pain will further aggravate the painful state. Therefore, the rule of thumb is to continue the pain medications through the pre-surgery period. One exception is nonsteroidal anti-inflammatory drugs (NSAIDs), such as ibuprofen, which generally should be discontinued three days prior to surgery to decrease the risk of bleeding. Anxiolytics may be indicated in patients with significant anxiety if other relaxation techniques have not been effective.

Smoking Cessation before Surgery

It is well known that smoking (cigarettes contain over 50 known poisons) can cause many health problems, including complications during anesthesia. It is highly recommended to stop smoking, at least for a few days before surgery. Smoking increases irritability and mucus production of the airway. It also increases blood nicotine and carbon monoxide levels that may lead to decreased oxygen delivery to tissues during and after surgery. Studies have shown that smoking may hinder wound healing. The benefit of discontinuing smoking can take effect rather quickly; within 12–24 hours after one stops smoking, the blood nicotine and carbon monoxide decrease to near normal levels.

The Day of the Surgery

On the day of surgery, you should allow yourself enough time to report to the hospital on time. As part of the patient safety campaign, your identity, type of surgery, site of surgery, allergies, and last time of food and liquid intake will probably be checked repeatedly. This is intended to ensure that you are the "right patient" for the "right procedure" at the "right site." You will have to dress in a hospital gown, and your vital signs will be measured and recorded. You will then be greeted by your surgeon, who usually will mark the site of the surgery after addressing your questions. Your anesthesia provider will meet you and take care of you until you are discharged from the hospital after surgery. He or she will explain to you the anesthesia plan and answer any questions you may have about anesthesia, recovery, or other matters. He or she may also do a brief physical exam, of your airway in particular. An intravenous (IV) catheter is then placed and fluid and medications, such as medications to help you relax or antibiotics, will be administered. In some cases, a catheter is inserted into one of your arteries, typically in the wrist, to continuously monitor your blood pressure. At times, a central venous line may also be placed typically in the neck vein for the purposes of monitoring your heart function and administering certain types of medications and fluids. These more sophisticated procedures are usually performed either in the pre-anesthesia waiting area or in the operating room, often after you have been given some degree of sedation.

IN THE OPERATING ROOM

Once in the operating room, you will be greeted by your surgeon, the OR nurse, and the surgical technician. You will be moved onto the operating table, positioned and fastened according to the surgical needs, and padded with foams or cushions to protect you against physical injuries. The OR staff will try their best to keep you covered with blankets for your comfort during the whole process. You will then be connected to a myriad of monitors for your heart (EKG), blood pressure, breathing, oxygenation (pulse oximetry), and body temperature. Use of these monitors is the standard of care to ensure your safety regardless of what type of anesthesia you may need.

TYPES AND CHOICE OF ANESTHESIA

There are several types of anesthesia that can be used to serve your needs. *Local anesthesia* involves application of local anesthetics (numbing medicine) directly into the surgical area to block the nerve endings and pain sensations. It is commonly used by the surgeon in combination with other types of anesthesia to achieve optimal surgical condition. When used as a sole method of anesthesia, it is usually for minor procedures such as biopsy, typically in an office setting. It normally does not affect your consciousness and does not require an anesthesia provider to administer.

Monitored anesthesia care, also referred to as "*conscious sedation*," involves anesthesia with a moderate level of sedation. Patients usually maintain spontaneous breathing and are arousable. It is typically achieved by intravenous administration of both sedatives and pain medicines (often opioids). This type of anesthesia is commonly used for less invasive surgeries and procedures.

Regional anesthesia involves the injection/infusion of a local anesthetic to a nerve or a plexus of nerves to block pain in a certain *region* of the body. The injection site is usually proximal to the surgical site. For certain surgeries of the low part of the body, epidural or spinal anesthesia can be used. It is typically achieved by injecting a local anesthetic through a needle or infusing the medication through a catheter from the back. For surgeries of the arm and leg, more specific nerves can be blocked by a trained anesthesia provider under the guidance of an ultrasound machine or a stimulator to precisely locate the injection site. Regional anesthesia can be combined with general anesthesia in many cases for best pain control and surgical conditions.

General anesthesia, as suggested by its name, renders the patient completely unconscious. It is accomplished either by receiving intravenous anesthetics or by breathing gas anesthetics. Under general anesthesia, a patient typically needs a breathing tube that is open to your windpipe/lungs at one end and connected to a breathing machine at the other end. Most major surgeries are performed under general anesthesia.

The choice of a particular type of anesthesia depends on the type and duration of the surgery, the patient's health status, and sometimes the preference of the patient and physician. For example, open heart surgery can be performed only under general anesthesia, while many other surgeries can be performed either under general anesthesia or regional anesthesia. Your anesthesiologist should work with you to determine which type of anesthesia fits your needs best. Also, different types of anesthesia are not mutually exclusive. In fact, local or regional anesthesia is commonly combined with general anesthesia for optimal surgical conditions and pain control. For instance, when you have abdominal (belly) surgery, you may have general anesthesia for the operation, in addition to an epidural (regional) anesthesia for pain control during and after the operation.

A TYPICAL GENERAL ANESTHESIA EXPERIENCE

Let's use general anesthesia as an example to walk you through a typical anesthesia experience. Once you are properly positioned on the OR table, and once all the monitors have been connected and are functioning properly, you will be asked to breathe pure oxygen through a face mask for a few minutes. Your anesthesia provider will then start delivering anesthetics through your IV (IV induction) or through the face mask. Within a minute or two, you will fall into deep sleep without discomfort. At this point, after you are asleep, your anesthesia provider will place a breathing device in your mouth or trachea and connect it to a breathing machine. Once your breathing is secured and you are well asleep, the OR staff will again adjust your position as needed to optimize surgical exposure and access. Your surgeon will prepare your skin for the surgical field, drape with sterile techniques to prevent bacterial contamination, and start the operation after getting a "go-ahead" from your anesthesiologist.

While your surgeons are doing your surgery, the anesthesiologist will vigilantly monitor your vital signs and your responses to the surgery and keep you under an appropriate level of anesthesia. He or she will also closely watch the progress in the surgical field and adjust the anesthetic to your surgical needs. The goal is to ensure your safety while providing optimal surgical conditions. Although you are unconscious at this stage, your body may still respond to painful surgical stimulation with increased heart rate and/or blood pressure. The anesthesiologist will read these signs and respond to these changes by constantly adjusting your depth of anesthesia or providing additional pain medications. As you can see, a good anesthesia is a combination of science and art. It makes it possible for your surgeon to perform the operation safely and efficiently.

The final stage of anesthesia is called "emergence." At the end of the operation, your anesthesiologist will gradually discontinue your anesthetics. You will emerge from anesthesia by gradually returning to spontaneous breathing and regaining consciousness. This process usually takes a few minutes, thanks to the advances in anesthetic drugs that take effect fast but also get cleared from your body fairly quickly. Your muscle strength will also recover fully so you can follow commands to lift your head or squeeze the anesthesiologist's hand. At this point, the breathing tube may be safely removed. Similar to induction, emergence is also a very dynamic stage. Many changes happen in a short period of time while you are under close monitoring.

Emergence does not necessarily mean you have completely recovered from all the effects of anesthesia. Certain effects may persist. It is not uncommon that you may feel very drowsy, confused, and disoriented immediately after the surgery. Therefore, you need a period of recovery. There is a special area designated to recovery from anesthesia. The area is often called "post-anesthesia care unit" or "recovery room." Your anesthesiologist will escort you from the operating room to the recovery room. He or she will report to the recovery nurse and direct further care in the recovery period. Your vital signs and overall condition will be monitored in the recovery room. You may need to be treated if post-anesthesia side effects do occur, such as nausea, vomiting, and pain. Your surgeon may also check on you and your incision. From the recovery room, you will be able to go home or go to your regular hospital room, depending on your surgery and the progress of your recovery. In some cases, you may be directly transferred from the operating room to the "intensive care unit" for recovery if you have a major operation such as a heart or brain surgery.

COMMON SIDE EFFECTS AFTER ANESTHESIA AND SURGERY

Side effects may occur, albeit major complications from anesthesia and surgery are less frequent. Common side effects include nausea and vomiting, post-surgery pain, feeling cold, urinary retention, sore throat, and aching muscles. Factors affecting the rate of side effects/complications include the type and duration of the surgery, choice of anesthetic and other medications, and individual variability. In general, local anesthesia is less likely to cause complications, although an overdose is possible if too much of it is injected in a short period of time. Regional anesthesia bears some risks of bleeding, nerve injury, local anesthetic overdose, and infection. In addition, spinal and epidural anesthesia may cause low blood pressure or headache, both of which are readily treatable. General anesthesia may have a wider range of side effects and/or complications simply because it has more profound impact on the entire body.

Post-surgery pain is common as the anesthesia wears off. Your anesthesiologist usually will treat you with IV pain medications, most commonly opioids. You may also be given the option of "patient-controlled analgesia" (PCA), meaning that you control your pain by pressing a control button to deliver pain medication through this PCA pain pump device. It is important to adequately control your pain to avoid restlessness and stress on your body and to promote a timely recovery. It is sometimes advantageous to have a regional anesthesia that usually offers excellent pain control in the post-surgery recovery period. It is particularly useful in patients with chronic pain conditions that require long-term opioid therapy because it is very difficult to use other methods to control pain in this patient population due to their high level of tolerance to pain medications.

Post-surgery nausea and vomiting can occur after any type of anesthesia, although it is more common after general anesthesia. You are more likely to experience this if you undergo a lengthy procedure, a procedure involving gynecologic, eye and middle ear, breast, and abdominal surgery, if you otherwise suffer from motion sickness, and if you are a young female. The anesthetic gas, opioids, and surgical stimulation may sensitize the part of your brain that controls nausea and vomiting reaction. Severe nausea and/or vomiting can be debilitating and can prolong the length of stay in the hospital. As a current standard of care, your anesthesiologist will give you antinausea medication to prevent or reduce this unpleasant side effect.

Low body temperature (the medical term is *hypothermia*) occurs as a result of disturbed temperature regulation of the body during anesthesia and surgery. A drop in body temperature is common during general anesthesia due to reduced body heat production and increased heat losses, if no adequate warming mechanism is applied. You may feel cold or even shiver when you wake up from anesthesia. A warm blanket usually makes you feel much better. A special warming device that looks like a blanket may be placed on top of you while you undergo anesthesia and surgery.

Urinary retention (inability to urinate even though you have a full bladder) may occur as a result of residual effects of anesthetics. Post-surgery pain and use of opioid medications may also cause urinary retention. Urinary catheter may be needed in such patients. The patient should not be discharged from the hospital before the urinary retention has been resolved. Injury to your teeth and lips may occur during to insertion of the breathing tube, even though it is rare. *Sore throat* is relatively common if you had a breathing device placed during general anesthesia. The throat discomfort usually goes away in a couple of days without any treatment. *Muscle aching* may be due to the use of a type of muscle relaxation medication during general anesthesia or may be due to a long surgery.

DISCHARGE FROM THE HOSPITAL

Most minor surgical procedures are done on an outpatient basis, which means that you will be discharged home from the recovery room on the same day you have your surgery. If you are not ready for discharge, you may be admitted for further monitoring or care, usually in a regular floor ward where your family and friends can visit. The length of hospital stay will depend on the type of surgery and your progress in recovery. When you meet the criteria for safe discharge, you will be given instructions on what to do and what to avoid, contact information in case any issues arise, follow-up plans, and discharge medications such as antibiotics and painkillers. In order to be discharged on the same day you have surgery and anesthesia, you will have to have a responsible adult to accompany you. You should not drive yourself home. It is important to have a reliable caregiver who can accompany you at least for the first 24 hours after discharge in case you need help.

ADDITIONAL RESOURCE

American Society of Anesthesiologists: http://www.asahq.org/PressRoom/anesthesia
    fastfacts.htm

29

PAIN MANAGEMENT AFTER SURGERY

Gulshan Doulatram, MD, and Vu Tran, MD

INTRODUCTION

Pain after surgery is often called acute or postoperative pain. It occurs immediately after surgery and may last for a period of two to four weeks. However, it may last for as long as several months. This is in contrast to chronic pain, which usually lasts for more than six months. Acute pain differs from chronic pain in several ways. Acute pain functions to signal that tissue damage has occurred and protects individuals from further harm. For example, not moving an arm or leg after surgery due to associated pain will aid in natural healing. However, a pain that continues on does not provide any additional benefits and may be harmful and requires to be treated. The goal is to reduce or eliminate pain and discomfort with a minimum of side effects. Acute pain can affect the skin, joints, bones, and ligaments. The medical term for this type of pain is somatic pain: it tends to be sharp and throbbing, and is localized around the operated area. Acute pain also can be classified as visceral, that is, coming from the internal organs. This type of pain tends to be diffuse, deep, achy, and poorly localized.

SYMPTOMS

Pain after surgery is a normal phenomenon and can be mild, moderate, or even severe. Furthermore, the perception of pain varies widely among individuals. Therefore, it is essential to properly diagnose and treat the various types of pain individually following surgery. It is very important to understand the precise reasons for the existing pain in order to be able to treat it successfully. Pain can be described in many ways, as discussed below.

Pain after surgery is composed of different types. Broadly, we can categorize pain into two classes: "nociceptive" pain and "non-nociceptive" pain (nerve pain).

The stimulation of specific pain receptors in the surgical area is called nociceptive pain. This pain involves specific receptors in our bodies that respond to heat, cold, stretch, and pressure. In contrast, non-nociceptive pain arises from within a nerve itself rather from direct stimulation of pain receptors.

There are two ways in which nociceptive pain presents itself: "somatic" pain and "visceral" pain. The source of somatic pain is from pain receptors located throughout the body tissues; for example, pain in the skin resulting from a surgical incision. Somatic pain is often described as sharp and well localized. The source of visceral pain, however, is the internal organs of the body like the gut, liver, gall bladder, and spleen. The characteristic most often associated with visceral pain is that it often presents as a poorly localized vague deep pain in the belly.

Non-nociceptive pain or "neuropathic" pain is often caused by the direct or indirect injury to the nerves themselves. The nerves do not have pain receptors on themselves and the non-nociceptive pain arises from the misfiring and improper function of these nerves. Such misfiring can be described or interpreted as tingling or burning along the body's geographic distribution of various nerves. These types of pains are often treated differently. The patients often describe this pain as follows:

- Medical term: *Allodynia*
  - Pain due to a stimulus that does not normally provoke pain, such as stroking the skin or when having clothes on increases the pain (similar to when one has sunburn)
- Medical term: *Dysesthesia*
  - An unpleasant abnormal sensation, whether spontaneous or evoked, like a tingling or electrical sensation
- Medical term: *Hyperalgesia*
  - An increased response to a stimulus that is normally painful, such as pinching the skin causes more pain than normal
- Medical term: *Hyperesthesia*
  - Increased sensitivity to stimulation when slightly touching the skin may feel like deep pressure on the skin
- Medical term: *Paresthesia*
  - An abnormal sensation, whether spontaneous or evoked, such as feeling of spiders crawling on the skin

Diagnosing the type of pain the patient may have after surgery is an essential first step to designing the most effective treatment and thus achieving better pain management and the desired relief.

Pain after surgery is usually described as throbbing, gnawing, pulsating, or sharp and can be either localized or diffuse, depending on the site of the pain. The pain may also be referred to an area far from the source of the pain, for example in the right shoulder after gall bladder surgery. The skin over the scar may have characteristics of burning and tingling. The site of the surgery generally has a profound effect upon the degree of postsurgical pain a patient may suffer. Surgical operations on the chest and upper abdomen are more painful than operations on the lower abdomen, which are relatively more painful than the operations on the limbs. However, any operation involving a body cavity, large joint surfaces, or deep tissues should always be regarded as painful. In particular, operations on the chest or upper abdomen may markedly decrease lung function and induce difficulty when taking deep breaths and inability to cough and clear secretions. Together, these may lead to further collapse of lung tissue and even pneumonia.

Pain also increases the stress response in the body with subsequent rises in heart rate and blood pressure. Prolonged pain can reduce physical activity and increase immobility, which can cause pooling of blood in the legs and an increased risk of blood clots both in the legs and lungs. Also, intense pain may reduce gut motility, which can, in turn, lead to constipation, nausea, vomiting, and inability to urinate. These problems are quite unpleasant for the patient and may prolong the hospital stay.

Diagnosis

Keeping in mind that pain is a symptom and not a diagnosis, all efforts should be made to find the inherent cause of pain. In some cases, it is obvious if the pain occurs at the exact surgical site and can easily be explained. Sometimes, however, the pain is due to other causes that are often missed, such as abdominal enlargement due to bleeding after surgery, which needs prompt investigation and treatment. The patient needs to be completely evaluated, including the current pain level, use of medicines, and their side effects. Previous experiences with postsurgical pain will help in predicting the need for pain medications. Potential difficulties associated with the language or culture, in defining the pain, are also assessed in evaluating the pain status. Expectations need to be discussed before surgery, which will avoid disappointment and anxiety after surgery. Special considerations need to be made if patients are using pain medications on a long-term basis to control their chronic pain. The nature and intended purpose of the surgery may also be important. If the proposed operation will lead to a restoration of normal function, for example, a removal of gall bladder or fixation of a fracture, it is likely to be seen in a positive way by the patient. However, where the outcome is not clear, for example, an operation for cancer or to investigate an unknown pain, the patient's fear and anxiety may lead to high levels of pain. Patients who are afraid of anesthesia or surgery may report more pain, which can be very difficult to manage or treat.

Adequate time must be allowed to explain the surgery, and patients need to be reassured that all steps will be taken to ensure the pain relief afterwards. It is important to establish the expectations of the patient before surgery. An adequate and friendly explanation in simple terms will often reduce anxiety and minimize misunderstandings about the nature of the proposed surgery and pain that will be expected for the nature of the surgery.

Controlling pain before the onset of surgery either with use of pain medication or use of local anesthetic blocks establishes a level of pain control and provides for better pain management after surgery. This is called preemptive analgesia and has become one of the preferred methods of controlling pain especially in patients who have a high degree of pain even before surgery.

There are several pain rating scales used by doctors and other health care providers that will help measure and quantify pain. These scales help to determine the severity, type, and duration of pain and are useful in making a treatment plan and also in evaluating how effective a specific treatment is for a patient. Verbal rating scales consist of words commonly used to describe pain. You read the words and choose the one that best describes the pain you are experiencing. A score (e.g., from 0 to 3) that is assigned to each word is then used to measure pain levels.

Numerical rating scales usually consist of a series of numbers ranging from, for example, 0 to 10. The ends of the scale are labeled to indicate "no pain" and the "worst pain possible." You choose the number that best corresponds to the level of pain you are experiencing.

Visual analogue scales commonly consist of a vertical or horizontal line, 10 cm in length, with end points labeled "no pain" and the "worst pain," or similar words. You are asked to place a mark on the line that corresponds to the intensity of the pain you are experiencing.

These are simple, minimally intrusive tests that are effective and easy to administer and score in most cases. However, verbal, numerical, and visual analogue scales cannot be used in all patients. They may be ineffective in patients who have trouble following instructions, in patients who are unresponsive (e.g., due to injury), and in young children and elderly patients. The Wong Baker FACES scale has been used in these cases with good success. You circle the face that represents your pain. Also, some observations (for example, sighing, groaning, sweating, ability to move) have been used as indirect measures of pain. This has the advantage that it does not rely on the patient to any great degree. Vital signs such as heart rate and blood pressure are indirect measures of pain. It is important to emphasize that pain should be assessed and measured when the patient is active to obtain the true functional status of the patient and to obtain an accurate measure of pain.

There are seven features of a pain symptom, namely, location, severity, duration, onset, quality, and exacerbating and relieving factors. Pain distant from the operative site may indicate complications not associated with the procedure, which may require separate treatment. Complaints of generalized pain all over the body may represent stress, anxiety, or in some cases, fever. The description of the pain may indicate the cause. For example sharp, stabbing pain is associated with surgery, whereas numbness or tingling may mean that there is nerve compression or irritation.

It may still be difficult to assess pain in the few days after surgery by any of the methods described above. It should be emphasized that you should be evaluated at regular intervals and symptoms of pain be asked as a routine part of the check every day. Nurses, ancillary staff, and physicians should be encouraged to make assessment of pain a routine part of the examination. By checking on you regularly, we can look to see if pain is improving, worsening, or staying the same and also look to see the response to medications and other therapies.

TREATMENT

Treatment of pain after surgery actually may start before surgery. A variety of different techniques can be implemented to avoid the side effects from one modality or medication alone.

Intravenous Patient-Controlled Analgesia (PCA)

Patient-controlled analgesia (PCA) is a machine that safely permits the patient to push a button and deliver small amounts of pain medicine into an intravenous (IV) line. PCA provides stable pain relief in most situations. Many patients like the sense of control they have over their pain management. Since this mode is regulated by the patient, it is much safer and causes stable level of the medication in the bloodstream compared to intermittent intramuscular injections. If family members push the button for the patient, then the patient can get higher doses and have side effects, neither of which is desirable. Morphine is the typical drug used in PCA, although occasionally other drugs such as hydromorphone (Dilaudid) can be used as well.

Patient-Controlled Epidural Analgesia (PCEA)

Patients are familiar with epidural anesthesia because it is frequently used to control pain during childbirth. PCEA uses a PCA pump to deliver pain-control medicine into an epidural catheter that is placed in the back in the epidural space. A mixture of numbing medication and opioid (narcotic) medications is infused through this epidural catheter. An epidural is usually more effective in relieving pain than intravenous medication. Patients who receive an epidural typically have less pain when they take deep breaths, cough, and walk, and they may recover more quickly. For patients with medical problems such as heart or lung disease, epidural analgesia may reduce the risk of serious complications such as heart attack and pneumonia.

Epidural is safe, but like any procedure or therapy, not risk free. Sometimes the epidural does not adequately control pain. Nausea, vomiting, itching, and drowsiness can occur. Occasionally, numbness and weakness of the legs can occur, which disappear after the medication is reduced or stopped. Headache can occur, but this is rare. Severe complications such as nerve damage, bleeding into the epidural space, and infection are extremely rare.

A spinal may be an alternate method of pain control in which pain medication is directly injected into the spinal space to mix with the spinal fluid. The medications will bind to pain receptors in the spinal cord, thus providing very effective relief with small doses.

Nerve Blocks

Peripheral nerve blocks are very effective methods to control pain after surgery. Whereas an epidural controls pain over the abdomen or legs, a nerve block is used when pain from surgery affects a smaller region of the body, such as an arm or leg. Sometimes a catheter similar to an epidural catheter is placed for prolonged pain control. There are several potential advantages of a nerve block. It may allow for a significant reduction in the amount of pain medication that you may need to take. This may result in fewer side effects such as nausea, vomiting, itching, and drowsiness.

Injection of Medication at the Surgical Site

Medication such as local anesthetics (numbing medications) can be injected into wound or joints by the surgeon at the time of surgery. Depending on the type of medications, they can provide up to 24 hours of relief.

Medications

A so-called "balanced" analgesic approach uses a combination of opioid and non-opioid painkillers such as nonsteroidal anti-inflammatory drugs (NSAIDs) and acetaminophen (Tylenol). The choice of pain-relieving techniques will depend on the kind and location of surgery. *Opiates* are drugs like morphine, and they work directly on the pain receptors in the brain and spinal cord. Some of the side effects of these opioid medications include nausea, vomiting, itching, drowsiness, and slowing of the gastrointestinal system causing constipation. The general principle is that the first line of treatment is medications such as aspirin, acetaminophen, and nonsteroidals. If these are not effective, then weaker opioids such as hydrocodone (Vicodin) can be utilized. The next rung of the treatment ladder is the use of stronger opioids such as morphine, hydromorphone (Dilaudid), and fentanyl. An important consideration for pain management after surgery is that patients sometimes cannot take medications by mouth in the first couple of days. In that case, the treatment modality may require to be modified so that pain medications can be given intravenously. These medications can be slowly titrated down as the pain intensity decreases and patients can begin taking medications by mouth. Aspirin is an effective medication that can be utilized. However, aspirin may cause gastrointestinal bleeding which may limit its use. *Acetaminophen* (Tylenol) has pain-reducing and fever-reducing properties, though it may not help treat the inflammation of surgery. It has few side effects at normal doses and is widely used for the treatment of minor pain. High doses can cause damage to the liver. *Nonsteroidals* (NSAIDs) reduce pain and inflammation. All NSAIDs work in the same way, and thus there is no point in giving more than one at a time. They have a high incidence of side effects with prolonged use, and caution should be exercised. NSAIDs should be used cautiously in people with stomach bleeding, kidney problems, bleeding problems, or people who are sensitive to NSAIDs. Using a combination of different medications is ideal because these work through different mechanisms and they will exert a synergistic effect in the treatment of pain. The doses of these various medications can be decreased to minimize the side effects.

PROGNOSIS

The prognosis for acute pain is extremely favorable, and it usually abates within a few weeks after surgery. Usually, the intensity of pain sequentially decreases over time. Persistent pain will interfere with optimum recovery during this period and also leads to increased health care costs. Patients who have chronic pain prior to surgery have a much higher chance of having persistent pain after surgery. This subset of patients needs a more aggressive approach to pain management utilizing a "balanced" approach of medications and regional anesthetic techniques (nerve blocks, spinal, or epidural). If acute pain is not controlled adequately, 2–10 percent of these people may develop long-term chronic pain. Good, aggressive control of acute pain may improve long-term recovery such as quality of life and return to function. In addition, adequate control of acute pain may facilitate timely and active participation in rehabilitation. The benefits of effective pain control include return to work; decreased disability; prevention of complications like pneumonia, blood clots, and suppression of the immune system; and prevention of painful memories. This will prevent the likelihood of developing chronic pain and long-term disability.

ADDITIONAL RESOURCE

Pain after surgery: Managing and treating post surgery pain: http://www.webmd.com/pain-management

30

REHABILITATION PROGRAMS

Rinoo V. Shah, MD, MBA, and Alan D. Kaye, MD, PhD

Our society is suited for mobility. Whether you board a taxi, drive a car, or visit a library, painless movement is better than painful movement. Pain interferes with a person's mobility and daily activities. Chronic pain patients become distressed and alter their behaviors. They become apprehensive and avoid movement. They can no longer enjoy recreation. They may not be able to work or earn money. These patients have to adjust their daily schedules to accommodate pain. Simple activities may be frustrating and fatiguing. Although pain is an invisible disease, patients require aids that inadvertently announce their disability to the world. Pain does not respect privacy. They may become socially isolated. Many of our patients, for better or worse, consider a cane as a sign of weakness. Limitations on mobility, motivation, and drive can be unforgiving and humiliating. Restoring mobility is as important as pain relief.

Pain physicians recognize that pain treatment must be accompanied by functional improvement. The patient and physician can set goals to improve mobility. Physicians may refer a patient to an allied health provider, such as a physical or occupational therapist. These providers engage in face-to-face interactions with patients, in order to improve function and rehabilitate patients. A comprehensive rehabilitation program has several components: exercise (stretching, strengthening, aerobic); specialized equipment (braces, splints); modalities (hot, cold, electricity); massage; and walking aids. Rehabilitation programs use nonsurgical methods to relieve pain, restore function, modify abnormal pain behaviors, and educate patients. Patient motivation and physician input is essential to make this program a success.

Therapists are licensed, nonphysician health providers. They use several approaches for pain relief, motivation, and mobilization. Modalities are noninvasive tools to reduce pain. They are typically considered "passive." The patient doesn't have to actively participate—they just lie there and the modality can help with the pain.

Cryotherapy (cold) is used to relieve pain. This is applied to the surface of the skin, overlying the painful area. Cold may reduce blood flow, metabolism, swelling, muscle spasms, and nerve activity. This reduces pain. Cryotherapy methods are cheap: ice, cold water, refrigerated units, and chemical packs. Frostbite is an important concern. Skin application should be limited to 20 or 30 minutes. Temperature is about 59 degrees F (15 degrees C). This should not be used by patients with nerve damage and blood flow problems.

Heat is used to relieve pain. Our body temperature is about 98.6 F (37 C). A hot water faucet is typically 110 F, with a safety limit of 120 F. Human pain threshold is about 106 F (42 F). Nerve damage can occur at 113 F (45 C), with prolonged exposure.

Patients can tolerate temperatures ranging from 109 to 113 F (43–45 C). The heat is generally tolerable for 3–30 minutes. In general, the higher the temperature the shorter the duration. The temperature will rise in the skin and deeper tissues. Heating should not be carried out over insensate or poorly visualized areas. Patients can develop burns, discoloration, or permanent darkening over the areas treated. This is why heating should be conducted under the supervision of a specialist.

Heat can be delivered in different ways. Heat can be delivered to the outer or deeper surfaces in the body. The most common method is known as conduction: hot pack, hot water bottle, or heating pad. They are applied for about 20 minutes at a time. They are low cost and easy to use. For the hands and feet, a paraffin or mineral oil bath is used. If you have attended a wedding banquet, paraffin is used to keep the food in a foil tray heated. Paraffin and mineral oil have different heating properties, as compared to water. Paraffin can be heated to 125–130 F (52–54 C). A patient then dips their fingers into the paraffin for pain relief. A similar temperature in water would scald the skin!

Convection is a way of transferring heat with moving fluids or air. Convection is best visualized as a Jacuzzi, heated swimming pool, or sauna. Temperatures in a heated pool or Jacuzzi must be within a narrow range. The whole body can tolerate 91 to 98 F (33 to 36 C) and the limbs can tolerate 109 to 114 F (43–46 C). Patients must be carefully monitored during this type of heating.

Conversion is another method of heating. One type of energy, such as sound, is converted to another type of energy, heat. Conversion allows a provider to heat deep tissues. Ultrasound is a type of sound, above the hearing range for humans. Ultrasound can be used to heat deep tissues. Certain types of radio waves, such as microwaves, cause quick rotation of small molecules in the body. This molecule flips back and forth, very fast. As a result, this motion generates heat. This type of heating should not be used in people with implants or electrical devices. This device should not be used near fluid-filled structures in the body or on pregnant women.

Electricity can be used for pain relief. Small pads with a conducting gel can be applied to a painful part of the body. These pads are then connected to a small electrical box. The electrical current is usually of a small voltage or current. The shape of the electrical current can be adjusted. This can alleviate pain. Electrical fish and eels have been used in ancient times to treat all kinds of maladies. The modern view is that electricity can help shut a "gate" to the nervous system. This can conceptually block pain fibers. This is a major oversimplification, but a useful rule of thumb to help visualize how electricity can help with pain. The "shape of the wave form" is a controversial area of debate. In simple terms, a lower frequency is useful for muscle spasms. A higher frequency is used for nerve problems. Many of the textbooks discuss changes in blood flow, retarding muscle atrophy, improving healing, and restoring proper nerve inputs/signals. Electricity is most commonly delivered as a transcutaneous electrical nerve stimulation (TENS). Your therapist may request a home TENS unit. Electricity can help drive certain topical medications through the skin into a muscle or joint. This is known as iontophoresis (movement of molecules through a medium). Anti-inflammatory medications are most commonly used by physical therapists.

Massage therapy involves manipulating the surface of the body to relieve pain and improve well-being. Secondary goals are to reduce swelling and to mobilize a joint. Origins of this word stem from Europe and the Middle East. These origins refer to "kneading," "dough," "touch," "feel," and "handle." The therapist will manipulate and move the superficial muscles and connecting tissues. Massage can be applied to most regions of the body. There are a variety of styles of massage therapy. Massage therapy should not be applied to patients with recent burns, infections, inflamed vein clots, certain skin diseases, and certain types of cancer.

Massage has mechanical effects. Adhesions can be stretched; fluids can be mobilized; and return of blood or lymph facilitated. There are different methods for massage. In fact, there are multiple schools and styles of massage that are available. Simply, the methods involve stroking, compressing, tapping, or sustaining pressure on soft tissues. Myofascial release is a manual massage technique for stretching the soft tissues and improving range of motion. Patients should discuss these techniques with a massage therapist. A physical therapist may employ this technique as part of an overall treatment. Massage has many beneficial effects. For example, one of the authors of this chapter (also one of the editors of this book, Dr. Kaye) demonstrated that there is a significant drop in blood pressure and heart rate after deep tissue massage.

Active rehabilitation involves patient participation. Thus far, the aforementioned methods are passive—the patient simply has to lie there. Active therapy requires the patient to be a participant. The mainstay of active therapy is exercise.

The goals of exercise are to strengthen muscles, to improve flexibility, to increase endurance, and to restore the normal patterns of motion. The long-term goal is to relieve pain and maintain a state of well-being.

Exercise can focus on range of motion (ROM). Physicians and therapists use cryptic language about the type of ROM exercise: passive, active-assist, and active. Passive means the therapist moves your body for you. Active-assist means the patient and therapist work together to move the body or joint. Active means the patient moves by themselves and the therapist coaches and supports. ROM exercises typically do not use weights. As the patient makes improvements, resistance weights can be used in the exercise. The goal is to improve strength in the muscle. Stretching is an important part of exercise. Aerobic exercise is necessary to improve a patient's overall fitness. When a patient is in chronic pain, they may become deconditioned and their stamina may be reduced. Aerobic training may help to improve this stamina. A specially trained and licensed health care provider is necessary for exercise. For instance, a physical therapist will be familiar with precautions such as heart disease, high blood pressure, thin bones (osteoporosis), and breathing problems. Other providers may not have this background.

There are subsets of exercise programs that can be useful for pain control. Yoga is an effective low-impact exercise that can help with pain and mobility. Yoga can be tailored to one's specific age, sex, and physical limitations. Yoga has a rich and diverse history. In principle, yoga refers to control of body, mind, and speech. Hatha yoga is a commonly practiced form of yoga. This incorporates specific physical postures, poses, breathing, and meditation. Yoga in a distilled form is practiced as an exercise, devoid of religious connotations. The focus is on physical fitness, deep breathing, and relaxation. Interest in yoga has grown over the past few decades. When yoga is coupled with aerobic exercises, patients can reach an optimal level of fitness. Both aerobic and yoga exercises, however, are not specific to a pain condition.

Exercises specific for a pain condition include coordination training, fall prevention, desensitization training, postural control, mobilization, manipulation, and proprioceptive neuromuscular facilitation. The goals of these techniques are to reduce pain, enhance safety, and a graded return to mobility.

Manipulation deserves special mention. Osteopaths and chiropractors may engage in this practice. High velocity and low-amplitude techniques are synonymous with a forceful thrust. The joint is moved beyond its physical barrier. Patients who have osteoporosis, instability of the spine, infections, fractures, or a poor blood supply to the upper spinal cord (vertebrobasilar insufficiency) should not undergo manipulation.

Traction is a manual technique. Most commonly, traction is used for neck pain. Various devices can accomplish this. In the simplest form, a strap is placed around the base of a patient's skull. The strap is connected to a pulley that is connected to a weight, in turn. The weight places gentle traction along the neck axis. The weight is typically 5–10 percent of a patient's body weight, generally about 10–20 pounds. Patients may be seated or lying flat. The neck must be slightly flexed. The treatment lasts about 10–20 minutes. Lumbar traction has gained increased popularity, due to the development of specialized machines.

A force of about 25–50 percent of the patient's body weight is necessary. This type of force is difficult to generate. A harness can be used to induce manual low back traction. Patients lie on their stomach, and their hips are flexed. The degree of hip flexion will determine which segment in the lower back is stretched. Automated lumbar traction devices are available. There continues to be controversy about the role of these devices. Patients are encouraged to discuss the safety, costs, and effectiveness of these devices with providers. Some insurance companies may not cover these treatments. Patients are encouraged to negotiate the best deal possible under these circumstances.

An initial visit to a rehabilitation professional will typically consist of an evaluation, treatment recommendations, and goal setting. Several subsequent sessions over the next 4–6 weeks will use the previously mentioned approaches. Patients will have one-on-one encounters with the allied health professional, unlike a membership gym or exercise facility. The patient will then transition to an unsupervised and independent fitness program. These programs are not work specific, but may be used to rehabilitate an injured worker in pain. This is known as work conditioning.

Some centers focus on work-specific activities. This is known as work hardening. The therapist simulates work activities and focuses on physical and emotional work demands. Ergonomics is a science of designing equipment and devices that fit the human body, its movements, and its cognitive abilities. The goal is to improve how a patient interacts with his or her physical work and home environments. Simple strategies include keeping a wrist straight with the elbow down for wrist pain. Rotating (swivel) chairs with arm rests and rubber floor mats may help with back pain. These therapists look for ways to reduce force, movement frequency, holding time, and extreme postural motions.

Chronic pain rehabilitation is primarily concerned with improving function, reentry into the community, mobility, and pain relief. Physicians and allied health professionals evaluate the patient to decide which nonsurgical approach would be best. Face-to-face interactions with a patient and the application of various modalities subserve the goal of restoring function. The patient is coached and monitored over time to meet these goals.

Additional Resource

American Academy of Physical Medicine and Rehabilitation: http://www.aapmr.org

PART IV

SPECIAL POPULATIONS

31

PAIN IN CHILDREN

Galaxy Li, MD, and Christine Greco, MD

INTRODUCTION

Pain is an important signal that warns us that something is wrong. Whenever we are sick or injured, our brain sends out pain signals as an alarm. Everyone experiences pain differently, including children. Children can experience pain from many different causes, such as a bruise, an earache, a sore throat, a broken bone, or just having had an operation. Even though we now consider treating pain very important in children of all ages, for many years, pain in children was undertreated. There were several myths that led to this undertreatment of pain in children. It was believed that the nervous system of infants was not mature enough to actually perceive pain. The belief that infants could not feel pain was the reason why little or no pain medicines were regularly used for circumcisions and other minor operations. Another myth was that children rarely need pain medications because of the notion that they tolerate pain better than adults. This myth was based in part on the lack of understanding of how to measure the amount of pain an infant or young child has. Many also thought that some children were just "too sick" to be able to receive pain medicines. We now know that nerve pathways that transmit pain signals exist even in premature infants, just as there are these pathways in older children and adults. In fact, some think that infants may be even more sensitive to pain than older children. Pain scoring systems have been developed for children of all ages, even for premature infants, so that the amount of pain a child is experiencing can now be measured.

Over the past 25 years, research studies have led to a better understanding of how to treat pain in children. Research has also shown that it is important to treat pain, since untreated pain can sometimes cause the nervous system to become more sensitive to pain. The management of pain in children is now considered a basic and important part of caring for children. In this chapter, we will outline how to assess pain in children and what treatments for pain are available in the context of some specific pain conditions in children.

Assessing Pain in Infants and Children

Determining whether a child has pain and how much pain a child has can be challenging for parents and for doctors and nurses. Pain assessment can be particularly difficult in infants and young children, since they are not able to communicate as well as older children. It is important to be able to assess pain, since this is the first step in treating it. Children should be asked where they have pain and how much pain they have. Sometimes it is helpful to give a child choices in assessing their pain. For example, young children are often able to tell whether they are having a little bit of pain, medium pain, or a lot of pain. Using the words that a child uses for pain can also be helpful—for example, using familiar words such "boo-boo" or "ouchie." Parents' observations about their child's pain can be important in helping doctors and nurses to understand how to treat the pain. Older children can sometimes use the adult 0–10 scale, where 0 is no pain and 10 is the worst pain you can imagine. It can also be helpful to ask older children to describe what their pain feels like, if possible.

The child's description of pain can help doctors and nurses decide what kind of pain the child is having and the best treatment for it. For example, if a child who describes his or her pain as feeling like "pins and needles" or as if "it's asleep" can sometimes suggest nerve pain. On the other hand, a sprain or muscle pain can sometimes cause pain that is throbbing. It is important to realize, however, that older children who are sick or in the hospital may not be able to describe their pain well, and they might need to use simpler methods of assessing pain rather than the 0–10 scale. A child's fear and anxiety may complicate pain assessment and may cause children to seem like they are having much more pain or much less pain than they actually are having. For example, a two-year-old who is distressed, crying, and afraid of a relatively painless ear exam may appear to have severe pain. In contrast, an eight-year-old with severe pain may say that they have no pain in order to avoid receiving a "pain shot." The meaning that pain has for a child can also change how they report their pain. For example, a child who has had a disfiguring birthmark removed may report pain differently from a child who has had a cancerous mass removed. Because it is sometimes hard for children to express how much pain they have, doctors and nurses often use pain scales to help measure pain. Many pain scales for children use faces or different colors to measure pain.

Ways to Treat Pain in Children

Treating pain in infants and children generally involves combinations of pain medications with non-medication techniques such as ice, distraction, guided imagery, and acupuncture. For some painful conditions, nerve blocks that numb the nerves are also used to treat pain. It is important to treat pain and stay ahead of it, since sometimes more medication is then needed to feel comfortable again if the pain gets out of control.

For minor aches and bruises, the use of ice, comfort measures, and distraction techniques work very well. Comfort measures such as hugging or cuddling allow a child to feel protected and less anxious about their pain. Helping a child feel less anxious is important in managing pain, since anxiety tends to worsen pain. Distracting a child when they have pain helps them to focus their attention away from their pain. Playing with a favorite toy, reading together, or singing together are types of distraction techniques that are easy and work well.

Allowing children to feel that they have some control over their pain is also helpful. For example, a child can be allowed to help wash and bandage a skinned knee, apply their own ice pack to a bump, or choose which finger for a blood draw.

Medications are used for some types of pain that are not easily relieved by comfort measures and distraction. Acetaminophen and nonsteroidal anti-inflammatory drugs (NSAIDs) are medications that are commonly used to treat pain in children. Narcotic medications are also sometimes used. Acetaminophen (Tylenol) is one of the most commonly used pain medications and is used to treat mild to moderate pain and to treat fever. It can be helpful to treat pain from ear infections, mild headache pain, and other common types of pain. Although acetaminophen is safe for most children, it is important to stay within recommended daily dosing guidelines since too much acetaminophen could cause liver damage. Parents should check with their child's doctor if they have questions about how much pain medicines to give. NSAIDs such as ibuprofen are also used to treat mild to moderate pain and to treat fever. Unlike acetaminophen, NSAIDs help reduce inflammation, which helps to reduce pain and swelling. NSAIDs are particularly useful for pain that occurs with swelling and inflammation, such as pain from arthritis, sprains, or muscle strains. NSAIDs can sometimes cause stomach upset and bleeding problems. Most children, however, have little or no problem when they take NSAIDs. In many cases, NSAIDs are not used in children who have recently had surgery because of the possible increased risk of bleeding. As with acetaminophen and all other medications, it is important to stay within the recommended dosing guidelines and check with your child's doctor if you are unsure how much NSAIDs to give your child.

Narcotic medications are sometimes used to treat moderate to severe pain and include medications such as morphine and oxycodone. Narcotic medications are often used to treat more severe types of pain—for example, pain after an operation, pain from a bone fracture, or cancer pain. Narcotics are often combined with acetaminophen or sometimes NSAIDs, which can help improve pain relief and help to reduce how much narcotic medication is needed. In addition to providing pain relief, narcotics also cause other effects such as slow breathing, drowsiness, itching, upset stomach, and constipation. It is helpful to start a stool softener if a child is going to need to take narcotics for more than just a couple of days. Parents should let their child's doctor know if they have an upset stomach, vomiting, or itching, or are too sleepy while taking a narcotic medication, because switching to a different one or decreasing the amount may be necessary. Infants are more sensitive to narcotics compared to older children, since narcotics are more likely to affect their breathing and consciousness. Finally, ask your doctor about the different types of preparations of pain medications that are available for different age groups.

Many parents are concerned about whether their child might get addicted to narcotic medications. It is very rare for children to become addicted to narcotic medications when these medications are used appropriately. If a child who has been taking narcotics for a long period of time no longer needs them, then the narcotics will need to be gradually reduced instead of stopping them all at once so that the child does not have unpleasant withdrawal symptoms. This does not mean that the child is addicted to the narcotic medications, but rather that the child's body has become tolerant to them. Children should never be given pain medications that were prescribed for other family members. As soon as the pain is lessened, any remaining medication should be safely discarded.

Pain from Needles

Many children worry and are afraid that they will have pain from a needle during IV placement or another procedure. Distraction and relaxation techniques can be very helpful to reduce anxiety and lessen the pain. There are different types of numbing creams and patches that can be placed on a child's skin to help lessen the pain from needles. Numbing creams and patches are used to temporarily numb the skin shortly before a needle stick, a blood draw, or other minor needle procedure. Parents can place the cream or patch on their child's skin themselves before coming in for the procedure, as it usually takes about 30–45 minutes for the cream to numb the area.

Pain Right after Surgery

For severe pain, especially in hospitalized children, pain medicines such as narcotic medications are often given intravenously (in the vein) so that pain can be treated quickly. Narcotic medications are also given intravenously when children are not yet able to eat or drink after an operation. A common way to give narcotic medications to children who experience severe pain is through a system called patient-controlled analgesia (PCA). This type of system gives a small dose of narcotic medication such as morphine whenever the child pushes the PCA button. PCA is often used to treat pain after surgery, pain from sickle cell, and cancer pain. Most children over the age of six years are able to use the PCA well because most are able to understand that they can receive pain relief by pushing the PCA button. Nurse-controlled analgesia (NCA) can be used for children who are not able to use the PCA button.

Once children are able to eat or drink after surgery, then intravenous narcotic medications are usually switched to narcotic medications that are taken by mouth. Oxycodone combined with acetaminophen or NSAIDs is commonly used and gives good pain relief for many children. Codeine used to be commonly prescribed to treat pain. However, we discourage the use of codeine because research has shown that it is not effective in relieving pain for some children and also seems to cause nausea in many cases.

Depending on what kind of operation a child has, medicines might be given to numb the nerves so that pain can be blocked. An epidural block is one way that doctors can numb the nerves and block pain. Sometimes the numbing medicine is placed directly around the nerves. Since most children are afraid of needles, nerve blocks are usually done after a child is already anesthetized for the operation. Once the medicine that numbs the nerves is stopped, then the numbness wears off in a few hours.

CANCER PAIN

Children with cancer can experience pain from the cancer itself, or pain can result from treating the cancer. Cancer can cause pain wherever it is located, particularly if it involves bones or nerves. The treatment of cancer often involves the use of chemotherapy drugs and sometimes radiation, which can be associated with pain. Many children with cancer will need frequent needle procedures for the treatment of their cancer, such as lumbar punctures, bone marrow biopsies, blood draws, and operations. Pain that is due to needle procedures is a significant source of distress to children with cancer. Again, numbing creams and patches should be used for brief needle punctures; sedation or general anesthesia should be used for more painful procedures. Non-medication therapies such as guided imagery and hypnosis can also be effective for pain due to procedures.

The World Health Organization created a stepwise analgesic "ladder" for adults with advanced cancer, which can often be applied to children with cancer pain. Mild pain is typically treated with acetaminophen or NSAIDs, sometimes combined with small amounts of narcotic medications when necessary. Moderate to severe pain is treated with increasing amounts of narcotic medications, such as morphine. For many children, the pain medications can be taken by mouth. Intravenous narcotic medications are needed when pain is severe or when a child is unable to eat or drink. In addition to pain, children with cancer can experience other symptoms that can cause suffering. Children can experience low energy, shortness of breath, poor appetite, and depressed mood, and it is important for caregivers to recognize these symptoms and treat the cause whenever possible.

Recurrent Pain in Children

Children and adolescents commonly experience recurrent types of pain, such as headaches, abdominal (belly) pains, and arm, leg, and chest pains.

Recurrent abdominal pain is a common problem among school-age children, with some estimating that as many as 10–25 percent of all school-age children will experience recurrent abdominal pain at some point. Most of the time, children with recurrent abdominal pain say that their pain comes and goes and that it is usually located around the belly button. Most of these children are between the ages of 4 and 16 and are otherwise healthy with no signs of illness. A careful evaluation is important to find out if there are other reasons for abdominal pain, such as inflammatory bowel disease or appendicitis, to name just two. Children who have fevers, weight loss, other worrisome signs, or a family history of inflammatory bowel disease should be more thoroughly evaluated. Treatment of recurrent abdominal pain often includes relaxation and distraction techniques to reduce pain and teaching a child good pain-coping skills so that the pain has less of an impact. Children with recurrent abdominal pain often miss much school, which seems to cause children to focus more on their pain and feel that their pain is even more intense. Learning good coping skills, relaxation, and other similar techniques can help a child attend school more regularly even if they have pain.

Chest pain is frequently experienced by children and teenagers and accounts for at least 65,000 physician visits per year. It is often a source of worry for parents because of the ominous association with chest pain in adults and having a heart attack. In otherwise healthy children and teenagers, chest pain is more commonly caused by inflammation of the cartilage that connects to the ribs, called costochondritis, and from muscle strain from coughing. Many children with chest pain from costochondritis and muscle strain have good pain relief with NSAIDs and by learning muscle relaxation techniques.

Nerve pain occurs when nerves become abnormally sensitive. Injury to nerves from physical injury and irritation of nerves from certain chemotherapy medicines, for example, can cause nerves to become abnormally sensitive and cause pain. Sometimes there is no cause for having nerve pain. Causes of nerve pain seen in adult patients, such as pain after shingles or from diabetes, are not often seen in children. Nerve pain most commonly occurs in the arms or legs. Many children find it difficult to describe their nerve pain, since it is not like any pain they have experienced before. Children with nerve pain will sometimes say that their pain feels like pins and needles, burning, or shock-like, but some children will simply say that their pain is "weird" or "strange." Sometimes the skin is very painful when it is lightly touched. The skin can also have a purplish discoloration, and there can be either too much or too little hair growth. Children with nerve pain will often avoid having anything touch their painful skin, such as wearing shoes and socks or using a blanket at night. One possible diagnosis could be reflex sympathetic dystrophy, which is discussed in Chapter 21. Sometimes they will not be able to walk because the pain is so severe. Medications can sometimes be helpful in treating nerve pain. Distraction, guided imagery, relaxation techniques, and physical therapy can also help reduce pain.

NON-MEDICATION PAIN THERAPIES

Many non-medication therapies are sometimes helpful in reducing pain in children, whether they are used alone or along with pain medicines. Even if a child is taking narcotic medications for pain, non-medication therapies can still be helpful. These therapies are generally considered safe and effective for children. Common non-medication therapies that children use include acupuncture, distraction, guided imagery, hypnosis, and biofeedback. Some of these techniques are discussed in Chapter 8.

Acupuncture is widely used in children for treating a variety of pains, especially headaches, back pain, and stomach pains. As part of this technique, special hair-thin needles are placed in specific sites of the body. Acupuncture is thought to relieve pain by restoring the balance of energy flow in the body. Most children over the age of seven are able to use acupuncture. Even though acupuncture is relatively painless, some children are afraid of trying it because it involves needles. Acupressure, which uses mild pressure instead of needles, can be offered to children who are afraid of the acupuncture needles. Distraction techniques help a child to focus their thoughts and attention on something other than pain. Simple distraction techniques such as play therapy, talking to or playing with friends, or playing a game can be effective for a wide range of children of different ages. Guided imagery is a technique in which children are taught to focus their thoughts on a pleasant situation. It allows children to feel relaxed and less anxious, which helps to relieve pain. Biofeedback is a technique for older children and teenagers that uses sensors to measure and detect changes in the bodies' responses to pain, such as muscle tension, heart rate, and temperature. Biofeedback is based on the idea that our mind and our bodies interact and that it is possible to change our bodies' response to pain. Reiki is a bioenergetic therapy based on Japanese tradition in which one transmits invisible healing energy through contact by hands. Reiki practitioners undergo training and through various levels by a Reiki master. For some children and families, spiritual well-being can be important for overall health.

In summary, pain is a common sensation that children as well as adults experience. Since the feeling of pain is different for everyone, children should be involved in describing their pain. There are a variety of medication and non-medication therapies that can be used to help treat pain. Parents are the best source of information about their child and can be helpful in determining what kind of pain their child has and the best way to treat it.

32

PAIN AND THE ELDERLY

Michael Harned, MD, and Paul Sloan, MD

INTRODUCTION

What does it mean to be old? Does it mean that one is retired with fewer responsibilities and more time to travel, or does it mean failing health, many physician visits, and a feeling that the best years are now behind you? Because we see vast differences in physical makeup among people of similar age, being old is no longer based solely on chronological age. We now know that as people progress toward the later years of life, there is a continued increased risk of experiencing pain. Effective pain control can improve quality of life in one's later years.

With baby boomers swelling the ranks of retirees, persons over 80 years of age are now one of the fastest-growing population segments. Pain in this age group is common and often undertreated. It is reported that half of persons over 70 years old experience pain at any given time. This percentage further increases among the nursing home population. A variety of root causes are to blame. With increasing age, musculoskeletal conditions are the most common cause of painful disease states. In addition, surgical procedures, with their associated pain, often become unavoidable as we age. When pain persists beyond its expected course, a whole new disease state can develop, called *chronic pain*. This type of pain is often misunderstood by the patient, and if left untreated, it can adversely affect many different aspects of a person's life, resulting in social isolation, depression, and functional decline. These associated psychological factors will, in turn, exacerbate pain, leading to further psychological distress and an overall decrease in quality of life.

Pain among the elderly is often undertreated for several reasons. First, the elderly are less likely to self-report pain to their physician because of the belief that pain is a normal part of aging. Second, elderly persons in pain sometimes feel they are bothering the health care provider, taking time away from consideration of more important medical problems. Third, patients may fear the diagnosis of the chronic pain and wish to avoid this distress in their life. Fourth, patients sometimes fear there is little to be done for the pain and so resist reporting the symptom. Fifth, health care providers do not always ask appropriate questions to diagnose a chronic pain condition among their patients. For example, elderly patients who deny having pain may admit to having "discomfort" or "aching." Finally, health care providers often feel uneasy about prescribing additional medications to an elderly patient, since many people already exhibit multiple medical problems and extensive medication lists.

SYMPTOMS

There are two broad categories of pain: *acute* and *chronic. Acute pain* begins suddenly and is usually the result of an obvious event such as surgery or a fractured bone. This pain will begin as sharp, stabbing pain, but as the body heals, the pain will quickly subside. Since acute pain is associated with a specific cause, it is self-limited and rarely lasts more than three months.

Chronic pain is less well understood and often more confusing, both to the patient and the treating physician. The onset of chronic pain is frequently more insidious, and the specific cause of the pain may not be obvious. Chronic pain by definition is pain lasting longer than three to six months; it may start out as acute pain that fails to resolve in spite of adequate treatment of the acute problem. Chronic pain is further broken up into two broad categories, *mechanical pain* (nociceptive) and *nerve pain* (neuropathic). Mechanical pain will present as a dull ache and may be worsened with movement. This type of pain is typically seen with arthritis of the musculoskeletal system. Patients suffering mechanical pain may avoid certain positions or activities that increase their pain, such as walking down stairs, which may be difficult for a patient with an arthritic knee. On the other hand, the symptoms of nerve pain differ from the symptoms of mechanical pain. Nerve pain is usually described as a burning, shooting, or electric pain along the course of the nerve. It may be the result of injury to a nerve from compression or stretching. Sciatica, for example, with its shooting pain going down the back of the leg, is a classic example of neuropathic pain.

Elderly patients may develop pain from cancer. Cancer is more common in the elderly compared with younger people. Patients may experience dull abdominal pain from cancer invading the liver or kidney, or may experience colicky abdominal pain from obstruction of the intestines within the abdominal cavity. Cancers that spread to the bone may result in a deep, boring, and aching pain within the bone itself.

In addition to the physical symptoms of pain, patients often suffer psychologically as a result of persistent pain. As patients reduce life activities in order to minimize their pain, they suffer from the resulting social isolation. The network of family, friends, and life activities that had previously provided support may begin to dissolve. Second, with this decreasing activity, a physical deconditioning occurs, which in turn makes previously non-painful activities difficult. It is no surprise, therefore, that there is a high prevalence of depression within the elderly population with chronic pain. Furthermore, the depression itself can intensify the pain and may limit the effectiveness of analgesic treatments.

DIAGNOSIS

Elderly patients should be prepared to discuss and explain their painful conditions to their health care providers. The provider may use different pain scales and surveys to help characterize and quantify the degree of pain you are experiencing. Often a simple numeric scale, with 0 being no pain, and 10 being the most intense pain possible, allows patients to rate their pain severity. During the office visit, the provider will perform a pain history including attention to the onset, quality, intensity, location, and duration of the pain. The provider will ask you questions regarding what previous treatments, especially medications, have been tried in the past and whether they were effective. The provider should also question you regarding changes in sensation, motor strength, or bowel and bladder function. Additional factors such as disturbed sleep, change in activity level, or worsening mood can provide additional clues as to how the pain impacts your overall quality of life.

During the office visit, the provider will also perform a general physical examination while concentrating on a focused neurological examination of the painful area in question. For example, if you present with a history of chronic low back pain, it will be important for the provider to examine the strength of the lower extremity muscles as well as the sensation and reflexes in this area. A detailed physical examination should address not only the area of complaint, but also the entire body. The examination should include overall inspection, palpation (touching), and manipulation of the body part. Examination of the musculoskeletal and neurological systems specifically checks for the presence of sensation (feeling light touch), symmetric motor strength, and reflexes, assuring there is no serious underlying condition requiring immediate intervention.

Chronic pain is commonly associated with depression; there is a strong correlation between higher levels of pain and more significant depression. The physician should consider the whole individual when treating chronic pain by looking for associated psychological conditions associated with the physical cause of the pain. Therefore, you may need to answer questions about symptoms of anxiety, depression, altered sleep, and social isolation.

Finally, additional studies may be needed to help make or confirm a diagnosis. Often practitioners will start with plain x-rays, as these are inexpensive and easy to obtain. Next, depending upon the pain complaint, a *computed tomography* (CT) scan or *magnetic resonance imaging* (MRI) scan may be ordered. Both are painless tests that provide information about the structures of the body. MRI is especially useful in detecting abnormal changes in the nerves of the brain or body. Another diagnostic tool that may reveal the cause of neuropathy (a medical term for nerve damage) is called *electromyography* (EMG) and *nerve conduction velocity* (NCV). These two tests are usually done in combination. The EMG portion uses a fine needle inserted into the muscles, while the NCV measures stimulation along the surface of the skin. The EMG portion measures the amount of electrical activity present when muscles are at rest and when they contract. This helps your doctor differentiate whether a muscle or a nerve disorder is the cause of your pain. The NCV portion can determine where along the nerve the damage has occurred, which can help the provider determine the cause of the pain. In addition to the above tests, standard blood work may be ordered to look for the many different possible reasons for your painful condition.

The elderly have increased frequency of dementia and Alzheimer's disease, both of which present additional diagnostic challenges for the clinician. Special surveys are available to help evaluate both acute and chronic pain conditions in patients who are unable to adequately verbalize their symptoms. In these situations, physical cues such as facial grimacing, protection of extremities, social withdrawal, or sudden behavioral changes will provide information to the health care provider about untreated pain.

TREATMENT OPTIONS

The treatment of pain will depend in part on whether the pain is acute or chronic, and mechanical or neuropathic (related to nerve injury). For the treatment of acute pain, short-term symptomatic relief is usually sufficient while the acute injury is healing. While acute pain is, by definition, self-limiting, it may be severe, requiring prescription medications. Pain medications for the short-term management of acute pain are rarely associated with any significant complications.

For chronic pain sufferers, the first component of any treatment plan is to educate patients about their pain. When patients understand that physical damage has resolved and that only pain signals continue, they show an improved outcome in the overall management of their pain. Educational programs thus empower the patient to take an active role in their care and help in the selection of a treatment plan based upon diagnosis.

Medication regimens for the treatment of painful conditions should be kept as simple as possible, and the risk-to-benefit ratio for each therapy must be carefully assessed. *Analgesics* (pain medications) are used frequently in the United States, with 20 percent of all elderly people taking at least some form of pain medication on a weekly basis. In addition, the average 70-year-old has three medical conditions and takes an average of seven different medications.

Therefore, the elderly are more likely to have an adverse event from an analgesic medication, and careful titration of the pain medication is always required. It is often prudent to start with a single analgesic medication, as the addition of multiple new analgesics simultaneously may be confusing for the patient and result in increased risk of side effects. It is helpful for the patient to receive both verbal and written instructions for analgesic use, both provided in a simple, understandable manner.

Acetaminophen (Tylenol) is a common and well-tolerated pain relief medicine for mild to moderate pain. It is especially useful for mechanical pain secondary to bone and joint pain. While usually well tolerated, recent guidelines have cautioned that acetaminophen dosing on a chronic basis should not exceed 2,000 mg per day, due to its potential to cause liver damage. In persons with a history of liver problems or high levels of alcohol consumption, further reduction in daily dose or even complete abstinence may be necessary.

Osteoarthritis is the most common arthritic complaint among the elderly. *Nonsteroidal anti-inflammatory medications* (NSAIDs) are analgesics that often work well when inflammation is the cause of the pain. NSAIDs should be used cautiously among the elderly because of increased risks of side effects, which may also be more severe in the elderly. The most common side effect is stomach upset (*gastritis*). Newer selective COX-2 NSAIDs may cause less irritation to the lining of the stomach than older NSAIDs. Additional side effects include gastric ulcer formation, kidney dysfunction, and fluid retention. Congestive heart failure may limit the use of the NSAIDs among the elderly. Recent research raises additional concerns about the use of NSAIDs in patients with heart disease. It is important that the provider explain the risks and benefits of NSAIDs, as well as regularly reassess their use.

Despite potential side effects, NSAIDs do have advantages over other strong analgesic medications because they are not associated with sedation or respiratory depression, nor do they have the potential for abuse. NSAIDs may be combined with either acetaminophen or opioids for increased pain relief. Moreover, NSAIDs have been effective in helping to manage bone pain secondary to cancer. These medications are commonly taken by mouth, but are now available in a patch form that reduces side effects.

When simple analgesics such as acetaminophen and NSAIDs do not provide adequate pain relief, your physician may prescribe a stronger class of analgesics called *opioids*. Opioids are drugs with morphine-like properties that provide pain relief for a wide variety of conditions. First used routinely on the battlefields of the U.S. Civil War to provide pain relief from injuries, opioids continue to be used today for pain relief following surgery. In recent years it has become common to provide surgery patients with a programmable device that releases small doses of opioids at the touch of a button. This *patient-controlled anesthesia* (PCA) device empowers patients to manage their own pain. The health care team controls the settings of the computerized pump system to limit toxicity such as overdose.

Since the late 1960s, long-term opioid use has been recognized as effective in the treatment of cancer pain. Many studies have demonstrated their safety and efficacy in controlling pain associated with many forms of cancer. The elderly undergo many body organ function changes associated with aging, which makes them more sensitive to opioid analgesics. Thus, often a low initial dose of opioid medication is prescribed; the dose is then adjusted (*titrated*) on an individual basis with careful follow-up. It is common for short-acting medications to be initially prescribed every four hours until adequate pain relief is achieved. Following this phase of treatment, the physician may change to a longer 12-hour or once-daily dose to provide sustained pain relief. If patients are unable to take medications by mouth, they may be prescribed a transdermal skin patch, rectal suppositories, or intravenous or subcutaneous administration.

Opioids in the treatment of cancer pain are generally safe; the most common side effects are constipation, nausea and vomiting, and sedation. Constipation typically requires ongoing treatment with a laxative. It is common for patients to accommodate to a mild degree of sedation or initial nausea, and not to require additional medication therapy for these side effects. While opioids can cause the serious side effect of respiratory depression, if carefully titrated among the elderly patient, this is extremely rare. It is especially important in an elderly patient with known liver or kidney disease that a gradual titration of medication is undertaken. It is common among the elderly for opioid doses to be reduced with a longer time interval between medication doses given.

The use of opioids for the treatment of chronic pain not related to cancer, such as osteoarthritis, has become more common in the past decade. A recent consensus statement issued by a panel of experts concluded that opioids are proven effective in the treatment of non-cancer pain. As with the treatment of cancer pain, initial doses of opioids for the elderly should be quite low, and should then be titrated slowly with constant reevaluation by the physician. Slow titration reduces the incidence of initial side effects such as nausea and vomiting.

All opioids show some efficacy in the treatment of chronic pain. Common opioids used include morphine, oxycodone (Oxycontin), hydrocodone (Vicodin), oxymorphone (Opana), methadone, hydromorphone (Dilaudid), and transdermal fentanyl patch. Elderly patients should be followed closely and their treatment should be adjusted for adequate effect. There is no upper limit of dose, and some patients may require quite high doses of opioid medication in order to achieve adequate pain relief. Methadone must be prescribed by an experienced practitioner because the drug can accumulate in the body, resulting in side effects that manifest several days after dose titration. When morphine is broken down in your body, the by-products may accumulate if you have kidney disease, and therefore this drug should be used with caution. Oxycodone is typically least likely to cause adverse reactions in the elderly; it can be used safely among patients with liver or kidney disease. Elderly patients may appreciate the simplicity of the transdermal fentanyl patch, which typically provides three days of pain relief per patch.

Because the elderly sometimes have preexisting thinking disorders (dementia, Alzheimer's disease) and psychiatric conditions, both the family and treating physician must be vigilant about any changes in mental health status. Opioid side effects such as confusion may diminish with a decrease in medication, or may be treated with a trial of a different opioid. It should be noted that a patient may respond well to one opioid with minimal side effects, while reacting poorly to a different opioid. The physician may, therefore, try several different opioids in succession.

In addition to the analgesic medications, there exist other classes of medications helpful in the treatment of certain types of pain, especially neuropathic pain. One such class is the *antiepileptic* (antiseizure) drugs, originally developed for the management of seizures but found to be an effective treatment for chronic pain caused by the abnormal firing of the peripheral nerves. Gabapentin (Neurontin) is the most widely used of these drugs. Gabapentin is more effective at higher doses, but its use may be limited by the side effect of drowsiness. A newer antiepileptic drug, pregabalin (Lyrica), is less sedating and appears to be better tolerated by the elderly. Again, trials of different medications may be required to determine the most effective pain relief approach for you.

The *antidepressant* class of medications has also been shown to have properties of pain relief. In particular, the *tricyclic antidepressants*, such as desipramine, have been useful in treating different forms of nerve pain. This pain relief effect is independent of any effect on mood or depression. The use of tricyclics can be limited by side effects such as dry mouth and excessive sedation. Another antidepressant, duloxetine, an SNRI (*selective serotonin and norepinephrine reuptake inhibitor*) provides relief for chronic nerve pain, especially in patients for whom depression is a coexisting condition. SNRIs are safe and cause only minimal side effects in the elderly. Their analgesic effects are the result of their ability to increase levels of *serotonin* and *norepinephrine* (chemicals that play a role in depression and mood) in the central nervous system.

Finally, there are a variety of drugs that are occasionally used to treat specific painful disorders. For example, mexiletine, developed as a heart medication, may be helpful in the relief of painful diabetic neuropathy. Calcitonin, a medication used in the treatment of osteoporosis, may provide pain relief in some patients with fractures of the spine due to osteoporosis. Transdermally, creams and patches may deliver medications such as local anesthetics, NSAIDs, or capsaicin.

There are other treatments for chronic pain besides medications. In addition to education, patients will benefit from regular exercise and weight reduction. Physical therapy is one of the most universally prescribed therapies for the treatment of both acute and chronic pain. A physical therapist will often use a combination of strengthening exercises, stretching, and hot or cold therapy. More advanced physical therapy techniques such as ultrasound and *transcutaneous electrical nerve stimulation* (TENS) can help improve function and reduce pain. TENS works by producing electrical current directly in the nerves in the affected area in order to reduce the sensation of pain.

Patients for whom traditional medical treatments have failed may seek out alternative therapies. Acupuncture, first recorded in ancient Chinese literature, involves inserting needles into various parts of the body in order to relieve pain. Vitamins, medicinal herbs, and natural remedies have been used by patients seeking relief from chronic pain. The efficacy of many of these treatments has been neither proven nor disproven, and further study is required. Because the FDA (Food and Drug Administration) is not involved in regulating supplements, except to say that the product labels may not make overt medical claims, the quality and safety of the ingredients may also be questionable. It is important for patients who use these supplements to tell their doctor about it, in order to avoid adverse drug interactions.

Finally, *interventional* therapy, involving surgically implanted devices that deliver medication directly into the body, can be used in the management of both acute and chronic pain. *Nerve blocks* or *epidural catheters* allow improved control of acute pain through the use of medication. Nerve blocks consist of injecting local anesthetics near the nerves that are likely to cause pain, rendering the area numb during surgery and reducing pain after surgery. An *epidural block* may be used to provide pain relief both during and after surgery of the chest, abdomen, or lower extremities. The epidural catheter delivers medication into the *epidural space*, within the bones of the back but outside the spinal cord. Studies suggest that pain relief and overall surgical outcomes are improved with the use of these interventional techniques. These techniques are further discussed in Chapters 26 and 27.

When more conservative measures fail in the management of chronic pain, interventional techniques may offer relief. These are termed *neuromodulation therapy.* Neuromodulation refers to medical technology that allows direct alteration of the nervous system to help control pain. The choice of therapy depends upon which type of pain is being treated. As a general rule, *spinal cord stimulators* (SCS) are more beneficial for neuropathic pain, while *intrathecal pumps* are effective for mechanical pain. SCS uses pulsed electrical energy applied near the spinal cord. The most common type of stimulation uses small electrodes placed into the epidural space. Next, an electrical pulse is sent to the leads via a small generator. The electrical pulse provides a pleasant vibratory sensation in the affected area, replacing the body's own painful nerve firings. This type of treatment has proven extremely beneficial for persistent neuropathic pain of the lower extremities in cases of failed back surgery syndrome, painful diabetic conditions, and peripheral vascular disease.

The second interventional technique, the intrathecal catheter, involves placing extremely small amounts of medication, usually opioids alone or in combination with local anesthetics and other medications, directly into the spinal fluid. This drug delivery route bypasses the oral or intravenous route, often reducing side effects and improving efficacy. The system is comprised of a small *catheter* (plastic tube) placed between the bones of the spine and a small pump placed below the skin. The device is refilled by placing a small needle through the skin about once every three months, but is otherwise maintenance free.

PROGNOSIS

Acute (new onset) pain, by definition, is short in duration. While acute pain, regardless of cause, may be severe in character, the pain should subside as the body heals. Acute pain is often the result of an accident, injury, or surgery. If pain does not subside but instead lasts longer than three months, it is considered chronic pain.

Chronic pain lasts longer than three to six months and is persistent, recurring, and difficult to treat. Regardless of the original injury or cause, chronic pain includes psychological as well as physical symptoms. Chronic pain is best thought of as disease much like diabetes; in both cases, treatment aims not for a cure *per se*, but rather for reducing symptoms and improving quality of life. Each medication or intervention is intended to help the patient, little by little, to manage the pain. Patients and clinicians alike must bear in mind that there may be no cure for the painful condition. The goal is to restore quality of life by providing as much pain relief as possible, with as few side effects as possible. This goal requires significant efforts toward teaching chronic pain patients to learn skills to cope with their pain. A behavioral pain psychologist may be able to help you with this aspect of treatment.

ADDITIONAL RESOURCES

Patients and families will find additional educational resources online at the following websites:

http://www.arthritis.about.com
http://www.everythinghealth.com
http://www.health.com

33

Pain during Labor and Childbirth

Raed Rahman, DO, and Magdalena Anitescu, MD, PhD

Introduction

The development of a new life is an ongoing excitement for soon-to-be new parents. However, during pregnancy, labor, and the delivery process, a woman undergoes many changes in her body, which can contribute to painful conditions during her pregnancy. This chapter will focus on a better understanding of the pain mechanisms involved in the labor and childbirth process. Hopefully, this will enable better coping with these potentially challenging times of pregnancy, and allow the soon-to-be mother, to enjoy the experience of carrying the child to birth.

Pregnant women may experience mild painful conditions, including back or buttock pains, typically during the latter part of their pregnancy. However, pain during actual childbirth can be significant and intense. The treating physicians, such as the anesthesiologists and the obstetricians, as well as midwives, nurses, and other health professionals, are trained to recognize and to address pain-related concerns. Therefore, increased pain during labor will be immediately evaluated for various methods of pain relief.

It is important to recognize that the healthcare providers actually attend to two patients, the mother and the fetus. Health care providers strive for a happy ending for both patients!

Sometimes, severe pain during labor can have psychological consequences resulting in post-delivery depression or the development of posttraumatic stress disorder (PTSD). Men are also affected during the labor process. A survey of first-time fathers demonstrated that men whose partners received a labor epidural felt three times as helpful and involved during the childbirth process.

They had less anxiety and stress as compared to men whose partners did not receive an epidural.

Symptoms

At the end of a 9-month period, approximately 38–40 weeks gestation, the human female gives birth to one or multiple babies during a process called labor and childbirth. The mechanism that signals the beginning of labor is unclear, but there are several hormonal and physical changes that may indicate the beginning of labor. These changes are divided into five sections: lightening phase, passing of the mucus plug phase, the contraction phase, the amniotic membrane rupture phase, and the cervical dilation phase.

1. *Lightening Phase:* This is the process by which the baby is settling low into the pelvis, just before the labor starts. It can occur a few weeks or a few hours before labor. This symptom cannot pinpoint the beginning of labor, but it is an early sign that things are moving in the right direction. Lightening appears more often in first-time pregnancies. While it relieves the uncomfortable symptom of breathing difficulty related to the high position of the baby underneath the rib cage, some women may feel pressure on their bladder during this period. This symptom together with the urge to urinate more frequently is related to the resting of the uterus low in the pelvis.

2. *Passing of the Mucus Plug:* During pregnancy, mucus accumulates in the cervix (which is the small, thick, and short portion of the uterus). With onset of the laboring process, the cervix begins to open and the mucus-like material is discharged into the vagina as clear, pink, or slightly bloody secretions. The contraction phase of labor can start immediately after the mucus discharge or one to two weeks later.

3. *Contraction Phase of Labor:* Contrary to the other phases, the contraction phase of labor is associated with pain, which progresses from mild at the beginning of this phase to very significant and intense toward the end of labor. The pain is primarily associated with contraction of the uterine muscles in the process of descending and delivery of the baby. During the contractions, the abdomen becomes hard. Between contractions, the uterus relaxes and the abdomen becomes soft. Labor contractions usually cause discomfort or a dull ache in your back and lower abdomen, along with pressure in the pelvis. Contractions move in a wave-like motion from the top of the uterus to the bottom. The time between contractions includes the duration of the contraction and the minutes in between the contractions. Mild contractions generally begin 15 to 20 minutes apart and last 60 to 90 seconds. The contractions become more regular until they are less than 5 minutes apart. Active labor (the time to come into the hospital) is usually characterized by strong contractions that last 45 to 60 seconds and occur 3 to 4 minutes apart.

4. *Amniotic Membrane Break:* During the pregnancy, the baby is protected by a small membrane, the amniotic membrane and the amniotic fluid. With increase of the pressure inside the uterus due to the uterine contractions of the laboring

process, the amniotic membrane (the water bag that surrounds the baby during pregnancy) ruptures and the fluid covering the baby is spilled down the vagina. It may feel either like a sudden gush of fluid or a trickle of fluid that leaks steadily. The fluid is usually odorless and may look clear or straw-colored. Even though active labor may not start immediately after the water breaks, delivery of the baby will occur within the next 24 hours. Keep in mind that not all women will have their water bag break when they are in labor. Sometimes the doctor will rupture the amniotic membrane in the hospital.

5. *Cervical Dilatation:* During the final phase of labor, the cervix (opening to the uterus/womb) becomes shorter and thins out in order to stretch and open around the baby's head. The shortening and thinning of the cervix is called effacement, measured in percentages from 0 percent (no changes to the cervix) to 100 percent (cervix completely thinned out). The stretching and opening of the cervix is called dilation and is measured in centimeters, with complete dilation being at 10 centimeters. Effacement and dilation are a direct result of effective uterine contractions. Progress in labor is measured by how much the cervix has opened and thinned to allow the baby to pass through the vagina.

DIAGNOSIS

The process of a normal human childbirth through labor has three stages through which progression is monitored and evaluated. It starts with the first stage of labor, the shortening and dilation of the cervix; continues with the second stage, descent and birth of the infant; and finishes with the third stage of labor, the delivery of the placenta.

1. *The first stage of labor consists of two phases, latent and active.* It starts with the onset of uterine contractions (labor) and ends when the cervix dilatation is complete (about 10 centimeters).

   a. During the latent phase, irregular contractions become progressively better coordinated, discomfort is minimal, and the cervix effaces (thins) and dilates to 4 centimeters. Its duration is about eight hours in first-time pregnancies (primiparous), and approximately five hours in women with multiple births (multiparous).

   b. With the active phase, the cervix becomes fully dilated (10 centimeters), and the presenting baby part descends into the pelvis. The duration of the active phase lasts five to seven hours in primiparous women (who are having a baby for the first time) and two to four hours in multiparous (who have delivered at least one baby before). Pelvic examinations are done by the obstetrician every few hours (a one- to three-hour interval) to evaluate labor progress.

   Women may begin to feel the urge to bear down, as the presenting baby part descends into the pelvis. They should be discouraged from bearing down until the cervix is fully dilated so that they do not tear the cervix or waste their energy. During this period, the women experience the majority of their pain known as the labor pain. The pain signal travels from the stretched structures, such as the uterus, vagina, and cervix.

2. *The second stage of labor is the time from full cervical dilation to delivery of the fetus.* The average time is one to two hours in first-time pregnancies, and 30–60 minutes in women with past multiple births. Contractions may be monitored by palpation or electronically. There are nerves innervate and attach to the perineum, the area between the vulva and the anus. These nerves also innervate the surrounding tissues of the uterus, such as the ligaments, nerves, muscles, and joints. These tissues are stretched and can be exposed to pressure during labor, causing pain.

3. *The third stage of labor begins after delivery of the fetus and ends with the delivery of the placenta.* This stage is usually not very painful.

PAIN MANAGEMENT OPTIONS

There are multiple options for treating pain during labor and delivery. The options most commonly available to women today are covered. During the early stages of labor, various relaxation techniques can help with the increasing pain; when pain becomes very severe in the late stages of labor, intravenous medications may be an option together with regional analgesic techniques such as epidurals.

The pain relief for vaginal delivery and cesarean delivery (C-section) are overlapping and depends on the progression of your labor. Pain relief for vaginal delivery can involve non-pharmacologic (no medications) options and/or pharmacologic options (medications, epidural, combined spinal/epidural). If concerns arise during the vaginal delivery labor process affecting either the mother or the fetus as determined by the obstetrician, then a cesarean delivery may be needed. A cesarean delivery will necessitate epidural, spinal, or general anesthesia. Regional anesthesia (nerve blocks, epidurals, spinals) and general anesthesia can be used to handle urgent obstetric complications, such as entrapment of the fetal head, fetal breech presentations, and shoulder dystocia.

Pain relief during the cesarean delivery performed under regional anesthesia is achieved by the injection of the medicine closer to the spine. During cesarean delivery performed under general anesthesia, the mother is asleep. During this time, the anesthesiologist will monitor vital signs closely.

Pain relief after the vaginal delivery often involves medications such as acetaminophen (Tylenol) or ibuprofen (Motrin). If the pain is moderate to severe, then opioid medications, either given through the vein during your hospitalization or orally as pills when leaving the hospital, can help with acute pain control. Additional cold packs applied to the hurting areas can add to the pain relief.

Pain relief after the cesarean delivery that was performed either under regional anesthesia (spinal or epidural) or general anesthesia can be effectively treated with a combination of nonsteroidal anti-inflammatory drugs (oral: ibuprofen, intravenously: ketorolac). In addition, an opioid self-administering pump known as Patient Controlled Analgesia (PCA) can be used for adequate pain relief related to pain around the incision. A relatively new procedure, called a TAP block, can also provide postoperative relief for a C-section. This procedure involves injecting local anesthetic directly within the abdomen after C-section. However, it is now offered in every hospital.

Adequate pain management is an essential goal for delivery. Below are many pain relief options that are available.

Pain Relief without Medications: Some women prefer to avoid pain medication during childbirth. They can still try to alleviate labor pain using psychological preparation, education, massage, hypnosis, or water therapy in a tub or shower. In some instances, delivering the baby in a squatting or crawling position allows effective push during the second stage of labor and permits easier, gravity-aided descent of the baby through the birth canal. Meditation techniques are also used for pain control during labor and delivery. These techniques are used in conjunction with progressive muscle relaxation, like hypnosis, to aid in pain control during childbirth. Additional options to manage pain may involve water immersion therapy. This involves sitting in warm water up to your chest area, and it is believed this therapy helps enhance relaxation and reduce labor pain. Also, a continuous support person can be a trained person providing supportive companionship during labor and to help the parturient cope with anxiety and pain. Application of cold and heat to the low back areas of the body can help ease the labor pains. These temperature applications can help decrease muscle spasms and decrease joint stiffness. Most childbirth and education classes present relaxation techniques to provide a distraction from the pain. Audio analgesia is the use of music to decrease the perception of pain. Another approach is aromatherapy, which is the use of essential oils to decrease labor pains.

Transcutaneous electrical nerve stimulator (TENS) is a device that can be applied to the area of discomfort—for instance, the low back—and transmit low electrical impulses to the skin through surface electrodes. This TENS device can be placed at the mid-to-low back area. A buzzing sensation may reduce your awareness of contraction pain.

Pain Relief with Medications: There are many options available. They consist of intravenous (injected into the vein) or oral pain killers to relieve anxiety and pain during labor and childbirth. In fact, when the non-pharmacological (no pain medications) approaches fail to provide adequate relief, then pain medicines given through a vein or by mouth can be highly effective to provide relief.

Medications used intravenously for pain relief are sometimes requested by patients who prefer less invasive techniques or if the patient cannot obtain an epidural or a spinal. The reason the epidural was developed and is so valuable in obstetrics is that it can be reinjected, or an infusion of medication can be delivered through it, over many hours and even days. This is particularly useful in obstetrics because there is no certainty as to how long it will take for the baby to be born. There are a wide variety of medications aimed at pain relief during labor and childbirth. The medications commonly used for moderate and severe pain in labor are the natural or synthetic opioids (narcotics).The most common medications are nalbuphine (Nubain), fentanyl, and morphine. Opioids produce their pain-relieving effects by binding to the mother's pain receptors in the brain. However, it is important to realize that there is a small portion that may cross the placenta and affect the fetus. This can potentially affect the baby's respirations after delivery, and it may affect the baby's heart rate before the baby is delivered. Therefore, the baby must be continuously monitored during labor. A thorough discussion should be undertaken involving this choice and other alternatives in the overall management of pain. The other, negative side effects of opioids include nausea, vomiting, and sedation.

Epidurals, Spinals, and Other Pain Blocks

These are more "invasive" options that involve a procedure and include spinal blocks, epidural blocks, combined spinal and epidural blocks, and, much less commonly, paracervical and pudendal nerve blocks. An epidural is the most common nerve block performed for straightforward labor and delivery. For the majority of cases, these options provide an effective pain relief for the parturient and allow a relaxed environment for the birth of the new baby.

All interventional techniques involve delivering local anesthetic (similar to novocaine used in the dentist's office), sometimes mixed with a small amount of narcotic, to the nerves involved in pain during labor. Whether it is an epidural catheter, a single application spinal or a local anesthetic injection around the cervix during a pudendal nerve block, these interventions provide superior pain relief with minimal side effects and minimal adverse events for the baby.

Epidurals and spinals generally provide better pain relief than opioids injected into the vein. Opioids can lead to respiratory problems of the mother and baby. If an epidural is being used during labor, one goal is to maintain muscle strength and sense of pressure during the second stage of labor. If there is too strong of an epidural block, the ability to push and pressure sensation will be decreased. If this happens, the mother may not feel the contractions and labor can be prolonged, increasing the chance of an instrumental delivery (e.g., forceps) or even C-section. Some obstetricians prefer to discontinue epidural medications late in labor to decrease the chances of instrumental delivery, but this may lead to inadequate pain relief in the second stage of labor.

Labor epidural is the most frequently used nerve block procedure. It consists of placing a small catheter close to the spine (between two spine segments known as vertebrae) in a virtual space (the epidural space) occupied with fat and veins. This space becomes a true space by infusion of local anesthetic (with or without opioids) which then bathes the spinal nerves involved in the labor pain. It should be noted that for a typical anesthesiologist, the placement of an epidural takes only a few minutes.

Figure 33.1 gives a schematic representation of a typical epidural catheter placement procedure.

The placement of the epidural catheter is performed under a sterile technique by identifying first the epidural space with the help of a needle and a special syringe, and then threading a small plastic catheter through the needle into the space. After the catheter is placed, the continuous infusion of local anesthetic is initiated and maintained by an electronic pump programmed to deliver a certain amount of medication to the epidural space. A specific function called Patient Controlled Epidural Analgesia (PCEA) can be employed as well. This technique involves patient self-administration of extra medication through the epidural catheter, by simply pressing a button, in addition to the continuous infusion. The epidural catheter can be placed early in labor and has the advantages of providing pain relief for the majority of the labor.

Complications Related to the Catheter Placement

Although the procedure is generally safe, patients should be aware of the risks associated with the placement of the epidural catheters. The possible complications that can arise during an epidural catheter placement can be related to the placement technique or to the medication.

Since the needle breaks the continuity of the skin, the risk of bleeding and infection around the insertion area is slightly increased; however, these complications are fortunately extremely low, with an incidence of approximately 1 in 100,000 epidural placements.

Figure 33.1
Epidural catheter placement procedure for pain control during labor.

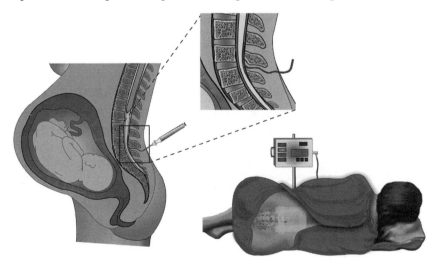

Another possible complication of the epidural catheter placement is post-dural puncture headache (PDPH), also known as "spinal headache." This unpleasant condition occurs when the epidural needle perforates the outer-most membrane that covers the spinal cord (called the *dura mater*). The head-ache is due to continuous leak of the spinal fluid through the dura mater hole. It has a positional character (worse in upright position and better while lying down), and it is usually located in the front and back of the head. The PDPH is usually self-limited, disappearing in up to one week. The incidence of this complication is 0.5 to 3 for every 100 epidural placements. The common treatment of this spinal headache includes intravenous fluids, caffeine, and sometimes weak oral opioid medications. If the conservative treatment fails, another procedure called epidural blood patch can be used to treat the head-ache; it involves harvesting blood from the mother's vein and injecting it into the epidural space.

Medication Complications

Commonly used medications for the epidural infusions are local anes-thetics and opioid medications (painkillers). The common side effects associ-ated with the opioid medications in the epidural space are nausea and itching. Oral or intravenous medications can also be used to treat these conditions.

A common side effect associated with the use of local anesthetics in the epidural or spinal catheter is the decrease of the blood pressure in the mother, which can affect the delivery of the nutrients and the oxygen to the baby. If there is a decrease in the blood pressure, the anesthesiologist will give medica-tion to bring it back to a safe level. In very rare circumstances, excessive deliv-ery of local anesthetic in the epidural or spinal spaces can cause the mother to stop breathing, since muscles involved with breathing become temporarily anesthetized. The anesthesiologist maintains the respiration and the heart func-tion using a mechanical ventilator to assist the mother until the effect of local anesthetic fades away.

Since there are rare side effects, all labor epidurals are continuously moni-tored in the hospital with frequent (every 30 minutes to 1 hour) visits from health care professionals to identify any potential side effects related to the medications used for epidural infusions.

An epidural is often used for delivery, primarily for vaginal deliveries but also for C-section. It has essentially replaced older regional techniques such as the pudendal and paracervical blocks. Other methods include caudal injec-tion (into the sacral canal), which is rarely used because of its own rare poten-tial complications related to needle misplacements and spinal injection.

Other Pain Relief Options

a. *Spinal injection* may be used either for vaginal delivery as part of a procedure called combined spinal and epidural (in which the initial spinal injection is followed by placement of an epidural catheter used for continuous pain relief for the reminder of the labor and childbirth) or alone as is the case of anesthesia for cesarean section.

   This technique involves perforating the dura mater (the membrane covering the spine) and depositing the medication, usually local anesthetic and opioid, in the spinal fluid. The advantage of this technique in cesarean section is that it provides immediate (5–15 minutes onset) anesthesia below the breasts. The patient will not be able to feel anything other than pressure, and will not be able to move the legs for a duration of 2–6 hours (depending on the local anesthetic used) after the spinal injection. When spinal injection is used, patients must be constantly watched and vital signs must be checked to detect and treat possible low blood pressure.

b. *Other local anesthesia techniques:* pudendal block, a perineal injection, and a paracervical block. Pudendal block involves injecting a local anesthetic solution through the vaginal wall so that the anesthetic bathes the pudendal nerve, which provides sensation to the lower vagina, perineum, and posterior vulva. This method is a safe, simple method for uncomplicated spontaneous vaginal deliveries if the woman wishes to bear down and push or if labor is advanced and there is no time for epidural injection.

   The perineal block involves infiltration of the perineum with a local anesthetic, although this method is not as effective as a well-administered pudendal block. Paracervical blocks are rarely used today. This involves injecting medication around the cervix, through the vagina, during stage 1 of the labor process.

c. *General anesthesia:* Regional techniques are routinely preferred in uncomplicated vaginal or cesarean deliveries. However, in urgent or emergent situations, a general anesthesia is used for delivery of the baby. This technique involves an anesthesiologist putting the patient to sleep, in a state of unconsciousness, while the obstetrician is delivering the baby through a cesarean section. General anesthesia is maintained with potent vapors administered by the anesthesiologist through a special tube placed in the trachea (windpipe). These vapors can have unwanted effects on the mother and the fetus; therefore, general anesthesia is not recommended for routine vaginal deliveries and is reserved for emergency/urgent situations requiring immediate delivery of a newborn.

Summary

Discuss your wishes and expectations with the doctor. It is important to review pain control options with the individuals involved in the delivery of the baby: the obstetrician, midwife, nurse, and so on. Find out which pain control methods are available at the institution where the delivery will occur. Many women make decisions about labor pain relief during the labor process. The best advice is to take the time and get educated about all the options for pain relief.

When true labor is suspected, call the health care provider. Also call if water has broken, for bleeding (more than just spotting), or if the baby seems to be moving less than normal. Inform the health care provider when contractions become very uncomfortable and when contractions are coming every five minutes for an hour.

While many consider it an invasive procedure, and despite possible complications associated with its placement, labor epidurals have radically changed the way childbirth is viewed in recent years. Delivery of the baby under labor epidural dramatically decreases the anxiety, provides effective pain relief, and allows for a more enjoyable experience for mothers and their support partners. The prudent patient who is pregnant should survey the site of delivery and the accessibility and options provided in a hospital setting. Knowing that an anesthesiologist is available within the hospital 24 hours a day will reduce anxiety and help provide the best care for the mother and child.

34

THE FUTURE OF PAIN MANAGEMENT: WHAT IT MEANS FOR YOU

Carl Noe, MD

Pain management is an immature field with less scientific basis to guide decision making than one would desire. Around 1990, pain began to receive increased attention by physicians and patient groups. Progress has been made in certain areas but practicing the art of medicine still applies to pain management to a large degree. One of the variables regarding the future of pain treatment is related to the future of the health care system in the United States and other countries. If the U.S. system changes to a more evidence-based (where treatments prescribed are based on research showing true effectiveness) and central control model, shifts in physician practice patterns could occur that result in changes in patient treatments unless patients are willing to pay out of pocket for treatment they desire. The theoretical advantage to a new system would be to maximize the benefit of limited resources and reduce the costs of delivering unnecessary and ineffective care. The future of our health care is still unraveling.

Let's review current treatments and the likely future of these treatments, emerging technology, and finally, where more research is needed. Medications are common pain treatments, and several types of drugs are available and they work in different ways.

As discussed in previous chapters, acetaminophen is an over-the-counter medication, which is helpful for some patients and some pains. It has stood the test of time, but high doses can cause liver damage and the same dose for chronic treatment is controversial. The future of this drug will probably include the use of the lowest effective dose and avoiding using a dose that is no more effective than a lower dose as well as staying within recommended doses. An intravenous form (injected into a vein rather than swallowed as a pill) of this type of drug is becoming available soon.

Anti-inflammatory drugs such as ibuprofen are over the counter, and many prescription medications exist. These medications are helpful for many patients but they can cause kidney damage, bleeding, and stomach and intestinal ulcers. The more selective "COX-2" drugs (Celebrex) have some advantages with regard to bleeding and ulcers, but concerns about heart attacks have led to some of these drugs being taken off the market. Hopefully, these problems can be resolved with new drugs in the future.

Anticonvulsants (antiseizure medications) are commonly used for chronic pain, especially abnormal nerve pains. Gabapentin (Neurontin) and pregabalin (Lyrica) have been heavily prescribed and have been shown to be helpful for several specific conditions. The future of these drugs will depend on additional research in other specific conditions in comparison to other available drugs such as the older, less expensive tricyclic antidepressant drugs. Antidepressants are also used for abnormal nerve pains, but not all antidepressants have an analgesic effect that is independent of the antidepressant effect. The tricyclic antidepressants such as amitriptyline, nortriptyline and desipramine have been shown to be about as effective as any drug for many nerve pains. The future of these drugs may be the development of newer-generation drugs with fewer side effects.

Opioids (narcotic pain relievers) face a future of increased scrutiny due to drug diversion problems, habituation, and overdose problems. New preparations are being developed with new safety features such as an additional drug to counteract an overdose if the drug is injected rather than taken as prescribed. The increased documentation requirements for some of these drugs will be significant for patients and their physicians.

Cannabinoids (marijuana-like drugs) do have some pain-relieving effect. However, the side effects and the stigma associated with them may limit the use of these drugs in the future due to legal and political restrictions.

The future of drugs for pain will likely include drug combinations that are proven to be more effective than individual drugs. Little is known at this time about combinations that really work, and many patients end up on too many drugs in an attempt to achieve better relief.

Procedures for pain relief include surgery and minimally invasive treatments such as injections, acupuncture, and manipulation. There is evidence that surgery is effective for joint replacement and specific spine problems. However, spine fusion for degenerative disk disease is going to be less common in the future based on existing outcome data. Joint injections are also likely to be less common, since data of cost-effectiveness is lacking for many of these procedures. Acupuncture seems to be effective for pain after dental surgery, but it is unclear if it is effective for back pain and arthritis, so it may fall out of favor for some conditions unless convincing evidence of effectiveness emerges. Manipulation seems to be effective for acute back pain, but it is unclear if it is effective for other conditions, so the future of third-party (insurer) reimbursement may be restricted.

Interdisciplinary—that is, involving different types of specialists—pain management is a comprehensive, integrated model of medical, psychological, and rehabilitative treatments for pain. Good research data exists for the use of interdisciplinary care; however, the use has been limited due to multiple factors. The future will likely include a growing role for interdisciplinary treatment since it improves quality of life, function, and coping ability more than many other existing treatments.

Hypnosis may be helpful for some patients, but many patients are not psychologically oriented to benefit from hypnosis.

Herbal remedies are relatively unregulated, even though about one-third of our drugs have a botanical origin (for example, the willow bark is the origin of aspirin). Many herbals have active ingredients that potentially can provide a beneficial effect; however, because of lack of regulation similar to that required by drugs, most formulations are at best questionable in terms of preparation and efficacy, and are largely unproven. Research is ongoing to critically determine positive effects of these substances, and most likely there will be more regulation in the future. This can already be seen in Europe.

A number of emerging tests and treatments for pain are likely to be available in the reasonable future. Functional MRI tests are used in research to learn about areas of the brain involved with pain and responses to treatments. In the future these tests may be used for diagnostic purposes.

Quantitative sensory testing (QST) is used to measure sensations to heat and pressure and may be useful in the future for classifying patients who may respond to particular drugs. Screening questionnaires are being developed to aid in diagnosis and prognosis for many conditions. In the future, you may be able to answer questions on a website and get an accurate diagnosis for some conditions. Patients who are at risk for chronic pain may also be identified and directed to early interdisciplinary treatment.

Genes have been identified that are associated with several chronic pain conditions including low back pain. Other conditions, such as migraine, arthritis, and cancer, clearly run in families and have some genetic component to their probability to occur in an individual. New treatments may become available as more is learned about genetics and pain, and genetic testing may be able to identify patients who are at high risk for developing conditions so that preventative measures can be taken to minimize the risk and severity of a condition that may develop later. With new technology such as stem cell research, new ethical dilemmas arise, and we will work our way through those. Also, genetic testing may identify patients who will respond to certain drugs or metabolize drugs differently and need higher or lower doses.

New classes of drugs may emerge that work by different mechanisms than currently available medications. This may allow for combinations of medications that are more effective than single drugs. New drugs that are more selective for analgesia may produce better pain relief at lower doses and consequently may have fewer side effects and drug interactions.

New procedures are being developed to help back pain and arthritis, which are less invasive and have less recovery time. However, these new techniques need to be studied and proven to be not only safe, but more effective than existing treatments and cost-effective as well.

Interdisciplinary pain management may have applicability for patients who are at increased risk for developing chronic pain. In the future, you may be screened with acute pain and treated with interdisciplinary care in order to prevent chronic pain, disability, and medication dependence.

Future clinical research will focus on cost-effectiveness to a greater degree than in the past in order to find the "biggest bang for the buck." Additionally, research measurement tools will become more standardized so that comparisons can be made more easily. Research of new commercial products will receive increased scrutiny in the future to minimize bias based on the funding source for the research. Also, much unpublished data exists from negative research trials. This data is valuable, but it frequently goes unpublished because it doesn't show a positive effect from a treatment. In the future, this data will be made publicly available in order to enhance the common good.

Basic science research in neurosciences, immunology, and genetics will undoubtedly discover new opportunities for treatments; however, in the future, we will relearn that basic science research is not product development. Basic research, for the sake of knowledge itself, will gain support.

The future of pain management is as unpredictable as any other attempt at foretelling the future, but it is important for you to remain hopeful, yet avoid putting your life on hold waiting for a dramatic breakthrough. Many patients have chronic pain despite large expenditures of time and money for treatment. Clearly, treatments for many conditions are ineffective and therefore, part of the future of pain management will be related to eliminating or reducing the utilization of these ineffective and costly treatments.

Back pain, for example, is a very common chronic condition that is often overtreated. This overtreatment not only gives patients false hopes, but also exposes them to complications beyond the high cost of ineffective treatments. A better approach for the future would be to direct you toward treatments proven to be effective and direct you away from unproven treatments associated with high risk and/or high cost.

In the future, we will not be able to afford cafeteria-style, consumer-driven health care utilization. It is the reason that there is so much talk and discussion about health care reform at present. Limiting the "treatment menu" will not only help the system; it will help the individual patient find appropriate care sooner and avoid wasting time and money on futile treatments made attractive by marketing campaigns or Internet websites.

Most patients are interested in high-tech solutions such as new devices, surgeries, and drugs. In the future, we will have treatments to better take advantage of our own ability to heal or treat ourselves without the help of a health care system. Many painful conditions are self-limited and intermediate, and long-term outcomes are not improved with increasing doses of health care. In the future, improved education will help patients make better decisions regarding the pain treatment they choose.

INDEX

Note: Page numbers followed by "t" refer to tables.

About the Editors and Contributors

Editors

ALAN D. KAYE, MD, PhD, has been a tenured professor, Director of Pain Services, and Chairman of the Department of Anesthesiology at Louisiana State University School of Medicine in New Orleans since 2005. He is also a Professor of Pharmacology. Prior, he was Program Director and Chairman of the Texas Tech Department of Anesthesia in Lubbock from 1999 to 2005. Dr. Kaye trained at Massachusetts General Hospital under the auspices of Harvard Medical School and Tulane Medical Center, where he was Chief Resident. He completed a specialized interventional pain fellowship at Texas Tech Health Sciences Center in Lubbock and is double board certified from the American Board of Pain Medicine and the American Board of Anesthesiology, with a special certificate in Pain Management. He attended the University of Arizona for college and medical school. Dr. Kaye was a state winner and national runner-up for a Rhodes Scholarship, among his many awards. He has been selected for Best Doctors, Super Doctors, Consumer Research Outstanding Doctors, and is regarded as one of the top anesthesiologists and interventional pain doctors in the world. He has been inducted into the New Orleans Anesthesia, Texas Tech Department of Anesthesia, and the Sahuaro High School Halls of Fame.

RICHARD D. URMAN, MD, MBA, currently serves as Assistant Professor of Anesthesia at Harvard Medical School and is a practicing anesthesiologist and Director of sedation services at the Brigham and Women's Hospital in Boston, Massachusetts. He also codirects the Center for Perioperative Management and Medical Informatics. He is a cofounder and Chief Executive Officer of the Institute for Safety in Office-Based Surgery, an independent nonprofit organization advocating safe practices in physicians' offices. His organization was recently featured in the *Wall Street Journal*. Dr. Urman received his MD from Harvard Medical School and an MBA from Harvard Business School. His academic interests encompass patient safety, education, and new medications. His many honors include being recently named the Morgan-Zinsser Fellow of the Harvard Medical School Academy and receiving the American Medical Association Foundation Leadership Award. Dr. Urman has coauthored several books for students and professionals in the fields of anesthesia and pain management. He is an active member of several professional societies and has served on many nonprofit boards.

CONTRIBUTORS

MAGDALENA ANITESCU, MD, PhD, is Director, Pain Management Fellowship Program, and Assistant Professor, Department of Anesthesia and Critical Care, University of Chicago Medical Center.

CHRISTOPHER ANNIS, MD, is Anesthesiologist and Pain Medicine Specialist, OSMC Pain Management Center, Elkhart, IN.

ARASH ASHER, MD, is Director, Cancer Survivorship and Rehabilitation, Samuel Oschin Comprehensive Cancer Institute, Cedars-Sinai Medical Center, and Assistant Clinical Professor, Health Sciences, University of California at Los Angeles.

GRACE CHEN, MD, is Assistant Professor and Associate Pain Management Fellowship Director, Department of Anesthesiology and Perioperative Medicine, Oregon Health and Science University.

JIANGUO CHENG, MD, PhD, is Professor of Anesthesiology, Cleveland Clinic Lerner College of Medicine of Case Western Reserve University, and Director of Cleveland Clinic Pain Medicine Fellowship Program, Departments of Pain Management and Neurosciences, Anesthesiology Institute, Cleveland Clinic.

JOE COOK, MPH, is a medical student at the University of Mississippi School of Medicine, University of Mississippi Medical Center.

SARETA COUBAROUS, DO, is Attending Physician at Mid Atlantic Spine and Pain Physicians, Temple University Hospital.

BRIAN DERHAKE, MD, MSc, is a Clinical Fellow of Pain Medicine, Department of Pain Management, Anesthesiology Institute, Cleveland Clinic.

JIGNYASA L. DESAI, DO, is a Pain Medicine Fellow, Temple University Hospital, Philadelphia, Pennsylvania.

SUDHIR DIWAN, MD, is Executive Director at The Spine and Pain Institute of New York, Staten Island University Hospital.

GULSHAN DOULATRAM, MD, is Associate Professor and Pain Fellowship Program Director, Department of Anesthesiology, University of Texas Medical Branch at Galveston.

TAMER ELBAZ, MD, is Assistant Professor at Columbia University and Director of the Pain Medicine Fellowship Training Program at St. Luke's-Roosevelt Hospital Center, New York City.

IKE ERIATOR, MD, MPH, is Professor of Anesthesiology and Director, Pain Fellowship Program, Department of Anesthesiology, University of Mississippi Medical Center.

FRANK J. E. FALCO, MD, is Adjunct Associate Professor, Temple University Medical School, Philadelphia, Pennsylvania; Director, Pain Medicine Fellowship Program, Temple University Hospital, Philadelphia, Pennsylvania; and Medical Director, Mid Atlantic Spine & Pain Physicians, Newark, Delaware and Elkton, Maryland.

DAVID E. FISH, MD, MPH, is Chief, Division of Interventional Physiatry, and Associate Professor, Department of Orthopedics, The UCLA Spine Center, David Geffen School of Medicine at UCLA.

JONATHAN GEACH, MD, is Assistant Professor of Anesthesiology and Co-Director of Acute Pain Management, Loma Linda University Medical Center and School of Medicine.

CHRISTINE GRECO, MD, is Assistant Professor of Anesthesia and Director of Acute Pain Services, at Children's Hospital, Boston, MA.

MATTHEW HANSEN, MD, is Clinical Fellow of Pain Medicine, Department of Pain Management, Anesthesiology Institute, Cleveland Clinic.

MICHAEL HARNED, MD, is Assistant Professor of Anesthesiology and Interventional Pain Associates Medical Director, University of Kentucky.

JUSTIN HATA, MD, is Assistant Clinical Professor, Departments of Anesthesiology & Perioperative Care and Physical Medicine and Rehabilitation; Medical Director, UC Irvine Center for Pain Management; and Co-Director, UC Irvine Comprehensive Spine Program, The University of California, Irvine.

SYED A. HUSAIN, DO, is a Pain Medicine Fellow, Temple University Hospital, Philadelphia, Pennsylvania.

RAJESH JARI, MD, is a Pain Medicine Fellow, Temple University Hospital, Philadelphia, Pennsylvania.

YOUSSEF JOSEPHSON, DO, is a Pain Medicine Fellow, Temple University Hospital, Philadelphia, Pennsylvania.

ADAM M. KAYE, Pharm.D., FASCP, FCPhA, is Associate Clinical Professor and Pharmacy Practice Experience Coordinator, Thomas J. Long School of Pharmacy and Health Sciences, University of the Pacific.

JUNG H. KIM, MD, is a Pain Medicine Fellow, St. Luke's-Roosevelt Hospital Center, New York City.

PAMELA LAW, MD, is a Resident Physician at the David Geffen School of Medicine at UCLA.

VANNY LE, MD, is a Pain Medicine Fellow, Department of Anesthesiology, St. Luke's Roosevelt Hospital Center, New York City.

GALAXY LI, MD, is a Pediatric Pain Medicine Fellow at Children's Hospital, Boston.

KATHLEEN McALPINE, CRC, CDMS, is a Vocational Counselor at Southwest Rehabilitation Association, Tucson.

KATHRYN NIXDORF, MD, is a Pain Management Fellow at Oregon Health and Science University.

CARL NOE, MD, is Professor and Division Director Pain Division, and Medical Director, Eugene McDermott Center for Pain Management, University of Texas Southwestern Medical Center.

ZACH NYE, DO, is a Pain Management Fellow at Oregon Health and Science University.

C. OBI ONYEWU, MD, is Attending Physician at Mid Atlantic Spine and Pain Physicians, and Faculty, Pain Medicine Fellowship, Temple University Hospital.

JOHN C. PAN, MD, is a Pain Medicine Fellow, David Geffen School of Medicine at UCLA, and VA Greater Los Angeles Healthcare System.

NATHAN PERRIZO, DO, is a Pain Medicine Fellow, David Geffen School of Medicine at UCLA, and VA Greater Los Angeles Healthcare System.

DANIELLE PERRET, MD, is Assistant Clinical Professor, Departments of Anesthesiology and Perioperative Care and Physician Medicine and Rehabilitation, The University of California, Irvine.

RAED RAHMAN, DO, is Medical Director of Pain Management, Cancer Treatment Centers of America-Midwest Regional Medical Center, Chicago, Illinois.

DANIEL S. REYNOLDS, MD, is a Pain Medicine Fellow, Department of Anesthesiology, University of Mississippi Medical Center, Jackson.

LOWELL REYNOLDS, MD, is Professor of Anesthesiology at Loma Linda University School of Medicine, and Director of Acute Pain, Department of Anesthesiology, Loma Linda University Medical Center.

RINOO V. SHAH, MD, MBA is a Pain Specialist and Associate, Department of Anesthesiology, Guthrie Clinic, Corning Hospital, New York.

PAUL SLOAN, MD, is Professor, Vice-Chair for Research, and Program Director, Pain Fellowship, Department of Anesthesiology, University of Kentucky, Lexington.

DMITRI SOUZDALNITSKI, MD, PhD, is a Clinical Fellow of Pain Medicine, Anesthesiology Institute, at Cleveland Clinic.

DAMIEN TAVARES, MD, is a Fellow in Pain Medicine, Department of Anesthesiology & Perioperative Care, The University of California, Irvine.

VU TRAN, MD, is a Pain Management Physician at University of Texas Medical Branch, Galveston.

RUTH VAN VLEET, MS, CRC, CDMS, is a Vocational Counselor at Southwest Rehabilitation Association, Tucson.

RENATO VESGA, MD, is Adjunct Assistant Professor, Temple University Medical School, Philadelphia, Pennsylvania; Faculty, Pain Medicine Fellowship Program, Temple University Hospital, Philadelphia, Pennsylvania; and Attending Physician, Mid Atlantic Spine & Pain Physicians, Newark, Delaware and Elkton, Maryland.

HAIBIN WANG, MD, PhD, is a Clinical Fellow of Pain Medicine, Department of Pain Management, Anesthesiology Institute, Cleveland Clinic.

PHILLIP R. T. WEIDNER, DO, is a Resident in Anesthesia at Oregon Health and Science University.

KAY YEUNG, MD, is a Fellow in Pain Medicine, Department of Anesthesiology & Perioperative Care, The University of California, Irvine.

EUN JUNG YI, MD, is a Resident in Anesthesia at Oregon Health and Science University.

JIE ZHU, MD, is Attending Physician at Mid Atlantic Spine and Pain Physicians, and Faculty for the Pain Medicine Fellowship at Temple University Hospital.

3 7256 82915 7713